BIRTH TO MATURITY

BIRTH TO

A Study in Psychologica

JEROME KAGAN

New Haven and Londo

MATURITY

Development

HOWARD A. MOSS

with a new preface by Jerome Kagan

YALE UNIVERSITY PRESS

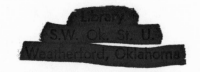

First published in 1962 by John Wiley & Sons, Inc.

Printed in the United States of America by
Edwards Brothers Inc., Ann Arbor, Michigan

Library of Congress catalog card number: 62–19148
International Standard Book Number: 0–300–02998–5
International Standard Book Number: 0–300–03029–0 (pbk.)

10 9 8 7 6 5 4 3 2 1

To the Fels children and their families

Contents

Preface to the Second Edition *ix*
Preface to the First Edition *xxvii*
1 Introduction *1*
2 Methods of Assessment *20*
3 The Stability of Behavior:
   I Passivity and Dependency *49*
4 The Stability of Behavior:
   II Aggression *85*
5 The Stability of Behavior:
   III Achievement and Recognition *120*
6 The Stability of Behavior:
   IV Sexuality, Social Interaction, and Selected Behaviors *156*
7 Maternal Practices and the Child's Behavior *204*
8 Sources of Conflict and Anxiety *229*
9 Summary and Conclusions *266*
   References *287*
   Author Index *293*
   Subject Index *297*

Preface to the Second Edition

The opportunity to reflect on an early work and mentally cut away the thickets of prose that a generation has shown to be debris permits a special pleasure, not unlike the one that accompanies a rare autumn visit to a favorite but distant forest. Although it is not possible to recall moods and beliefs that are now over twenty-two years old, it might be helpful for younger readers of this book to appreciate the web of suppositions that occupied the center of American psychology when Howard Moss and I were putting *Birth to Maturity* into first draft.

Environmentalism, the root premise, was sustained by a fruitful collaboration between closely reasoned elaborations on Pavlovian conditioning principles and ingenious transformations of Freud's ideas. This heady alchemy produced principles of psychological development that usually wound their way back to social interactions, replacing libido with motive, cathexis with acquired reward, symptom with habit, but more wisely leaving the displeasure of anxiety as a central incentive for thought and action. In this frame, the instinctively driven infant described by nineteenth-century observers was placed in a thick web of human relationships whose center was occupied by a mother who was the origin of both sanity and psychosis.

Erikson's reinterpretations of Freud's first two psychosexual stages capture the change in perspective that matured between the two world wars (Erikson, 1963). Trust and autonomy imply a relationship to others that is missing in the historically prior concepts of oral and anal stages. Freud imagined a hungry, nursing infant while Erikson, and later Bowlby, standing in the same nursery, perceived an affiliative, apprehensive one. Dissemination of the new metaphor for the infant—a baboon rather than a bear—had been completed when Howard Moss and I were gathering the data for *Birth to Maturity*. So it was almost reflexive for us, as it was for most students of development, to search for the formative forces in the close encounters between adults and children.

The origins of the second presupposition are more difficult to specify because fragments can be detected in Western writings about the child from the height of Athenian culture to the present moment. But the premise of connectivity in psychological growth had a major renaissance during the Enlightenment when mind, the immaterial descendent of brain, was conceptualized as a canvas gradually covered with indelible strokes whose only possibility for change was to become part of another pattern. This image of psychological growth implied a material connection between the present and all of the past, an idea that is axiomatic for the large number of scientists who assume that no memory engrams are ever lost. Failure to remember an event that has become part of long-term memory is due to interference with retrieval, not loss of the original treasure. Nothing is lost, nothing wasted.

The western scholar's assumption of the indefinite stability of early structures implies that every important disposition in the present contains enough of the past that one should be able to trace present behavior to its origins, no matter how far in the past the critical moments occurred. William Stern, a famous nineteenth-century observer of children, saw a connection between the babbling of the 5-month-old and the speech of the 2-year-old. Sigmund Bernfeld, an early disciple of Freud—who supposed that all adult cognition had its origin in early infancy—wrote, "Historically all phenomena of adult mental life must be traceable to birth" (Bernfeld, 1929, p. 213). Some early twentieth-century theorists held that the adult's proprietary motive shared elements with the grasp reflex of the newborn; others suggested that an adult's aesthetic sense was shaped originally by the opportunity to play with attractive toys. In one of the most popular psychology texts of the first decade of this century, Edward L. Thorndike (1905) ended his final chapter with a ringing affirmation of the permanence of early acquisitions.

> Though we seem to forget what we learn, each mental acquisition really leaves its mark and makes future judgments more sagacious. . . . Nothing of good or evil is ever lost; we may forget and forgive, but the neurons never forget or forgive. . . . It is certain that every worthy deed represents a modification of the neurons of which nothing can ever rob us. Every event of a man's mental life is written indelibly in the brain's archives; to be counted for or against him (Thorndike, 1905, pp. 330-31).

The possibility of a material connection between early and later phenomena takes two related forms. One requires only dependence of later structures on earlier ones. A second, stronger form holds that elements of the early structures are retained and participate in the later entities. It is the second, more materialistic assumption that has become a bit more controversial since the original publication of *Birth to Maturity*. Although there are as many instances of change as of preservation in development—a fear of snakes is extinguished; respect for a parent eroded—the assumption of early childhood determinism remains popular.

The supposition of connectivity imposes a nontrivial bias on what is seen and described. If an observer believes that a hidden structure is preserved over two points in time, he is prepared to search for actions on the later occasions that might be classified with those manifested earlier. Piaget grouped the newborn's grasping of a finger placed in its palm with the 18-month-old's imitative opening and closing of the hand and suggested that some residue of the reflex displayed on the first day of life participated in the more mature act.

> When we studied the beginnings of intelligence we were forced to go as far back as the reflex in order to trace the cause of the assimilating activity which finally led to the construction of adaptive schemas, for it is only by a principle of functional continuity that the indefinite variety of structures can be explained (Piaget, 1951, p. 6).

Piaget was not alone, for most nineteenth-century scholars—philosophers, historians, and natural scientists—were faithful to the connectivity premise, maintaining that in order to understand any phenomenon, one had to have access to its entire history from origin to present, a position Mandelbaum (1971) has called the bias of historicism. The nineteenth-century scholar, who had rejected the mechanical view of man held by Enlightenment philosophers, took biology as the most informative model and likened the history of society to the growth of plants and animals. This view assumed that any phenomenon that was part of a fixed sequence was a complex function of all that happened earlier. Each new stage grew out of a prior one, contained some of the past, and moved inexorably toward a stage that was better than the one before. Listen to E. B. Tylor on the history of civilizations:

> It is indeed hardly too much to say that civilization being a process of long and complex growth can only be thoroughly understood when studied through its entire range; that the past is continually needed to explain the present and the whole to explain the part (Tylor, 1878, p. 2).

Although a connected view of the history of civilizations and societies has lost popularity among twentieth-century historians, it still reigns in developmental pyschology. Faith in a connectivity between the deep past and the present continues to be, as it was for Howard Moss and me, an essential premise in theories of development. Many declarations of connectivity have been based on a single, superficial similarity between one component of the behavior of the infant and a quality noted in older children or adults. But observers are remarkably adept at inventing similarities between fundamentally different phenomena simply by detecting one feature that is shared, or seems to be shared, by the two events. A century ago the protesting cry of the 1-year-old in response to the mother's temporary departure was classified with the willful disobedience of the adult. Today the same act is grouped with the anxiety and sadness that follow loss of a sweetheart, spouse, or parent. As this century began, Havelock Ellis suggested a similarity between an infant's nursing and sexual intercourse, to which Freud referred in the *Three Essays on the Theory of Sexuality*.

> The erectile nipple corresponds to the erectile penis; the eager watery mouth of the infant to the moist and throbbing vagina, the vitally albuminous milk to the vitally albuminous semen. The complete mutual satisfaction, physical and psychic, of mother and child in the transfer from one to the other of a precious organized fluid is the one true physiological analogy to the relationship of a man and woman at the climax of the sexual act (Ellis, 1900, p. 250).

This analogy, which seemed reasonable in 1900, is less compelling today because nursing has become symbolic of trust rather than passion.

There are good reasons for our receptivity to the idea of connectivity in development. First, this doctrine renders original forms useful and rationalizes the maxim that one must prepare for the future. If the origins of important adult properties occurred during late childhood or adolescence, the first years of life would appear to have no future purpose, much like the embryonic notochord that vanishes after its mission is completed. The possibility that the products of a developmental era might be temporary is bothersome to those who want to believe that all psychological products are permanent and that everything we learn is permanently housed in the mind. If a child's future is determined by the present, tomorrow is to some degree knowable through careful attention to each day's actions. The hope that the adult's profile could be made a little more certain if one managed childhood properly became a creed for parents and social scientists, as it was for America's intellectuals prior to the Revolution, who urged mothers to care for their infants with the same conscientiousness they applied to gathering wood in August in preparation for December's frigid winds.

Additionally, arguments for connectivity have the illusion of being mechanistic. It seems easier to write cause-effect sequences if each new phenomenon is preceded by another that makes a substantial contribution to it than if a new behavior emerges rather suddenly as a result of endogenous changes minimally tied to the past. In the second instance the theorist is left with an explanatory gap, a state not unlike that of the eighteenth-century biologists who were troubled by the proposal of spontaneous generation of new life forms.

A third source of the persuasiveness of connectivity is more speculative. During each historical era there is a dominant philosophical view that most scholars avoid confronting—an intellectual electric fence. From the Renaissance to the nineteenth century, philosophers were reluctant to deduce or infer propositions that would refute or contradict biblical statements on man and nature. Although few contemporary scientists worry about the implications of their work for Christian teaching, many are concerned, often unconsciously, with the implications of their data for the doctrine of egalitarianism. The assumption of connectedness in psychological growth seems to be in greater accord with egalitarian principles than is belief in the possibility of occasional discontinuity in growth. Such discontinuity is often caused by maturation of the central nervous system, and acknowledging the influence of changes in the brain implies that an individual's biology has formative force. Since each person is biologically unique, except for one-egg twins, scholars are forced to assume that differences in rates of psychological growth have their roots in biological processes. This conclusion is regarded by some as inconsistent with egalitarian premises, although it need not be. Further, legitimizing discontinuities in development—due to either biological maturation, genetic variation, or new social arrangements—implies that the benevolent products of early experience might be abrogated later by peer groups, quality of schooling, social upheavals, or changes in physiology. Awarding power to these forces makes it more difficult to argue that arranging equally benevolent experiences for all young children will guarantee a generation that knows less shame, hatred, and dejection.

The belief in the permanence of early characteristics is also aided by our language habits, for there is a strong temptation to assume that entities with the same name must be of the same essence (sixteenth-century herbalists classified wheat, a grass, with buckwheat because both had *wheat* in their names). The adjectives in English that are used to describe human qualities rarely refer to the age of the actor or the context of the action but, like the names of colors, imply a permanence over time and place. Labels like passive, active, irritable, intelligent, or labile are applied to infants, children, and adults as if the meanings of these terms were not altered by growth. This practice is avoided in many languages. In Japanese, for example, different words describe the qualities of intelligence in an infant and in an adult. On the island of Ifaluk in the Western Carolines the feeling state called *fago*, which is only approximated by our word *compassion*, is never applied to infants and young children. The habit of using the same words to describe a characteristic in children and in adults predisposes us to believe in a hidden disposition that survives unchanged over the years.

The most valid reason for believing in the persistence of the consequences of early experience is based on our zeal for ranking children on valued traits, both in and out of school. This practice sensitizes every parent of a 3-year-old to the fact that his or her child will be judged at the end of the first grade, and that this evaluation will influence the quality of education the child will receive from that time forward. Few societies practice such a severe grading of young children. The American commitment to a meritocratic democracy forces us to select candidates for the limited number of responsible positions from the best trained, a decision that is made early, often by age 10 or 11. Most parents know this sequence, or sense it; hence, from their perspective, the goal is to guarantee that their child is ahead early in the race. The fact that the school-age child who gets off to a good start in reading and mathematics is likely, other things equal, to remain ahead of his or her peers persuades parents that the half-dozen years prior to school entrance determine that initial evaluation. Hence, they interpret the child's profile at age 7 as a complex derivative of all that has gone before.

Finally, nineteenth-century physiology and modern neuroscience have made a substantial contribution to the doctrine of infant determinism. A majority believe that psychological experiences can be translated into sentences with purely physiological content: quality of early experience affects the weight of the brain, and early sensory stimulation adds dendritic spines to neurons and alters the sensitivity of the visual cortex to vertical or horizontal lines. These findings are consonant with a picture of the central nervous system similar to Locke's tablet, a soft surface that accepts material marks that are difficult to erase. The belief that experience produces a permanent change in the brain, wedded to the premise that the brain directs thought and behavior, implies that the structures first established will monitor and constrain the later ones.

However, the most recent research on the nervous system indicates considerable inconstancy. Some cells and synapses vanish, some are replaced, and new ones are being established throughout the life span. Embryogenesis is characterized by many discontinuities, including the disappearance of major structures after their mission is accomplished. In the metamorphosis of the tadpole, for example, a particular class of sensory cell in the dorsal spinal cord vanishes, to be replaced by the more typical dorsal root ganglion cells. These new discoveries have led some biologists to suggest that each life stage requires special but temporary structures and functions that facilitate adaptation for that interval. When the next stage is reached and these cells, organs, or functions are no longer needed, they are either inhibited, replaced, or lost.

Similar discontinuities can occur in behavior. Although some believe practice of the responses that normally appear during infancy to be necessary for future functioning, this hypothesis is not always affirmed. The normal suckling of young rat pups appears to be of no consequence for the efficiency or quality of adult ingestive behavior. Similarly, even though play in juvenile squirrel monkeys might be expected to facilitate later social behavior, the absence of play among troops of juvenile squirrel monkeys does not prevent the appearance of normal social behavior. During the second year of life the child becomes strong enough to break expensive vases and pull down curtains and must become anxious about punishment by adults for such behaviors if order is to be preserved. Several years later the child will inhibit these same actions because of a desire to avoid shame and guilt. But there may be no dependent relation between the 1-year-old's anxiety and the 5-year-old's vulnerability to guilt. Similarly, the fear of strangers and of separation at 10 months, the single-word speech of the 18-month-old, and the absolute definition of right and wrong held by the 3-year-old may be temporary adaptations that disappear, along with their foundations, as development proceeds. They might even be omitted without affecting the child's development in any obvious way. Growth is not a relay race in which batons are handed in sequence from one runner to another.

The continued faith in a connected preservation of most early qualities resembles the pre-Darwinian belief in the fixity of species. Darwin's great insight was to treat species as dynamic entities, with some vanishing and new varieties always emerging. If the psychological development of an individual shares important metaphorical qualities with the branching tree of evolution, then we should expect structures and processes to be preserved only if they are adaptive. The demands of the first two years are so different from those at age four that many early reactions should disappear, as do the characteristics of the tadpole, because those early properties are designed to help the animal adapt to that special era of growth. Despite the attractiveness and seeming utility of regarding development as composed of a connected series of stages, we should remain open to the possibility of less connectedness than we have heretofore assumed. I do not claim there are no structurally preserved links among developmental phenomena—there must be some; I am only suggesting that it is unlikely that every actor in the first scene of the play has a role in the second act.

The twin presumptions of environmentalism and connectivity invited a concept of the older child as a patterned set of carefully crafted small pieces of jewelry, each with a different form, texture, and color, with tags labeled dependent, anxious, intelligent, and secure. Once forged, these gems could not easily be changed; the only way to get a necklace of the desired quality would be to begin again with a fresh set of unformed stones.

Although the stable psychological qualities were supposed to be acquired through social interaction, oddly enough they were conceptualized as residing totally within the person, and their expression was viewed as minimally dependent upon the context in which the child acted. Howard Moss and I accepted this Platonic treatment of human nature, and the qualities we quantified, with only a few exceptions, did not specify target or occasion. We rated the children for passivity, dependency, mastery, and spontaneity. We acknowledged context in a few instances—anxiety toward the observer who visited the home and physical aggression toward a peer—but these were exceptions. Evaluation of the adult interview also emphasized qualities that were free of links to particular settings. Achievement behavior, compulsivity, and ease of anger arousal were conceptualized as generalized traits. This was a serious error, not completely to be excused by pointing to the nature of the available material or the zeitgeist.

The hope that we might locate all the major sources of stable dispositions in environmental events, which was a second mistake, turned us away from attributing any formative influence to the maturation of the central nervous system. The appearance of anxiety in response to an unfamiliar adult or child was presumed to be the product of prior distressful experiences; the emergence of guilt was taken as based on prior parental punishments; frequent seizures of other children's toys must have grown out of earlier frustrations, together with the unselfconscious rewarding of such behavior by family members. We could not imagine an important response originating in structural changes in the central nervous system.

The most recent research with animals and young children embarrasses these ideas. There is a beginning consensus that growth of the central nervous system guarantees that cognitive competences appearing at fixed times in the opening years of life will lead all children, except the most isolated or organically impaired, to become afraid of strangers, to cry when separated from a target of attachment, and to become aware of their own talents (Kagan, Kearsley, and Zelazo, 1978). The source of these universal characteristics does not reside only in the interactive play between the child and its parents or playthings. Additionally, many investigators agree that children are born differentially prepared for qualities like distress, irritability, or joy that provoke accommodation by all but the most inflexible of parents. We did not appreciate then that our attempt to find the reasons for a 3-year-old's extreme timidity in a history of prior social exchanges was futile. Indeed, had we been wiser we would have searched for some of the incentives for the mother's behavior in the child's temperamental surface.

We also minimized the influence of the mind of the rater. Although recognition of observer error is not a recent insight, there is now greater sensitivity to the serious distortions induced by an observer's theoretical beliefs. Psychologists interested in human motivation, emotion, and conflict resisted then—as they do now—the serious implications of this limitation, because without qualitative evaluations of verbal reports or behavior many investigators believe they would not be able to do their work. And the first principle of empiricism demands that the work must go on. However, many investigations, especially the work of Richard Shweder, have made it painfully evident that each mind organizes its categories to minimize inconsistency—a least mean squares heuristic. Having decided that a particular child is anxious over maternal rejection, observers find it very difficult to regard that same child as bold, and easy to exaggerate any signs of weakness and uncertainty. Even though qualitative evaluations of interview and behavioral data are still used by investigators—and should be—there is a more sophisticated appreciation of the problem of observer bias than existed in the 1950s. I am not certain that we would have accepted the responsibility of *Birth to Maturity* if invited to do so this year.

The text of *Birth to Maturity* contains four major conclusions that have fared moderately well over a generation of research on human development. The most publicized generalization states that after 5 or 6 years of age there was a reasonable degree of preservation of differences in surface qualities like aggression to peers, dependency on friends, academic performance, and ease of social interaction with strangers. But, with one exception, there was minimal preservation of the differences observed during the first three years. This second conclusion represented one of the first factual bases for skepticism toward the doctrine of infant determinism. Because I was less confident then that the profile at age 3 was not a sensitive predictor of the future, this result was not highlighted by us or by our readers. Rather, the fact of preservation from age 6 forward was celebrated because we and our audience wanted empirical affirmation of the doctrine of connectivity.

The intervening years have added credibility to both the positive and the negative results (Brim and Kagan, 1980; Kagan, 1982; Moss and Susman, 1980). There is now a coherent set of reports, on both normal samples and populations at risk, that fails to support the supposition, so strongly held in the 1950s, that the behavioral profile and implied states ascribed to the 3-year-old are preserved. Winick and his colleagues, for example, followed 229 orphaned Korean girls who had been adopted by middle-class American families when they were between 2 and 3 years of age. These malnourished and in some cases retarded children were divided into three groups on the basis of the degree of malnutrition at the time of admission into the study. Six years later the average IQ of the group that had been severely malnourished was 40 points higher than the scores of similar Korean samples who were returned to their original home environments (Winick, Meyer, and Harris, 1975).

Studies of normal populations also reveal that behaviors displayed during the early years of life are altered with time. The behaviors of the young children in the University of California longitudinal studies were not very predictive of variations in culturally significant characteristics ten to twenty years later (Macfarlane, 1963). In a longitudinal study implemented in the Boston area after *Birth to Maturity* my colleagues and I found that, with only one exception, behavioral variations observed during the first year were not predictive of a small set of theoretically related qualities evaluated when the children were only 27 months old (Kagan, 1971). These children were seen again when they were 10 years old in order to determine if variation in the infant qualities might predict intelligence test scores, reading ability, or a tendency toward reflection-impulsivity. The educational level of the family was the only robust predictor of the child's intelligence and reading skill, and most of the variation noted during the first two years had no predictive power for the qualities observed at age 10 (Kagan, Lapidus, and Moore, 1978).

Even among laboratory-reared animals there is minimal preservation of differences noted during the period of infancy. The variation in aggressiveness, activity level, and excitability among infant monkeys is not preserved over periods as short as 18 months (Stevenson-Hinde, Stillwell-Barnes, and Zunz, 1980). After an extensive review of the relevant evidence, Cairns and Hood (in press) concluded that stability became obvious only as the animals approached reproductive maturity: "The findings offered meager support for the idea that significant features of social interactions at maturity are fixed by experiences in early development

... the qualities that are predictable are not in the organism but in the developmental context; its relationships and its likely course of subsequent development."

In sharp contrast to the failure of an infant's qualities to predict his or her future, the education and income of the parents are excellent predictors of many of the older child's characteristics. This means that discovery of a relation between variation in a quality seen during infancy and in one observed in a 10-year-old does not necessarily mean that some aspect of the original characteristic was preserved. Rather, it might indicate that the same forces that produced the behavior in the 1-year-old continued to operate for the next decade. For example, infants who are very attentive to unfamiliar events have higher IQ scores 10 years later. This fact seems to imply that a quality related to intelligence is preserved. However, both the pattern of protracted attention to the unusual during infancy and a high IQ later are characteristic of children from better-educated families, suggesting that the continuous experiences associated with rearing in middle-class homes form the bases for the relation between the two phenomena (Kagan, Lapidus, and Moore, 1978).

Consider an analogy. Well-nourished, healthy infants play with more vitality than malnourished or sickly ones, and healthy adults are likely to engage in more athletics than those who are ill. Yet few would posit a quality called *playfulness* that is preserved from the first year through adulthood. The relation between the two qualities is due to the continuous operation of specific external influences. If a marble released from the top of a narrow trough rolled in a straight line, we would not attribute to it a sense of direction. Although children's inherent qualities present different surfaces to their environments, each child accommodates to the pressures imposed from without and is altered in accord with those forces.

The important constraints imposed by gender and class represent a second conclusion that has resisted erosion. The differential continuities that began to appear at age 6 were seriously constrained by sex-role standards. Aggressive behavior to peers was better preserved among the males because traditional sex-role standards were more permissive of this quality in boys than in girls. Longitudinal studies of the stability of aggressive behavior in older boys, from both American and European laboratories, suggest stability of this behavior over a two- to four-year period, even though there is a gradual drop in the magnitude of preservation as the age interval increases. By contrast, passivity to attack and dependency on adults were better preserved for girls because in the period between the two world wars traditional American values treated these characteristics as more acceptable in females.

It is now common practice, although twenty years ago it was not, for investigators to perform separate analyses for boys and girls and to collapse data only when gender is not an interacting variable. Scientists have moved closer to the recognition that males and females may march to different pipers, although both missions have equal virtue. Although the two agendas originate in and are mainly supported by culture, there is beginning evidence suggesting that some parts of the two profiles may originate in the organization of the central nervous system.

Howard Moss and I also argued, with others, that class of rearing had a serious influence on the child's development. A family's social class was correlated with autonomy and competitiveness in adult women, with a more admiring attitude toward fathers among men, and, of course, with level of intellectual accomplishment and less traditional sex-role typing for both men and women. The psychological significance of class of rearing is now affirmed as a major correlate of many phenomena of interest, among them locus of control, quality of performance in school and college, occupational status, expectations, aspirations for success, and probability of serious mental illness. Class of rearing is a better predictor of future intelligence scores than any early psychological quality and most biological ones. Robert McCall (1977) has reported that the social class of a boy's father is a more powerful predictor of the son's eventual educational and occupational attainment than the boy's IQ during childhood. And class surpasses evidence of pre- and perinatal risk as a predictor of school achievement and IQ during later childhood (Werner and Smith, 1982).

Class is potent because it represents a coherent set of influences, including how a child is treated, the beliefs he or she acquires, the readiness for school tasks, and the child's profile of identifications. As early as the third birthday boys and girls from middle-class American families are more autonomous, more verbally proficient, and more concerned with failure on intellectual tasks than are working-class children of the same ethnic group. These class-related profiles are created, in part, from different patterns of parental behavior that are derived partially from each parent's unarticulated philosophy. The working-class mother sees herself less as a sculptor of an expensive marble block and more as a patron of and companion to her child. The well-educated mother is more reflective when she disciplines and more conscious of a philosophy that celebrates autonomy, responsibility, and intellectual talent.

The most provocative finding in *Birth to Maturity* was the preservation of inhibition and fearfulness of the unfamiliar from the first three years forward, especially in boys. There was a small group of extremely timid, shy, quiet, inhibited boys who withdrew to their mothers when the Fels visitor came to the home, were social isolates during the nursery school years, and were reserved with peers as they approached adolescence. These boys avoided male sex-typed activities, were reluctant to date girls during adolescence, and chose less traditional masculine vocations.

The behavioral style to which we refer can be seen in the 9-month-old but is displayed in clearest form after the first birthday. Most 2-year-olds will stop playing, become quiet, or occasionally cry in response to some events that are surprising or puzzling. But 1- and 2-year-olds differ in their threshold for this profile and in the consistency with which it is displayed across situations varying in familiarity. About 10 percent of American 2-year-olds show extreme degrees of behavioral inhibition when confronted with a variety of nonthreatening but unfamiliar events, like the presence of an unfamiliar child. They will become quiet, assume a facial expression most would call wary, and retreat to their mothers. Other infants of the same age, class, and cognitive ability will smile, talk to the peer, and offer a toy. The inhibited child may recover after 10 minutes and talk and play with the stranger with zeal and obvious pleasure. Even though the inhibition is temporary, it is a reliable characteristic during the second and third years.

In a recent longitudinal study, we filmed the behaviors of over 100 21-month-old children faced with a variety of uncertain incentives. The resulting records led to the selection of the 28 most-inhibited and 30 least-inhibited children. When these children were 31 months old they were observed at home and in the laboratory while playing with an unfamiliar peer of the same age and sex but of the opposite behavioral style. The children previously classified as inhibited at 21 months were inhibited with the visitors to the home as well as with the unfamiliar peer (Garcia Coll, Kagan, and Reznick, in press).

When these children were seen at 4 years of age, the majority had retained their characteristic style. The formerly inhibited children were initially self-conscious with the examiner, rarely made irrelevant, interrupting comments during the testing, and spoke in soft, hesitant voices. The uninhibited children were relaxed, smiled and laughed, spoke with confident and vital voices, and frequently interrupted the examiner with questions or irrelevant comments. When observed with an unfamiliar child of the same age and sex, the inhibited child rarely approached the peer and typically was passive to attacks from the less inhibited child.

These findings affirm other investigations revealing moderate preservation of this quality over the opening years of life in children and in animals. Longitudinal observations of small groups of laboratory-reared Macaque monkeys over a period of four years revealed that fearfulness of novel situations was the only one of three behavioral categories to show signs of stability. Excitability and sociability showed minimal preservation across the same interval (Stevenson-Hinde, Stillwell-Barnes, and Zunz, 1980).

In searching for a few concise adjectives that might capture the differences between the two classes of children, recognizing that any term distorts the phenomenon, *restrained, quiet,* and *gentle* come closest to capturing the behavioral surface of the inhibited child, while *free, energetic,* and *affective* capture the style of the uninhibited child. When an inhibited 3-year-old throws a ball, knocks down a tower of blocks, or hits a large toy clown, the action is tentative; the same behavior in the uninhibited child seems unchecked.

The heart-rate patterns of these children reveal that about one-third of the extremely inhibited ones show a loss of respiratory sinus arrhythmia when they are processing information that is discrepant and difficult to understand. Inhibition of vagal tone by the sympathetic nervous system can be one basis for the loss of sinus arrhythmia and the accompanying reduction in heart-rate variability. We hope it is not a coincidence that the small number of adult men in *Birth to Maturity* who had been the most inhibited children during the first three years of life showed the most stable heart rates during an initial 10-minute relaxation period prior to the administration of test procedures.

The dimension we call inhibition to the unfamiliar involves at least two different qualities that need not be associated. The first is a cognitive set for subtle discrepancy in experience; the second refers to the behavioral reactions that follow a state of uncertainty. Some children have a lower threshold for detecting the unexpected and unfamiliar and persist longer in trying to assimilate these events. This quality, which we call vigilance, is likely to provoke a state of uncertainty. Behavioral inhibition is a probable response to the state of uncertainty, especially in the young child. Hence, theoretically all children with this cognitive characteristic should be behaviorally inhibited. But parents differ in their acceptance of extreme behavioral inhibition in their children. Those who value a bold, fearless, adventurous child are threatened by the opposite qualities and socialize the child toward the more desirable profile. Consistent reward of an uninhibited style and punishment of an inhibited one can, to some degree, alter the child's surface so that, on occasion, a child who was initially inhibited becomes behaviorally uninhibited. It is still not clear whether the basic quality of vigilance to the unfamiliar is preserved, despite the change in overt behavior.

An initial inhibition or lack of inhibition to the unfamiliar, one of the few dispositions preserved from early childhood forward, may persist because it has a partial base in the child's biology. A basic principle in physiology is that each animal species is characterized by a small number of complementary systems that compete for dominance. The competition between the two cerebral hemispheres is one example: for most people, the temporal lobe of the left hemisphere is dominant over the comparable area of the right hemisphere for language functions, although for a small number of people the dominance relation is reversed. The competition between the sympathetic and parasympathetic arms of the autonomic nervous system provides another example. It is possible that genetic or prenatal influences create conditions that, in some children, create a dominant sympathetic tone. Such children might be prone to become the behaviorally inhibited youngsters we have been describing.

A final productive result that originated in *Birth to Maturity* became the basis for the later research on reflection-impulsivity. We invented a picture-sorting task designed to evaluate individual differences in degree of conflict over sexual, aggressive, and dependent behaviors. Our hypotheses seemed reasonable enough then; they do not now. We argued that if a group of figures suggestive of conflict were shown to the adults with an instruction to sort them into similar groups, those who were conflicted over the content areas suggested by the figures would not place together those figures representative of the conflict—a mechanically direct effect of conflict upon cognitive function. It was too simple an idea. The performances bore no relationship to any index of conflict, whether derived from the childhood information or the adult interview. Frustrated, I took the data home night after night, trying to determine why our strategy failed. Late one evening I noted a lawfulness that was to be the seed of the construct of reflection-impulsivity. Some of the adults sorted the figures into categories on the basis of physical properties alone—the dark figures, the figures holding something in their hands, or the figures with bent arms. Most important, these responses, which we called analytic, were produced with longer response latencies than the other classifications. That unexpected discovery led to the invention of the construct of a reflective style and the creation of the Matching Familiar Figures test, which has become a popular method to evaluate the individual-difference characteristic called reflection-impulsivity—a dimension that has proved to be of some utility to developmental and educational psychologists.

It is reassuring that a small proportion of the suggestions in *Birth to Maturity* have fared moderately well in the empirical arena. Psychologists are a bit more skeptical of the doctrine of infant determinism but more confident of the importance of gender and of social class, the preservation of individual differences in inhibition, and the relevance of reflection-impulsivity to cognitive functioning. Fine-tuning the validity of these ideas has required longitudinal information and extensive research on the infant and young child. Unfortunately, the expense of longitudinal studies and the pressure they impose on young scientists who believe they must have a long list of publications in order to gain tenure have made this research strategy less popular. Equally unfortunate is the conclusion of some psychologists that if early infancy does not provide a relatively efficient predictor of the future, perhaps investigators should shift their interest to later phases of the life course. That decision is vulnerable.

I assume, with good historical justification, that the basic aspects of complex forms are revealed more clearly in simpler organisms. Studies of drosophila and *E. coli*, which were critical for unraveling the structure of the gene, have led to the industrial use of bacteria in the production of hormones for clinical application. Beadle and Tatum could not have known that their investigations of molds over forty years ago would have contributed to discoveries with such extraordinary pragmatic implications. Psychological study of the infant holds the same promise.

The basic human functions—orientation to unfamiliar events, perceptual inference, classification, retrieval memory, inhibition, anxiety, shame and guilt, and awareness of the self's ability to act—all appear in their first and relatively unencumbered forms during the opening years of life. The form of their emergence and the qualities that accompany their display provide clues to their biological bases and essential character. Such knowledge is vital if we are to understand the essence of human psychological functioning. A theory of representation is at the heart of modern cognitive science, and a firmer understanding of how the infant represents experience before language is in place is critical for the invention of a relevant theory of representation. Similarly, awareness of standards of conduct, which a nineteenth-century observer would have called a moral sense, emerges in most children by the second birthday, suggesting that evaluation is, as Charles Osgood claimed so many years ago, a fundamental human characteristic (Kagan, 1981).

There are also pragmatic reasons for studying the opening years of life. Progress in pediatric diagnosis will be inevitable if psychologists develop more sensitive assessment devices for cognitive, social, and emotional development. But perhaps the most important consequences of research with the young child rests with its beneficial effects on the uncertainties of parents, most of whom hold strong, unreflected views about the infant's basic nature and act on those beliefs, usually unselfconsciously. During the period after the First World War pediatricians told middle-class American mothers that infants should be placed on four-hour feeding schedules. Mothers who were faithful to that advice placed their infants under distress for periods that were much longer than necessary. Today, mothers wonder whether their infants have to be bonded to them through skin contact in the first hours after birth. If that idea proves false, many thousands of mothers will not have to worry that, for whatever reason, they could not be close to their baby on the first postnatal day. Further, if the claims about the loss of plasticity after the third birthday are exaggerated, parental apprehension about a temporary retardation in speech or memory functioning of a 3-year-old will be muted. Research on the infant will prune the folk theory that usually dominates the first phases of investigation in the natural sciences.

Howard Moss and I remain grateful for the opportunity that became *Birth to Maturity*. As I have said publicly and privately on many occasions, most of my research during the past twenty years can be traced to that enriching experience. I continue to feel indebted to Lester Sontag and the staff of the Institute over its long and vital life, to John and Beatrice Lacey, and, of course, to the Fels adults who, with such generosity, allowed us to enter their lives.

JEROME KAGAN

Cambridge, Massachusetts
September, 1982

References

Bernfeld, S., 1929. *The psychology of the infant*. New York: Brentano's.

Brim, O. G. and Kagan, J. (Eds.), 1980. *Constancy and change in human development*. Cambridge: Harvard University Press.

Cairns, R. B. and Hood, K. E., in press. Continuity in social development: A comparative perspective on individual difference prediction. In P. Baltes and O. G. Brim (Eds.), *Life span development*, vol. 5. New York: Academic Press.

Ellis, H., 1980. The analysis of the sexual impulse. *The Alienist and the Neurologist, 21*, 247–262.

Erikson, E. H., 1963. *Childhood and society*. New York: Norton.

Garcia Coll, C., Kagan, J., and Reznick, J. S., in press. Behavioral inhibition in young children. *Child develpm.*

Kagan, J., 1971. *Change and continuity in infancy*. New York: John Wiley.

Kagan, J., 1981. *The second year*. Cambridge: Harvard University Press.

Kagan, J., 1982. *Psychological research on the human infant*. New York: W. T. Grant Foundation.

Kagan, J., Kearsley, R. B., and Zelazo, P. R., 1978. *Infancy: Its place in human development*. Cambridge: Harvard University Press.

Kagan, J., Lapidus, D., and Moore, M., 1978. Infant antecedents of cognitive functioning. *Child develpm. 49*, 1005–1023.

McCall, R. B., 1977. Children's IQ's as predictors of adult educational and occupational status. *Science, 157*, 42–43.

Macfarlane, J. W., 1963. From infancy to adulthood. *Childhood Education, 39*, 336–342.

Mandelbaum, M., 1971. *History, man, and reason*. Baltimore: The Johns Hopkins University Press.

Moss, H. A., and Susman, E. J., 1980. Longitudinal study of personality development. In O. G. Brim and J. Kagan (Eds.), *Constancy and change in human development*. Cambridge: Harvard University Press, pp. 530–595.

Piaget, J., 1951. *Play, dreams, and imitation in childhood*. Trans. C. Gattegno and F. M. Hodgson. London: Routledge and Kegan Paul.

Stern, W., 1930. *Psychology of early childhood up to the sixth year of age*. 6th German ed., trans. A. Barwell. New York: Holt Rinehart.

Stevenson-Hinde, J., Stillwell-Barnes, R., and Zunz, M., 1980. Individual differences in young rhesus monkeys: Consistency and change. *Primates, 21*, 498–509.

Stevenson-Hinde, J., Stillwell-Barnes, R., and Zunz, M., 1980. Subjective assessment of rhesus monkeys over four successive years. *Primates, 21*, 66–82.

Thorndike, E. L., 1905. *The elements of psychology*. New York: A. G. Seiler.

Tylor, E. B., 1878. *Researches into the early history of mankind*. New York: Holt.

Werner, E. E., and Smith, R. S., 1982. *Vulnerable but invincible*. New York: McGraw Hill.

Winick, M., Meyer, K. K., and Harris, R. C., 1975. Malnutrition and environmental enrichment by early adoption. *Science, 190*, 1173–1175.

NOTE: References in the text to appendixes should be disregarded; the appendixes have not been retained in this edition.

Preface to the First Edition

This book is the result of more than thirty years of prodigious effort by many people. It is a summary of a comprehensive assessment of a group of young adults who have been members of the Fels Research Institute's longitudinal population since their birth.

Although explanation of many facets of development requires continuous observation of the child, there has been an understandable resistance to the initiation of longitudinal investigations. The reasons for this resistance are obvious. Longitudinal research is expensive, time consuming, and usually does not provide immediate results. Moreover, longitudinal programs suffer from changes in staff and data collection strategies over time.

However, these handicaps are trivial compared to the potential dividends of a longitudinal approach. If we are to understand adult behavior, we must learn more about the process of its construction over time.

The potential contributions of this longitudinal investigation fall into four categories. The findings of this study point to islands of continuity amidst the changing response patterns of the growing child and suggest that some popular hypotheses about development need revision.

This investigation uncovered several new and provocative ideas about developmental sequences that are not emphasized by current theorists and that deserve careful empirical attention.

Finally, we attempted to test the validity of some contemporary personality assessment techniques by studying the relations between the test protocols produced by our subjects and the rich and extensive behavioral information available on each of them.

There is one set of issues that this book does not presume to evaluate. The gathering of the early longitudinal data was not guided by a consistent theoretical orientation, and it is impossible, therefore, to comment on the validity of psychoanalytic or behavioral theory as they refer to cause-effect sequences in development. Correlatively, this book does not contain any elaborate theoretical integration of psychological development. We would have liked to assume this responsibility but the data prohibited such an ambitious undertaking.

Whatever degree of success this project has achieved is clearly attributable to Dr. L. W. Sontag and the Fels staff, who assiduously gathered the longitudinal information on our subjects. Dr. Sontag has been the Institute's director since its birth in 1929. His insistence on continued observation of the child in natural settings provided the foundation for this investigation, and his support was of great value during the assessment program. Our debt to the Institute staff during this 30-year period is inestimable, and a complete list of authors should include Drs. Alfred L. Baldwin, Horace Champney, Thomas W. Richards, Virginia L. Nelson, Glen Heathers, and Vaughn J. Crandall; assisted by Frances Best, Faye Breese, Grace Harrison, Mary Frances Hartson, Joan Kalhorn Lasko, Frances Leuba, Leah Levinger, Helen Marshall, Marjorie Powell, Anne Preston, Alice Rabson, Margaret Slutz, and Margaret Sperry.

The current assessment required preparation of test materials and hundreds of hours of data analysis, and we express our gratitude to many hands and hearts, especially Carl Black, Edris Bright, Edmund Churchill, Meredith Dallas, Cele Kagan, Dorothy Laming, Judith Lemkin, Marcia Lord, Gay Meyers, Bernice Rosman, Barbara Hosken, and Miriam Young.

The data presented in Chapter Eight are the product of a joint research effort with John and Beatrice Lacey, who collaborated in the planning of the experiment and collected the autonomic data. Their advice and encouragement throughout all phases of the project are gratefully acknowledged. We are particularly indebted to William Kessen and Halbert Robinson for their careful reading of the entire manuscript and many constructive suggestions.

Wesley Becker of the University of Illinois has performed a factor analysis on the ratings involved in this study and has prepared a mimeographed summary of these results. Anyone interested in this summary may write to Dr. Becker for this report.

The opportunity to spend a semester in the Department of Social Relations at Harvard University allowed one of us (JK) to complete the manuscript under the most ideal conditions—away from administrative duties and surrounded by friendly critics.

Mrs. Leah Johnson typed all of the verbatim test protocols and draft after draft of our longhand scrawl, but managed to retain both her humor and sanity. Finally, we wish to thank Ruth Bean, the Institute's field secretary. Her continued contact with the Fels subjects over the years and her efficient arranging of research appointments made our task easier and contributed not only to the success of this investigation but also to the entire Fels program.

Financial support for the project came from the Fels Fund of Philadelphia and the National Institute of Mental Health of the United States Public Health Service in the form of research grants M-1260 and M-623.

JEROME KAGAN
HOWARD A. MOSS

Yellow Springs, Ohio
Bethesda, Maryland
August, 1962

CHAPTER ONE

Introduction

The search for stability in physical and biological systems is a lure that attracts much scientific inquiry. The stability of that system we popularly call human behavior has long whetted the curiosity of most men, be they scientists *qua* scientists or scientists *qua* parents.

Many of the behaviors that characterize childhood have transient lives and are either replaced or dropped long before maturity. Egocentric speech, faulty articulation, and fear of the dark are each associated with specific developmental periods, and we are not surprised when they vanish from the behavioral scene. There has always been, however, an explicit and rather dogmatic conviction that selected adult motives, attitudes, and behaviors begin their growth during the first 10 years of life. Once established during the childhood years, these responses are likely to remain permanent aspects of the individual's behavioral repertoire. Retrospective impressions of childhood gathered from psychotherapy sessions, anecdotal reports, and private introspections support this belief, but more substantial evidence has been difficult to obtain. Only systematic longitudinal observations can discover those behaviors that are marked for future use and those that will be lost along the way.

This book summarizes an investigation of the personality development of 89 white children (45 females and 44 males) from the Fels Research Institute's longitudinal population. These children, with their parents, have been participants in a longitudinal study of their psychological development from birth through early adulthood. The initiation of this project was coincident with the birth of the Institute and its multidisciplinary study of human development. In the fall of 1929 the first Fels child joined the longitudinal program, and during the next 10 years the 89 subjects in the present investigation followed suit. Dr. Lester W. Sontag, who has been the Institute's director since its inception, has guided its growth during the last three decades. The success of this project is due, in large measure, to his insistence on direct observation of the child in natural settings, repeated administrations of standard test procedures, and an implacable faith in the longitudinal approach to the study of man.

HIDDEN VALUES IN A LONGITUDINAL APPROACH

The link between child and adult behavior

One of the obvious reasons for continuous study of man's development is to discover classes of stable response systems and the developmental periods during which they become manifest. Is it possible to predict dependent or aggressive behavior in adulthood from the child's reactions with parents and peers? Does infant hyperactivity correlate with restlessness during the school years? These and similar questions require longitudinal observations of the developing child.

A related and equally intriguing question concerns the emergence of derivative behaviors, that is, behaviors that bear a lawful relation to early childhood responses but that have been transformed in the course of development. For example, it is generally acknowledged that fear of the dark or of animals in a 3-year-old is not highly predictive of similar fears in the adult. School-age children are pressured to suppress irrational fears, and these reactions usually disappear from the repertoire of overt behaviors. However, a substitute response may take its place. Avoidance of body-contact sports or reluctance to enter into competitive activities may be derived from early fear of environmental dangers. Similarly, the rage reactions to frustration that characterize some 2-year-olds may lead to derivative behaviors that, at a manifest level, appear unrelated to "tantrums" but are theoretically tied to the early behavior.

Adult behavior is a complicated code in which many responses bear a lawful relation to earlier behavior patterns. Insight into this code would provide important clues toward an understanding of human development and predictive power in forecasting adult reactions from childhood behavior. At present our knowledge of this cryptograph is meagre, and longitudinal information provides the opportunity to trace the connections between early and late forms of a class of responses.

The influence of the social environment and the sleeper effect

A second set of causal links in human development involves the specific influence of the family, peers, teachers, and other adults on the child's goals and behaviors. The significant social agents in the child's world direct his development through their actions. These agents establish contingencies for reinforcements (both rewards and punishments); they love and reject, restrict and ignore him. Furthermore, they serve as models for identification. The laws that describe how these actions influence the child's personality have not yet been established.

The economical, and therefore popular, strategy of attacking this problem has been to obtain simultaneous information on parent and child during a given developmental period and to relate these selected sectors of parent and child behaviors. This approach is most useful in those instances where we can be fairly certain that the parental attitude or practice is an antecedent rather than an effect of the child's behavior. For example, an association between maternal hostility and child aggression might well be the result of the child's aggression provoking a hostile maternal attitude.

There is a second instance in which simultaneous observations on mother and child may yield misleading or ambiguous relationships. Certain classes of maternal practices have a latent or sleeper effect and require several years before their influence is evidenced in the child's behavior. In a later chapter it will be shown that maternal acceleration of the child's developmental skills showed the highest correlation with adult achievement behavior when the measure of maternal acceleration was obtained during the first three years of life. Similarly, maternal protection of the child during the first three years was a better predictor of school-age passivity than the mother's protective behavior during later age periods. The correlations were considerably lower when the index of maternal protection was taken at the same time that the school-age child's passivity was assessed. Maternal reward of dependency in an 8-year-old has a different effect on the child than a similar maternal practice six years earlier. There is good reason to believe that other parental practices have similar "sleeper" effects. If this is true, only long-term, continuous study of parent and child will furnish a complete description of these delayed, developmental sequences.

A substitute for the experiment

Simultaneous observations of parent and child behavior are inadequate bases for deriving causal statements about the mechanisms of behavioral development. But the controlled experiment, which is admittedly the most potent weapon in the scientist's arsenal, is only amenable to selected problems in psychology. Many aspects of personality development are not subject to experimental manipulation. Aggressive children can not be transferred to loving homes; mothers can not be told to adopt a pattern of reinforcements so that the psychologist can have an aesthetically pleasing design.

A longitudinal investigation, however, might be viewed as a substitute for the powerful strategy inherent in experimental manipulation—a halfway house between the correlational and experimental investigation. One can hypothesize antecedent-consequent relations and assess, through continuous observation of the mother and child, the validity of the prediction. For example, a popular question asks whether maternal rejection leads to aggressive behavior in the child. The experimentalist avoids the problem because he can not assign children, at random, to accepting and rejecting mothers. The usual tactic of cross-sectional assessment of mothers and children at a given time is subject to the potential errors reviewed above. The longitudinal investigator assesses maternal rejection during the early years, follows the child over time, and evaluates him during the preschool and school years. A positive correlation between early maternal rejection and later aggression under these conditions is persuasive.

The longitudinal programs at Stanford University, University of California Institute of Human Development, University of Minnesota Institute of Child Welfare, Child Research Council, Harvard University, Menninger Foundation, and the Fels Research Institute are costly and unusual scientific enterprises. However, these projects address themselves to selected developmental questions that can be answered only through continuous study of the organism over a long period of time.

There are, of course, disadvantages and limitations in longitudinal work that are neither minor nor easily surmounted. Longitudinal samples are usually not representative. Parents with an interest in research or a desire for the prestige associated with being a part of a research project are most likely to enroll their child in such a program. This fact alone rules against a truly representative sample. A longitudinal regimen encroaches on the time and privacy of the parents, and the inevitable attrition in a longitudinal study is probably not determined by chance alone. Socioeconomic factors cause certain subjects to remain geographically close to the Institute, while others migrate to distant communities. Assurance of a random sampling in a longitudinal program is, therefore, practically unattainable. However, specification of the sample's characteristics can set the boundaries of generality that can be ascribed to the empirical results.

A RÉSUMÉ OF LONGITUDINAL STUDIES

Mental growth

Initially the major longitudinal centers in this country concentrated on those problems for which standard methods of measurement were available. Studies of morphological growth and mental development, therefore, comprised most of the research output of these programs. Historically, the Genetic Studies of Genius, conducted by Terman and his colleagues at Stanford, stand out as one of the first longitudinal studies directed at a specific class of psychological variables (Terman, 1925; Terman, Burks and Jensen, 1930; Terman and Oden, 1947; Terman and Oden, 1959).

The study, initiated in 1921, selected 661 California school children with IQ scores of 135 or higher for intensive study and follow-up at later age periods. The last follow-up occurred more than 35 years after the initial measurements, when most of the original subjects were in their forties. These investigations revealed that the original gifted subjects continued to maintain their superiority in intellectual activities. They attained considerably higher educational and occupational levels than the average person, and many of them achieved prominence in their vocations. They exhibited a lower incidence of physical defects, emotional disturbances, and asocial behaviors than a random sample of the population. Terman and his associates concluded that early intellectual superiority remained relatively stable over a 30-year period and that gifted children exhibited a cluster of behaviors that differentiated them from children with more typical mental ability. Terman's findings have negated the anecdotal view that giftedness is necessarily associated with deficiences in other areas and have formed an important base for prediction of the long-term consequences of superior intellectual ability in childhood.

There have been many studies on the constancy of mental test scores over the childhood years for more representative groups of children. This literature was reviewed by both Nemzeh (1931) and Foran (1926, 1929) for studies up to 1931, and by Thorndike (1940) for studies published between 1931 and 1940. Thorndike summarized over 100 reports on this subject.

Two conclusions emerge from the studies concerned with the stability of intelligence test performance. First, early IQ scores, particularly those obtained during the first two years of life, are not highly predictive of later test scores (Anderson, 1939; Bayley, 1949; Bradway, 1945; Ebert and Simmons, 1943; Honzik, 1938; Nelson and Richards, 1938).

Bayley and her associates at the University of California noted that mental growth proceeded at variable rates for different children and intelligence test scores obtained prior to 18 months of age were poor predictors of school-age IQ scores. Prior to 2 years of age, parental intelligence and educational level were better indexes of the child's intelligence at age 10 than the child's own test scores (Bayley, 1954; Kagan and Moss, 1959b; Moss and Kagan, 1958). Intelligence test scores obtained during the preschool and early school years, however, are fairly good predictors of adult functioning. In a recent study a correlation of +.59 was reported between Stanford-Binet IQ scores obtained during the preschool years and during young adulthood (Bradway, Thompson, and Cravens, 1958).

A second generalization derived from intelligence test data concerns the relation between rate of mental growth and personality. Sontag, Baker, and Nelson (1958) used the longitudinal data on the Fels population to investigate factors contributing to changes in Stanford-Binet IQ during the early school years. They found that some children exhibited substantial increases in test score (up to 40 points) during the years 6 to 10, while others manifested a steady decrease in test score over this period. During the first 12 years of life these children were interviewed and observed at Fels, at home, and in school. These naturalistic data formed the basis for ratings of the child on a number of personality variables. These ratings were related to their pattern of IQ change (i.e., whether the child was an IQ ascender or descender). Children who were overtly competitive and independent with peers and adults were more likely to show increases in IQ during the latency years than noncompetitive, dependent children. Bradway and Robinson (1961) have found that increase in IQ score during the elementary school years is also positively related to the social-class background of the child.

In sum, the application of the longitudinal method to the study of intellective function has yielded information on both the stability of IQ scores and some of the psychological correlates of change in intellective ability.

Personality development

Methods for assessing personality variables lack the degree of standardization possessed by intelligence tests, and for that reason longitudinal programs have not produced as impressive a set of findings for this more complex class of variables.

The early studies on constancies in personality were based primarily on anecdotal and biographical information. Smith (1952) studied a mother's diary descriptions of her three boys and three girls covering a period of eight years. These children were interviewed 50 years later, and their friends were questioned in an attempt to obtain a description of their adult personalities. Childhood differences in behaviors related to aggression, achievement, and intellectual competence appeared to remain stable for this small group of children.

In a similar study (Neilson, 1948), the personality sketches of 15 children (based on Shirley's observations during the first two years of life) were matched with personality sketches of these children during adolescence. The adolescent sketches were based on test and rating material and were prepared without knowledge of the earlier descriptive material. A group of judges were able to match the two protocols at better than chance, suggesting that some gross aspects of behavior remain stable from age 2 through early adolescence.

McKinnon (1942) evaluated the continuity of behavior over a five-year period for a small group of children who were of preschool age when first observed. The follow-up evaluation was based on behavioral observations, teachers' reports, and interviews with teachers and parents. McKinnon concluded, as did most investigators, that there were areas of behavioral consistency.

In a more objective study of behavioral continuity, Gesell (1939) compared motion-picture records of five children taken at 1 and 5 years of age. Ratings of behavior, based on the motion-picture material, yielded a remarkable degree of stability over the four-year period.

Unlike these early studies, which dealt with small numbers of cases, those that have appeared more recently are based on larger samples, survey a broader band of behaviors, and cover a greater proportion of the life span.

Tuddenham (1959) conducted a 19-year follow-up of those individuals who participated in the adolescent growth study at the University of California's Institute of Human Development. Ratings of the adolescents' personality were based on direct observations and cumulative impressions gleaned from years of contact with the subjects. In the follow-up, in which interviews were conducted with subjects who were approximately 33 years old, ratings were made on variables modeled after those used during the adolescent period. Stability coefficients were obtained between adolescent and adult ratings for each of the variables. Approximately one third of the variables for which reliable judgments could be made yielded significant stability coefficients over the 19-year period. A rating of aggressive motivation was most stable for men $(r = .91)$, whereas desire for social prestige was most stable for women $(r = .81)$. There were several methodological deficiencies associated with this investigation. The dissimilarity between the adolescent and adult rating situations and the low inter-rater reliabilities were two major sources of error in the study. Tuddenham points out that the stabilities obtained for some of the behaviors are quite remarkable, considering the potential sources of error.

Other investigations at the University of California explored the transmission of parental roles from one generation to the next (Bronson, Katten, and Livson, 1959). The investigators obtained retrospective descriptions, from the parents of the longitudinal subjects, of the degree of authority and affection they ascribed to their own parents (i.e., the grandparents of the children). Measures of degree of affection and authority shown by the parents toward their own children were also obtained. The results yielded negligible evidence for the direct transmission of affection and authority behavior between the two generations.

A seven-year longitudinal study was conducted in the community of "Prairie City" (Peck, 1958; Peck and Havighurst, 1960). The children were 10 years old when the project was initiated, and they were tested and interviewed by psychologists and rated by their peers, from 10 to 17 years of age. One of the central interests of the investigators involved the relationship between familial patterns and the child's developing personality, especially his character or conscience development. On the basis of the accumulated information, each subject was evaluated on a variety of personality and moral standard variables (e.g., ego strength, superego strength, spontaneity, friendliness, hostility-guilt, and moral stability). In addition, the families of these adolescents were rated for four kinds of practices: consistency, democracy, mutual trust, and severity.

The major findings suggested that ego strength was associated with a family milieu that was consistent and trusting. Friendliness and spontaneity in the child were related to democratic and trusting parental attitudes; hostility and guilt were associated with a severely autocratic and untrusting family milieu (Peck, 1958; Peck and Havighurst, 1960). Moreover, degree of conscience development and emotional independence at age 10 were highly correlated with similar variables at age 16, indicating the stability of these personality dispositions over a six-year period (Peck and Havighurst, 1960).

Escalona and Heider (1959), at the Menninger Foundation, attempted to predict the behavior of preschool children from observations of them during the first year of life. Degree of motor coordination and sex-role interests in the 5-year-old could be estimated from the infancy data. Other behaviors, such as shyness and achievement strivings, could not be predicted.

This brief summary is intended to give the reader a flavor of the research product from some representative longitudinal studies and should not be regarded as a comprehensive discussion of all the longitudinal research that has been published. For an annotated review of longitudinal studies, the reader is referred to Stone and Onqué (1959).

THE PRESENT INVESTIGATION

The study to be described is concerned primarily with the stability of selected motive-related behaviors, sources of anxiety, defensive responses, and modes of interpersonal interaction from earliest childhood through young adulthood.

A second and third objective are to consider the effect of a small group of maternal practices on the child's behavioral development and to assess the validity of some popular techniques in personality assessment. The sources of information used in this study comprise one of the most comprehensive bodies of longitudinal observations available. The next chapter contains a detailed description of our methods and analytic procedures. The present section summarizes the nature of the sample, the rationale of the investigation, and an overview of the sources of information.

The population

The 89 subjects studied were enrolled in the Fels longitudinal program during the period 1929 to 1939. The educational and vocational characteristics of the group placed the majority of the subjects within the popular definition of middle class. The fathers of these children were equally distributed among the following vocational groups: laborer, farmer, small businessman, white-collar worker, and professional. Table 1 summarizes the educational background of the parents of our subjects.

TABLE 1. AMOUNT OF FORMAL EDUCATION OF THE
PARENTS OF THE LONGITUDINAL SUBJECTS

(Numbers refer to per cent of group)

	Mother		Father	
Education	Boys	Girls	Boys	Girls
Eighth grade or lower	9.3	13.3	13.6	27.2
Part high school	11.6	11.2	11.4	13.6
High school graduate	32.6	33.3	25.0	13.6
Part college	30.2	17.8	2.3	16.0
College graduate	16.3	24.4	27.2	22.7
Postgraduate	0.0	0.0	20.5	6.9

There were no significant differences in educational level of parents of the boys or girls, and about 75 per cent of the parents were high school graduates.

The 89 children came from 63 different families, with 19 of the families supplying 45 of the children. Seven families each furnished three children and 12 supplied two children to the total sample. The remaining 44 families had only one child in the study. The religious backgrounds of the 63 families were 53 Protestant, 9 Catholic, and 1 Jewish. Two girls were adopted during the first year of life and remained with their adopted parents during the course of the study. The mothers of three girls were divorced during the early school years, and these children acquired stepfathers soon after. The mothers of two girls died while the girls were in elementary school; one father remarried; the second girl was cared for by her father and an older sister. One boy was adopted during his first year of life, and no cases of divorce or parental death occurred among the boys. There was one set of triplet boys in the group and no twins. The ordinal positions of the 89 children are summarized in Table 2.

TABLE 2. ORDINAL POSITION OF THE LONGITUDINAL SAMPLE

(Numbers refer to per cent of group)

Ordinal Position	Boys (N = 44)	Girls (N = 45)
Only child	11.3	4.4
Eldest	34.2	28.9
Second	25.0	37.8
Third	13.6	15.6
Fourth	2.3	8.9
Fifth	6.8	0.0
Sixth	0.0	2.2
Seventh	0.0	2.2
Triplets	6.8	0.0

Sources of data: Birth through adolescence

The major purpose of the project was to relate the functioning of the child to the psychological status of the adult. The historical data were collected during the period 1929 to 1954. During the initial years of the Institute's program (1929 to 1932), psychological information was sparse. By 1933, however, a fairly comprehensive program of mental testing and behavioral observations had been initiated, and by 1935 a variety of psychological material was being obtained on each subject. Observations of behavior of mother and child at home were gathered semiannually during the first six years of life and annually from 6 to 12 years of age. The children were observed at the Fels experimental nursery school semiannually from 2½ to 5 years of age, and annually from 6 to 10 years of age.

Children under age 5 were given mental tests twice a year. After age 5, intelligence tests were administered annually. During the school years, usually beginning at age 8, the Rorschach and selected TAT stimuli were administered every third year. Other personality tests were administered on a less regular schedule. School grades were collected, and many of the children were observed semiannually in their public school settings for half-day periods. The children from 6 to 14 were interviewed each year by a staff member, and the mothers of the children were interviewed annually either at home or at the Institute. These sources of information constitute the core of the longitudinal data available on our subjects. Table 3 summarizes the types of information obtained for the typical child in our current sample.

TABLE 3. SUMMARY OF LONGITUDINAL INFORMATION ON A TYPICAL CHILD

Type of Information	Setting and Method of Recording	Typical Frequency
1. Observation of child's behavior	(a) Half day of observation of child and mother in the home. Observations summarized in narrative style.	Twice yearly from birth to 6 years of age. Annually from age 6 to 12.
	(b) Observations of child in Fels Experimental Nursery School and Day Camp; half-day sessions for 3 weeks. Observations summarized in narrative style and ratings made on Child Behavior Rating Scales.	Twice yearly from 2½ to 5. Annually from age 6 to 10.
	(c) Interview with child. Interview summarized in narrative style.	Annually from age 6 to 12.
	(d) Observation of child in school with narrative summary.	Semiannually from 1st to 8th grade.
2. Testing—personality	(a) Thematic Apperception Test; selected stimuli from Murray's series (1943).	Every third year from age 8–6 to 17–6.
	(b) Rorschach.	Every third year from age 8–6 to 17–6.
	(c) Minnesota Multiphasic Personality Inventory.	Once during adolescence—age 17.
	(d) Kuder Preference Record.	Once during adolescence—age 17.
3. Mental development	(a) Gesell Developmental Schedule.	6, 12, 18, and 24 months.
	(b) Merrill-Palmer Infant Test.	18, 24, 30 months.
	(c) Stanford-Binet Intelligence Test.	2½, 3, 3½, 4, 4½, 5, 6, 7, 8, 9, 10, 11, 12, and 14 years.

TABLE 3 (CONTINUED)

Type of Information	Setting and Method of Recording	Typical Frequency
	(d) Wechsler-Bellevue IQ.	Age 13 and 17.
	(e) Primary Mental Abilities.	Age 17.
4. Observation of mother	(a) Half-day observation of mother in home with child. Observations summarized in narrative style and ratings made on Parent Behavior Rating Scale.	Twice yearly from birth to 6 years of age. Annually from age 6 to 12.
	(b) Interview with mother with narrative summary.	Annually from birth to adolescence.
5. Mental testing of mother and father	Otis IQ Test.	One administration.

Most of the personality information about the child consisted of narrative summaries of observations of the child at home, in school, or at the Institute. This was the richest and most accurate source of data on the child's behavior, and it was decided to attempt a quantification of these observational statements. The nature of the data precluded the inclusion of some variables that contemporary theory regards as important. For example, there was little information on the personality or attitudes of the father or the father's relationship to the child, and it was impossible to evaluate reliably the father-child or father-mother relationship. The final choice of variables was a function of the nature of the available material and the theoretical predilection of the authors.

RATIONALE FOR CHOICE OF CHILD BEHAVIOR VARIABLES

Current theory and research in personality development place considerable emphasis on four classes of variables: (a) behaviors aimed at attainment of culturally salient goals (i.e., motive related behaviors), (b) sources of anxiety and conflict, (c) defensive responses to anxiety-arousing situations and conflicts, and (d) modes of interpersonal interaction.

Motive-related behaviors

Motives, in contrast to primary needs or drives, are typically defined as learned desires for specific goal states, and the label applied to the motive is derived from the nature of the goal that is sought. It is generally assumed that the acquisition of a motive is a complex function of antecedent experiences and that the arousal of a specific motive is under the partial control of stimuli that have become associated with the relevant goal state (i.e., incentive stimuli). That is, the concept of motive arousal implies a learned association between a class of stimuli and a goal state. When this association is triggered, by internal or external stimuli, behavior directed at goal attainment is likely to occur.

The major motivational systems studied in the present research include the desire for social recognition, task mastery, nurturance and affection, sex-appropriate interests, sexual gratification, affiliation with peers, and perception of a state of injury or anxiety in others (aggression). It is difficult to specify the measurement operations used to assess each of these motives, and this is a topic of considerable controversy (Bolles, 1958; Littman, 1958; Malmo, 1958). One approach involves observation of changes in the ongoing behavior of the individual following elicitation of the motive in settings that have been designated as motive arousing situations. For example, if a child suddenly begins to cry when his mother leaves him at the Fels Nursery School, we assume that the desire for nurturance has been aroused. If the child seeks out tasks that are challenging and lead to an opportunity for task mastery, we assume the child has a need for achievement satisfactions. However, the intensity and frequency of goal-related behavior is not perfectly correlated with motive strength, for other response systems may interfere with the execution of behavior aimed at the satisfaction of a particular motive. In some cases a stronger competing motive may be present. In most cases, however, anxiety over goal attainment leads to inhibition of goal-directed responses. *For this reason we concentrated our efforts on quantifying overt goal-related behavior* and tried to avoid the more precarious task of assessing motive strength.

Sources of anxiety

Development is typically accompanied by various sources of anxiety that begin to be established during different age periods and that often have a long-term effect on future behavior.

During the first four years, anxiety over anticipated loss of parental love and nurturance is unusually strong and an important force in the socialization of the child. During the preschool years, anxiety becomes attached to the anticipation of physical injury and to expression of aggressive, sexual, and dependent behaviors. The intensity of each of these sources of anxiety is a function of the child's familial and extra-familial experiences. Finally, anxiety over failure to master socially valued skills, withdrawal from problems, personal inadequacy, and deviation from sex-role standards grow in strength during the latency and preadolescent years. We attempted to evaluate these sources of anxiety. Although this list is not exhaustive, it samples some of the important foci of anxiety that punctuate the developmental process among members of western culture.

The semantic definition of anxiety is less subject to debate than are the various proposals for an operational definition. There is consensual agreement that anxiety is an unpleasant, affective state. As with motives, however, there are no standard behavioral indicators that are acknowledged as valid indexes of anxiety. Changes in ongoing behavior in situations that are designated, *a priori*, as anxiety provoking provide one source of data for quantification.

Anxiety as a motive for defensive behavior

Anxiety has motivational properties, for it elicits responses aimed at a specific goal. The goal, in this case, is diminution of the unpleasant feeling state. Those learned responses that are instrumental in attaining this goal have been called defenses. The term defense has referred classically to covert thought sequences, such as repression, projection, and rationalization, which attenuate the anxiety resulting from conflictful ideas or commission of prohibited acts. It is reasonable, however, to extend the definition of defense to include overt reactions that are attempts to reduce anxiety. One popular defensive maneuver is withdrawal from situations where task failure or social rejection is anticipated. The developmental records of our subjects contained extensive evidence of differential preference for withdrawal, and we focused our attention on this class of behaviors.

Social interaction

Finally, we considered the quality of the child's interpersonal interactions as an important developmental variable. The tendency to approach or to avoid social objects, the degree of spontaneity or tension in social interaction, and the tendency to dominate or submit in peer interactions are tendencies that are clear in the 5-year-old child and that may preview the adult's orientation to others. It is possible to derive or to explain these social interaction patterns from a detailed consideration of the motive, anxiety, and defense constructs. However, considering the immature stage of psychological theory, it seems wise to use variables that are closer to the phenomena under study.

These, then, are the major classes of child-behavior variables we chose to investigate: motive-related behaviors, sources of anxiety, defensive responses, and modes of social interaction.

The behavior of the mother

Although there are a great number of dimensions that could be assessed in the mother-child interaction, investigators have concerned themselves with a limited number of maternal practices. The variables of hostility, restriction, protection, and acceleration are among those that are as popular today as they were 30 years ago. Both factor analyses of ratings of maternal behavior as well as current theory suggest that the above variables are of psychological importance in the child's development (Baldwin, Kalhorn, Breese, 1949; Schaefer, 1959). The Fels Parent Behavior Rating Scales (Baldwin, Kalhorn, Breese, 1945) emphasized these dimensions and directed the attention of the Fels observers toward assessments of these maternal practices. Thus the narrative summaries of the observers were particularly discursive in these areas but rather meagre in other aspects of the mother-child interaction. It was decided, therefore, to attempt a quantification of degree of maternal hostility, restriction, protection, and acceleration, during the first decade of the child's life. A more complete description of these variables and the rationale for their selection appear in Chapter Seven.

OVERVIEW OF THE PROCEDURE

The historical data covered the span birth through early adolescence, and we tried to construct variables that would be relevant for the first 14 years of life. This was impossible for child behaviors that have relevance only for specific age periods. Anxiety to the Fels visitor, for example, could only be assessed during the first few years, while an interest in intellectual activity could only be evaluated after the child had reached a certain degree of conceptual maturity. Aggression to mother or frustration tolerance, however, is an appropriate variable for both the 2- and the 12-year-old. A set of 48 variables was defined and the cue points established for a seven-point rating scale. The coding of the longitudinal data followed the following plan. The longitudinal material was divided into four age periods: 0 to 3, 3 to 6, 6 to 10, and 10 to 14. These divisions roughly parallel important developmental periods. The first three years deal with infancy and the early socialization training period. Years three through six, the preschool years, involve initial peer interaction and the child's attempt to resolve dependency on his parents. The next four years involve adjustment to school, establishment of interests and skills, and relationships with same sex peers. The preadolescent years (10 to 14) deal with the development of heterosexual interests, emergence of vocational choice, and the firm establishment of modes of defensive reaction to anxiety-arousing situations.

We would have preferred to divide these periods into finer age categories, but the material available for a one- or two-year period was insufficient to make reliable ratings for most of our variables. Once again the limitation of the data interfered with the best possible procedure.

Initially the material for each child was studied for the first three years of life and ratings made on those variables for which there was adequate information. After the ratings for ages 0 to 3, the ratings for ages 3 to 6, 6 to 10, and, finally, ages 10 to 14 were made, in that order. In general, a period of about 6 months intervened between the rating of a child for one period and the rating of that child for a subsequent period.

Howard Moss, who made the ratings, *had no knowledge of* any of the test information on these subjects (i.e., intelligence test scores, projective tests) or of their adult psychological status. Special precautions were taken to insure that he would not learn of any information about them except for what he read in the longitudinal reports. These four sets of ratings comprise the primary source of historical data on our subjects.

ADULT ASSESSMENT

Of the 89 subjects (Ss) for whom longitudinal ratings had been made, 71 participated in the recent adult assessment program during the period July 1957 through October 1959.[1] At the time of the assessment the subjects were between 19 and 29 years of age. Table 4 presents the age, marital status, education, and religious affiliation of the 71 adult subjects.

TABLE 4. AGE, MARITAL STATUS, EDUCATION, AND RELIGIOUS AFFILIATION OF THE SUBJECTS PARTICI- PATING IN THE ADULT ASSESSMENT

(Numbers refer to per cent of group)

	Males (N = 36)	Females (N = 35)
Age		
Mean	24–4	23–11
Range	19–29	20–29
Marital status		
Married	55.6	71.4
Single	44.4	28.6
Education		
Part high school	5.5	5.8
High school	19.5	28.6
Part college	50.0	51.3
College graduate	16.7	11.4
Postgraduate	8.3	2.9
Religious affiliation		
Protestant	72.2	82.8
Catholic	25.0	17.2
Jewish	2.8	0.0

Where possible, the older subjects were seen first and the younger subjects later in order to obtain a minimum age difference among the subjects at the time of assessment. The adult assessment contained two parts, interviews and a formal testing schedule. Two subjects completed only the interview sessions, leaving 69 who went through both procedures. The interviews always occurred first and were conducted by Jerome Kagan. *The interviewer had absolutely no knowledge of any of the longitudinal or test information on the adult at the time of the interview.* This precaution insured that the childhood data would influence neither the interview process nor the subsequent evaluation of these adults. Thus the longitudinal and interview ratings were completely independent of each other. Since the primary purpose of the research was to relate child and adult personality dispositions, this independence was mandatory.

After the tape-recorded interviews, each adult was rated on a seven-point scale for variables similar to those rated from the longitudinal records. The second part of the adult assessment consisted of a testing program which included a modified ink blot task, selected TAT stimuli, a self-rating inventory, conceptual sorting tasks, a tachistoscopic recognition task, Wechsler-Bellevue Intelligence Scale (Form I), and measures of autonomic reactivity. A detailed description of these procedures appears in the next chapter.

The research had two separate aims. The primary goal was to investigate the selective stability of behavior from childhood through early adulthood. It was hoped, however, that this rich source of information on a moderately large sample would lead to important conclusions concerning the meaning of some of the popular measuring instruments in personality research. Contemporary psychology is, in large measure, method poor. Most of our techniques are of unknown or questionable validity. We hoped that a detailed analysis of the test behavior of a sample of subjects for whom a comprehensive personality picture was available would help determine the validity of these instruments. The intriguing problem of developmental continuity in human behavior has not been empirically answered because of insufficient information. Since these longitudinal observations were unique, we felt free to speculate on many results that were of borderline significance. We view this research report primarily as a source of new hypotheses and not as an almanac of facts. It is an invitation to our colleagues to select ideas according to their taste and to submit to more rigorous testing the provocative hunches uncovered by this investigation.

Footnote

1. Of the 18 subjects not assessed, only two refused to cooperate. The remaining 16 resided far from the Institute and found it difficult to come to Yellow Springs.

CHAPTER TWO

Methods of Assessment

This chapter describes the methods and sources of data associated with the longitudinal and adult assessments. The longitudinal program will be considered first.

LONGITUDINAL INFORMATION

The longitudinal material was collected during the years 1929 to 1954. The first few years of data collection were unsystematic, but by 1933 a fairly comprehensive program had taken form, and the program that was established in the 1930's has remained the basic model for data collection up to the present time.

The longitudinal data that were used to make the childhood ratings included two major classes of information: (1) narrative reports and ratings of behavior observations and (2) interview protocols and interview summaries. The intelligence and projective test protocols were analyzed independently and did not enter into these ratings. All of these protocols were gathered according to the schedule outlined in Table 3 of Chapter One.

The intelligence and personality tests were administered through the use of procedures recommended in their respective manuals. The narrative reports and interview summaries were necessarily subjective and influenced by several uncontrolled factors. Since these reports were the basis of the behavioral ratings covering the first 14 years of life, a description of this material should provide the reader with a base on which to judge the results.

LONGITUDINAL OBSERVATIONS OF THE CHILD

The observations were based on visits to the home, visits to the public school, and the child's behavior in the Fels Nursery School and Day Camp. The interview summaries were based on discussions with the child, mother, and the child's teacher.

Naturalistic observations: Home visits

Naturalistic observations were made in the home semiannually for the first six years of life and were continued on an annual basis through age 14 for the majority of the subjects. The home visit was the most important source of information used in making the behavioral ratings for the first three years of life.

Most of the subjects were enrolled in the program during the last trimester of the mother's pregnancy. The first home visit usually occurred during the first three months after birth, and, during the first year, three or four home visits were made. Thereafter, a minimum of two visits a year was scheduled. In cases where there were sibs in the sample, each subject was seen twice a year regardless of how extensively his behavior may have been described in the reports of his sibs.

The visits were made by a professional worker who had psychological training. Typically, only one staff member made the home visits during any one period of time. However, there were periods when two staff members divided the cases or made visits to the same home to assess the inter-rater reliability of specific rating variables. The same home visitor continued to observe a particular family as long as that staff member remained with the Institute. The family's increased familiarity with the staff member led to good rapport and a relaxed atmosphere in the home. Over 90 per cent of the home contacts were made by a female home visitor.

Each home visit usually lasted from 3 to 4 hours during which the visitor observed the child, the mother, and the child's interactions with mother and siblings. When the visitor returned to the Institute, she wrote a lengthy summary of her observations and filled out the Fels Parent Behavior Rating Scales. The visitor rarely acted as a therapeutic or advice-giving resource. Within this relatively broad context the home visitor was flexible while in the home. She had to adapt to the way the family chose to interact with her. With some families she was seen as an intruder; in other families she was immediately assimilated into the ongoing activity of the home.

Verbatim excerpts from some representative home visits at different age levels are presented below. In these sections, S stands for child, M for mother, and F for father.

SUBJECT 006 AT 3 MONTHS OF AGE

"S was having her bath when I arrived. M handled her awkwardly and timidly, admitted that she was afraid that she would break. At the end of the bath, when she was being dressed, S started to cry, got very red, and shook in her anguish. M asked me if S cried more intensely than other babies. S was put to the breast for 10 minutes but did not nurse the entire time. She is a slow suckler; M had to tap her cheek to encourage her. She then drank eight ounces of milk, slowly also. By the end of the feeding, she was asleep. M puts her in a buggy in the library, the sun in her eyes. S slept until the home visitor left."

"Aside from a slight cold which she has now and some constipation and colic, S has been relatively well. M said that she called her father for 'every little thing' and annoyed him with her over-solicitude."

CASE 006 AT 5 YEARS, 3 MONTHS

"Characteristic of the relationship between M and S is a lack of warmth on M's part. M likes to dress S up and have her look cute—but makes no pretense above loving her. S fondled over me and sought my attention during the entire visit. For the most part this seemed to represent the desire for really close physical contact with an adult. She crawled up on my lap or snuggled close beside me whenever an opportunity presented itself. In one instance M was particularly negligent of S's welfare or feelings. M was washing dishes when S mounted a stool, sitting with the garbage can under her feet, and proceeded to help with the dishes. She stood up on the garbage can, at which point M commanded her to 'Get down off that garbage can.' S started to sit down on the stool again, but at the same time, M moved the stool and S took a hard tumble on the floor. She got up crying and threw herself against her mother, who did nothing to soothe her. M disengaged herself from S's clutches and went about her work without comment. Having failed with her mother, S came crying over to me and quieted down promptly after a minimum of sympathy and petting."

CASE 006 AT 9 YEARS, 5 MONTHS

"In regard to S's school work this past semester, M said that she came out very well. Shortly after my last visit M got busy with S, helping her to settle down to her studies. High grades are very important to both parents. M drilled S particularly with her arithmetic and spelling. 'We did college work for a month,' M said. (She meant they worked hard and untiringly.) Almost as soon as S got home from school they would begin their drill. They worked hard until dinner time, sometimes starting in again until bedtime. As a result of all this work S made marks of 100 on two or three of her exams. Therefore her final grades were excellent, mostly A's, which M was very proud of."

"S seemed tense and nervous to me today. She resorted to tight gesturing, hair twirling, and exaggerated responses to situations. One example of the latter occurred upstairs. I was watching S having her hair combed, holding the baby on my lap. The baby spit-up some undigested milk, got some on my skirt. S almost cried with concern saying, 'Oh, Mother! quick. It's all over her dress! Get something quick!' She was pretty close to tears."

SUBJECT 2640 AT 8 YEARS, 9 MONTHS

"M is a rigid disciplinarian, has fixed ideas of what is good and bad for the girls, and is convinced that their judgment is inferior to hers. She gave me a long discourse on how a girl of seventeen was too young to go away to college, 'co-educational colleges are dangerous for young girls (exposed to dangerous men without enough sense to know it),' etc."

"S called her mother after school, wanted to go home and play with a friend. M told her she could not, gave no reason: S didn't argue, as nearly as I could tell from the conversation. She was cheerful enough when she came home, asked if she might go out later in the afternoon. M very pointedly left us alone together, instructing S to entertain me. I asked *S* about her Christmas; she listed her presents, offered to show them to me, was quite poised in her artificial adult manner. She brought her dolls out for me to see, and when I admired them became enthusiastic and natural. She told me about her dolls and those of her friends, but when *M* joined us she was inhibited once more. *M* makes the children very conscious of their social position and manners and reminds them frequently of the 'correct' thing to do. This gloss over *S*'s personality, combined with her rather mature intelligence, makes her a child difficult to know or get close to."

NURSERY SCHOOL AND DAY CAMP

Each child in the study, with few exceptions, attended the Fels experimental nursery school and day camp. The nursery school and day camp consisted of half-day sessions for two- to three-week periods. The nursery school was held semiannually, for ages 2½ to 5, in the fall and spring. The day camp was held annually for children, ages 6 to 10, soon after the completion of the school year. The nursery school provided an unstructured, free-play situation for groups of 8 to 10 children. A large room within the Institute was specially equipped for this purpose. The available materials included dolls, household toys (e.g., ironing boards, tea sets); finger paints, clay, water colors, tinker toys, books, bead-stringing sets, tricycles, and other gross motor apparatus.

The day camp was a bit more structured. Competitive games were organized, and a standard battery of tests for mechanical abilities and physical skills was administered occasionally. The day camp was designed for the school-age children and was held in the same area as the nursery school.

A trained observer made detailed observational notes of the child's behavior in the nursery school and day-camp settings. The observer usually remained apart from the children and did not participate in the program. When the observation sessions were over, the observer wrote a comprehensive report on each child, organized according to several personality dimensions, such as aggressive tendencies, major interest patterns, reactions to stress, problem-solving behaviors, ease of frustration, social compliance, verbosity, and social participation. Two representative excerpts follow.

SUBJECT 213 AT 4 YEARS

"S looks like a little old gnome—large, pale eyes, often darkly shadowed, a colorless skin unrelieved by her light lashes and hair. She has a solemn monkey expression—of old wisdom, some strain, rather constant small worries. She frowns a lot, wrinkles her forehead, seldom smiles. Her facial expressions are those of a much older woman, and her pseudo-adult language and concepts further this impression; she looks like a midget of 50. She accentuated this adult-like appearance by her lack of vigor. She spent a lot of her time just sitting at times alone, dreamily holding a doll or patting at some clay, leafing through a book. She also did a lot of inert spectating—sitting on the sidelines watching the antics of the other children for long periods of time. She gave one the impression that she was amused by their activity—but just content to watch—like a tired mother. Even in her more organized social play she managed to sit down a lot and watch the other players or take a role where she could talk or work sitting down. Outdoors, too, she sat in the sand, in boxes, on the swing; dreamy, idling, listless. This sedentary attitude has been marked throughout her visits—and was even somewhat less obvious this time. When she did move she was often rather slow, deliberate, unforceful."

"Her most consistent interest was in doll and house play—of every variety. She liked to fuss around maternally, dressing dolls, cooking, and feeding them, taking them for buggy rides and walks, holding them. Much of this was done in the company of two other girls. She was quiet in this play but a full participant. When these girls moved on to other things she was frequently alone, and at these times she appeared to be indulging in a fantasy life of some kind. She ventured into books, puzzles, for brief periods but usually returned to the staple form of house play when all else failed. In her dramatic play, S often assumed an adult role, mother, teacher, etc., and her portrayal was amusingly accurate. She mimicked her own mother in speech and habit. Her phraseology was adult and her inflection was caricature of feminine speech. 'I just don't know what I'm going to do with this child!' She stood, postured, gestured, in a pseudo-adult manner. This dramatic fantasy of hers, whether overtly social or individual, almost always concerned family life, and she went through detailed reliving of everyday home life—always in the role of the managing

and dominant female, occasionally speaking for the child, too, of
course, but seemingly closely identified with the adult part."

SUBJECT 1240 AT 4 YEARS, 2 MONTHS

"S is a well-knit child. He was forceful and at ease on the apparatus.
However, it was his grace rather than skill that made him stand out
in the group; swift, easy-flowing bodily movements, diving and bound-
ing up again in one unbroken movement. There was a brief period
when S needed to get his bearings, a shrewd gaminish sizing-up of the
situation before he committed himself. From the first day he displayed exceptional social poise and made many contacts, but it was
not until the end of the first week that he definitely came out as one
of the masters of the situation and that his gaiety asserted itself.

The group really revolved around S. His leadership was outstanding, not only for his group but for older nursery school groups. S
seemed really to like others, and while the prestige of leadership may
have mattered to him when it was challenged, much more dominant,
I believe, was the fun of the whole group doing something together.

Many of the fights which S inveigled others into were of a shadow-
boxing or puppy-role wrestling variety, with lots of laughing; but
when the other kids got mad and fought hard, S would flare-up and
retaliate, so that adult interference was needed to prevent injury. He
would also fight viciously when his structures were wantonly destroyed
or a toy was snatched away from him. He was a great bargainer and
trader and seemed to get the best of most of his bargains. S did not,
on the surface, seem to have individual conflict with adults, or any
real hostility, but he acted most of the time as if there was a natural
schism between the world of children and of grown-ups. He seemed
well aware of all the adult-imposed standards, carelessly conforming
when they were irrelevant to his purposes and blithely violating them
when they got in his way. This was particularly true in regard to
fighting, where, when separated by an adult, he let himself be
pulled off and smiled responsively over the lecture and then, when
the adult was across the yard, renewed the fight. But both his failure
to get mad and let this become an emotional issue and his intelligent
reasonableness made S one of the easier children to direct. S was one
of the few 4-year-olds who seemed to really grasp the concept of a
deferred goal."

School visits

About 10 per cent of the subjects attended a private elementary school; the remainder were enrolled in public-school systems. Semi-annually, from the first to the eighth grade, a Fels staff member spent a half-day observing the child in his normal classroom activities and wrote a summary of her observations.

Interview summaries: Child interview

Children from 6 to 14 years of age were interviewed at the Institute each year. The interviewers had previous contact with the subjects, and an atmosphere of rapport was usually present. A summary of each interview was placed in the child's file. In most cases the summary did not follow a schedule but did emphasize the child's interests, relation to parents, and school adjustment.

Maternal interview

The mother of each child was interviewed at Fels each year from the child's birth through adolescence. These interviews were guided by a schedule that assessed the child's behavior and the mother's attitudes and practices with the child. Summaries of these interviews were also prepared.

Teacher interview

The child's public-school teacher was interviewed each year. The interview summary included salient characteristics of the child's behavior, general assessment of the child's skills, sociability, conformity to the classroom situation, and the teacher's sentiments about the child.

EVALUATION OF LONGITUDINAL DATA

The quality of these sources of information varied for different subjects and for different age periods. For example, some subjects missed some nursery-school sessions. Some of the mothers were employed for a time, and this interfered with the scheduling of home visits for those families. For most of the subjects in the present sample, the data were adequate. For those subjects for whom information on a specific variable was insufficient, ratings for that variable were not made.

As mentioned earlier, the longitudinal data were analyzed for the following age periods: age 0 to 3 (Period I), age 3 to 6 (Period II), age 6 to 10 (Period III), and age 10 to 14 (Period IV).

BEHAVIOR CLUSTERS: LONGITUDINAL MATERIAL

The major behavioral areas evaluated for the child included: dependence, aggression, achievement, recognition, heterosexual behavior, fear of physical harm, quality of social interaction, and passive withdrawal. In addition, a group of specific child variables not directly associated with the above content areas (e.g., sex-role interests, compulsivity, nurturance, hyperkinesis) and for categories of maternal behavior were assessed. Initially a rating manual containing definitions for 48 variables (seven-point rating scale) was prepared. Detailed behavioral referents were provided for scale points 1, 4, and 7. Nine of these variables were eliminated subsequently because of lack of clarity or similarity to other variables. The titles of the 39 remaining variables with their inter-rater reliabilities appear in Appendix 1.

The specific behavioral referents used in rating a variable varied for the different age periods. For example, aggression to mother for Period I was manifested in the form of a tantrum or resistance to feeding. For Period III, verbal aggression to mother and disobedience were typical indexes of aggression to mother.

Some behaviors were only relevant for specific developmental periods and, therefore, were not evaluated for all four age periods. For example, heterosexual interaction only had meaning once the child initiated peer interaction. On the other hand, direct physical aggression was frequent at the early years but was rare for this sample during age 10 to 14.

THE RATING PROCEDURE

Howard Moss first studied all of the longitudinal material for each subject for the first three years (Period I).[1] He then made his ratings for all variables for which he had sufficient information. After a period of interpolated work, he then studied all the material for each S for ages 3 to 6 (Period II) and again made all the ratings for this period. This procedure was repeated for ages 6 to 10 (Period III) and 10 to 14 (Period IV). A period of 6 to 8 months intervened between the evaluation of the material for any one child between age periods. The rater felt that the time interval and the large number of intervening ratings were sufficient to minimize memory of ratings for one period while making the ratings for subsequent periods. A second psychologist independently rated a sample from 50 to 60 cases for each age period in order to determine the reliability of the ratings. However, the ratings used in the analyses that follow were the ones made by Howard Moss. Appendix 1 lists the inter-rater reliabilities, using both product moment correlations and essential percentage of agreement.

Essential percentage of agreement was defined as the ratio of the number of instances in which the two raters agreed within one point of each other (agreements) to the total number of agreements plus disagreements.

The inter-rater reliabilities based on product moment correlations ranged from .32 to .97. Reliabilities determined by essential percentage of agreement ranged from 67 to 98 per cent. Table 1 presents the median inter-rater reliabilities for the four age periods.

TABLE 1. MEDIAN RELIABILITIES FOR LONGITUDINAL VARIABLES

	Period I	Period II	Period III	Period IV
Product moment correlations	.68	.76	.85	.83
Essential percentage of agreement	.83	.88	.91	.89

These reliabilities are sufficiently high to support the contention of independence of ratings between age periods.

SOURCES OF ERROR IN THE LONGITUDINAL RATINGS

There are at least three potential sources of error in the longitudinal ratings. First, the rater's theoretical conceptions about the interrelationships among the longitudinal variables may have influenced his ratings unconsciously. Second, the retroactive inhibition from period to period may not have been as complete as the rater believed. Evaluation of the child at age 10 may have been influenced to some degree by his earlier ratings. These two objections are negated, to some degree, by the pattern of results to be presented. For example, many relations that might be expected theoretically did not occur, while many unexpected relationships did occur. Further, there were striking sex differences in the pattern of stability correlations.

The relationships between child and adult behavior, however, are based on completely independent assessments and are, therefore, free from this potential source of error.

Finally, the fidelity of the original source material might be called into question. This source of error is controlled, in part, by the many staff members responsible for data collection. The observations of child and mother were made either by psychologists or by psychologically trained personnel who tried to describe what they saw rather than make clinically sophisticated interpretations of the child's behavior. Moreover, there were frequent staff changes during the 14 years that observations were made on any one child. There was no instance in which a child was consistently observed by the same person. The observations of the child in the nursery school were usually made by people other than those who made the home observations. Most of the home observations were made by five staff members: Helen Marshall, Joan Kalhorn Lasko, Faye Breese, and Mary Frances Hartson. A small number of home visits were made by Dr. Horace Champney. The majority of the nursery-school and public-school observations were made by Leah Levinger, Margaret Slutz, Marjorie Powell, and Frances Best. Interviews with the children were usually conducted by Drs. Thomas W. Richards or Alfred L. Baldwin. The typical child was observed by six different people during the four age periods, and this provides some insurance against observer bias in the protocol statements that were quantified.

ADULT ASSESSMENT

Since the relation between child and adult behavior was of primary interest, most of the adult variables were devised to correspond to the behaviors rated from the longitudinal records. Thus variables related to dependency, aggression, achievement, recognition, withdrawal, sexuality, sex-role interests, and characteristic social behavior were included in the assessment. Since contemporary psychology does not possess standard techniques that are valid indexes of most of these variables, the interview was chosen as a comprehensive measure with an acceptable degree of face validity.

One of the factors favoring the choice of the interview was the long-standing relationship and favorable rapport between the subjects and the staff of the Institute. A major methodological criticism of the interview is that subjects become defensive and evasive in order to avoid creating a bad impression on the interviewer, who is typically a stranger. This defensive maneuver leads to imperfect assessment of the subject's motives and behaviors. This source of error was attenuated, to some degree, for the majority of the adult subjects had a warm feeling for the Institute and its goals and were emotionally involved in the assessment. None of the subjects was paid for cooperating with the program, and all volunteered with minimal pressure. Only one man out of the 71 individuals interviewed was noticeably hostile, and only two adults refused to cooperate with any part of the adult program, suggesting the absence of volunteer bias in the selection of the adult sample. The subjects were interested in the purpose of the research and were willing and, in some cases, eager to talk honestly about their goals, fears, resentments, and conflicts.

THE INTERVIEW

All subjects were first contacted by the field secretary of the Institute, a woman who had established an informal and friendly relationship with the subjects over the years. Since many subjects had not been to the Institute in several years, this initial contact from an old friend made the interviewer's task easier. For those Ss who lived close to the Institute, the interview schedule was broken into three parts, each session lasting 1½ to 2 hours. For the subjects who came a long distance, the interview schedule was compressed into two successive sessions in one full day or two half-days. About 15 per cent of the sample underwent this more intensive interviewing procedure.

The interviews were tape recorded with the subject's permission, and no one seemed disturbed by the recording process. The interview was divided into 13 topical sections, the interviewer following a standard question order. The structure and language of individual questions were tailored to the background and intelligence of the subject. Appendix 2 contains an outline of the interview schedule, with major topics and the content of leading questions.

Initially a manual of 59 interview variables was constructed. These variables dealt with dependence, aggression, achievement, recognition, sexuality, sex-role interests, identification with parents, interpersonal behavior, compulsivity, impulsivity, and introspectiveness, and each was rated on a discrete seven-point scale. At the end of each set of interviews the interviewer studied his notes, listened to the recordings, and made a final set of ratings for all the variables. It will be recalled that the interviewer had no knowledge of the subject's early history or test protocols at the time of the interview. The ratings were based solely on the subject's behavior and verbalizations during the interview.

RELIABILITY OF THE INTERVIEW RATING AND
SELECTION OF INTERVIEW VARIABLES

Several of the interview variables were not regularly rated because of insufficient information. Other variables were eliminated because of a skewed or restricted range of scores. As a result of this initial screening, 44 variables were selected for an evaluation of inter-rater reliability. The reliability of the interview ratings was based on a sample of 32 tape-recorded interviews. In no instance were two subjects from the same family chosen for reliability ratings. After several practice cases were studied, a second psychologist made an independent set of ratings. Reliability was assessed with product moment correlations. Of the 44 variables rated by the second psychologist, 29 had satisfactory reliabilities and were related theoretically to the longitudinal variables.[2] These 29 variables were subjected to various statistical analyses. Appendix 3 contains a list of the interview variables to be described in this report, with their inter-rater reliabilities. The median inter-rater reliability was +.81, and 87 per cent of the coefficients were over .70.

TEST BATTERY

Although the interview was expected to yield a moderately valid picture of the personality of our subjects, special techniques were used to assess selected processes that were of particular interest. These special variables included areas of conflict and anxiety and preferred modes of conceptualization.

Assessment of conflict and sources of anxiety

Aggressive, dependent, and sexual motives are three sources of conflict that confront most individuals in our culture. All three of these classes of behavior were assessed from the longitudinal and interview material. An additional anxiety source involves the anticipation of physical harm or danger to one's bodily integrity. Anxiety over physical harm is quite evident in the nightmares of children, in the avoidance of dangerous activity, and in the reluctance to enter into rough, athletic games. This variable was rated from the longitudinal records, and we attempted to determine if derivatives of this form of childhood anxiety were present in the functioning of the adult.

It was assumed that conflict over dependency, aggression, sexuality, and anxiety over physical harm were present, in different degrees, in the adult sample. Test situations were devised to measure these potential differences. Two of the techniques included tachistoscopic recognition of pictures illustrating conflict areas, and autonomic reactivity following experimental arousal of these conflicts.

Tachistoscopic recognition

The rationale for this technique rested on the following set of assumptions. If the symbolic representation of a conflicted behavior elicited anxiety, there would be a tendency for the individual to show delayed recognition of stimuli that represented the anxiety-arousing action. Specifically, if a man did not regard himself as dependent on his wife and was anxious about manifesting dependent behavior toward her, he should not entertain thoughts of himself in a dependent relation with a woman (i.e., he should repress dependency motives and ideation). When presented with an illustration of a man on his knees in front of a woman, we would expect him to distort or show delayed recognition of the scene.

A man who is dependent on his wife and recognizes this tendency is more apt to experience images of men in a dependent relation with a woman and implicitly rehearse dependent phrases and images. When the dependent scene is flashed tachistoscopically, the hypothesis "That is a man on his knees in front of a woman" should be more readily available. This is not to say that a dependent man is not anxious over his behavior. However, awareness of his dependent posture should predispose him to recognize more accurately information that is only suggestive of this behavior.

The tachistoscopic task was designed to assess ease versus difficulty in the recognition of potentially conflictful behavior. It was assumed that this difficulty was diagnostic of a tendency to deny and repress the behavior in question.

The assumptions mediating the above predictions require that the individual be given sufficient information at each stimulus exposure so that his perceptual response is the result of distortion of input information rather than a fanciful guess of the content of the stimulus. That is, if the picture of the "man on his knees" were presented at exposure levels close to visual threshold, we might be measuring potential differences in the tendency to project dependent action onto the social environment rather than the tendency to distort cues suggesting dependency. Previous research (Kagan, 1956; Lesser, 1958) and the theory of approach-avoidance gradients (Dollard and Miller, 1950) suggest that conflict-related responses are regulated by different processes, depending on the ambiguity of the stimulus situation for the conflictful behavior. In order to measure distortion by conflicted individuals, the nonconflicted subject must receive sufficient information to allow for recognition of the conflictful behavior. For these reasons the conflictful scenes were presented at exposures above threshold.

Autonomic changes

Presentation of a conflictful communication and the recording of subsequent autonomic reaction was a second procedure designed to measure anxiety and conflict. Changes in heart rate and palmar resistance were made after an announcement that the subject was about to listen to a potentially conflictful tape-recorded monologue and while the subject listened to the monologue. The announcements and monologues dealt with aggression, sexuality, and physical harm. For methodological reasons, a dependency monologue was not used in this procedure.

Conceptual styles and intellective functioning

During the last decade there has been increased excitement over the renaissance of a class of psychological phenomena that had been buried for 50 years by the overwhelming impact of a motive-biased psychology. These phenomena deal with the ways in which individuals organize their environment—the characteristic ways they form concepts and interpret novel stimuli. This class of behavior has acquired the name "cognitive style" (Gardner, 1953; Gardner et al. 1959; Holzman and Gardner, 1959; Kagan, 1961). A cognitive style is a preferred mode of organizing and labeling various stimulus situations. A person's style is related, in part, to his command of the language and the richness and imaginative quality of his verbal products. Styles exert an influence on the content and organization of all language behavior and, therefore, are involved in most psychological test procedures.

Because style variables were not popular prior to 1950, there were no specific tests of cognitive styles in the longitudinal data. It was hoped, nevertheless, that exploration of these variables would be profitable. We had reason to believe that cognitive styles were intimately associated with quality of intellective functioning, interpretive approach to projective stimuli, and selected personality dimensions. Thus tests of conceptual styles, projective stimuli, and a standard measure of intelligence were included in the adult assessment program.

This completes a summary of the major variables assessed with this unique group of young adults. The interview was used to gather comprehensive information on goals and goal-related behaviors, modes of interpersonal interaction, sources of conflict, and defenses. Additional indexes of conflict were obtained through a tachistoscopic perception task and measures of autonomic reactivity. Styles of conceptualization and intelligence were measured with appropriate instruments.

Administration of test battery

The test information was gathered after the interviews were completed. Several sessions were required to complete the test battery and the intersession intervals varied from one day to six months, with the most frequent intersession interval being four weeks. A brief description of the tests in the order in which they were administered follows. A detailed description of the variables scored from these tests and their relation to the child and adult behavior ratings will be presented in Chapter Eight.

Modified Rorschach ink blot stimuli

A modification of the standard Rorschach ink blots was prepared, which has been called the Modified Rorschach. In this modified series, a part of the standard stimulus was covered with a template of white cardboard, leaving only a part of the original stimulus visible. The 32 stimuli in the series were common D or d areas, each tended to be perceived as unitary Gestalt, and, with one exception, all the stimuli were totally achromatic or chromatic. This instrument had two methodological advantages. First, it guaranteed an equal and fairly large response pool for all subjects, since most subjects gave a response to each blot. The statistical problems associated with unequal protocol length have long plagued Rorschach investigators, and this instrument was used in an attempt to overcome this thorny problem. Second, these stimuli gave the investigator considerable control over the stimulus input to the subject and allowed for specification of those aspects of the stimulus upon which the response was based. The 32 stimuli in this series were congruent with the following Klopfer areas (Klopfer et al. 1954, pp. 70–79).

Rorschach Plate	Klopfer Areas
I	(D1) (D2) (d3 symmetrical)
II	(D1) (D2 symmetrical)
	(D3 symmetrical) (d1)
III	(D2) (D1) (D3)
	(D8 symmetrical plus D3)
IV	(D1) (d2) (whole blot minus D1)
V	(d2) (whole blot minus d3 and d1)
VI	(D2) (D4) (d4)
VII	(D4 symmetrical) (d1)
VIII	(D2) (D1 plus D3 plus D4)
	(D3 the center) (D4 the bottom)
IX	(D2 symmetrical) (D5) (D7)
X	(D8) (D17) (D3) (D1)

Thematic Apperceptive Test stimuli

Each adult was asked to tell a story about each of 13 pictures from the Murray (1943) Thematic Apperception Test stimuli. This was the only test in the battery in which males and females were given different stimuli to which to react. The males were administered Cards 4, 8BM, 7BM, 6BM, 12M, 17BM, 13MF, 13, 3BM, 5, 1, 3GF, and 18 GF. The females were administered Cards 4, 6GF, 12F, 2, 8GF, 17BM, 13MF, 13, 3BM, 5, 1, 3GF, and 18GF. Nine of the 13 cards were identical for both sexes, and the order of these nine cards was the same for men and women. Seven of the cards (17BM, 6BM, 13, 3BM, 5, 1, 3GF) were familiar to the subjects, for they had told stories about these pictures during early adolescence.

Self-rating inventory

A self-rating inventory containing 110 items was filled out by each subject. The inventory was devised by the authors and dealt with motives, attitudes, and overt behaviors related to dependency, aggression, physical harm, sexuality, compulsivity, recognition, and relation to peers. The subject was required to place a number (1 through 4) by each item, indicating the degree to which the printed statement was characteristic of his personality. The inventory items appear in Appendix 31.

The preceding three tests (Modified Rorschach, TAT, self-rating inventory) were completed in two sessions. The following tests were *all* administered in one 3½-hour session during which two male examiners were present (JK and HM).

Figure sorting task: Array 1

In order to evaluate the subject's preferred conceptual style, three separate arrays of cardboard figures were devised. Each figure was about 3½ inches high, and some of the stimuli were taken directly from the Shneidman Make-A-Picture-Story Test (1949). Each of the arrays contained 22 figures, and Figures 1 and 2 illustrate two of the three stimulus arrays.

The first task in this session involved the conceptual sorting of the figures in Array 1. The array was placed on a table in front of the subject, and the following instructions were given:

We are now going to show you a group of human figures that are arranged in no special order. We would like you to pick out one group of figures that go together on some common basis, any basis you like. The number of figures in your group can be any size you like. Just pick out a group of figures that go together on some common basis and tell us the basis upon which you grouped these figures.

After the first sort, the figures selected were replaced in the original array and the subject was asked to produce another grouping that went together on a different conceptual basis. This procedure was repeated until the subject had produced six different sorts.

The French Insight Test

Each subject was then administered 10 items from the French Insight Test (French 1955; French 1956) for achievement and affiliative preoccupations.

Figure sorting task: Array 2

Each subject was presented with the second array of human figures and given the same instructions that held for Array 1. Each subject produced six different conceptual sorts from this array.

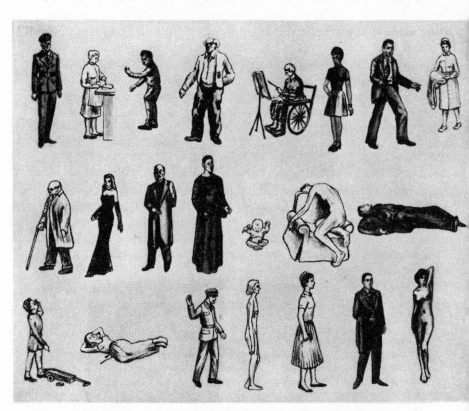

FIGURE 1. ARRAY 1: FIGURES USED IN SORTING TASKS.

Tachistoscopic recognition task

At this point in the schedule each subject was taken into a light-proof room and dark-adapted for several minutes. He was then shown a series of 14 line drawings of people in various situations. The pictures were presented at seven different exposure speeds ranging from

0.01 to 1.0 seconds. The 14 stimuli contained 4 aggressive scenes, 3 dependency scenes, 2 romantic scenes, 2 physical harm pictures, and 3 motivationally neutral situations. Separate sets of stimuli were drawn for the sexes so that the central figures in the conflict pictures were the same sex as the subject. In the brief description of the pictures that follows, the central figure is the first one described.

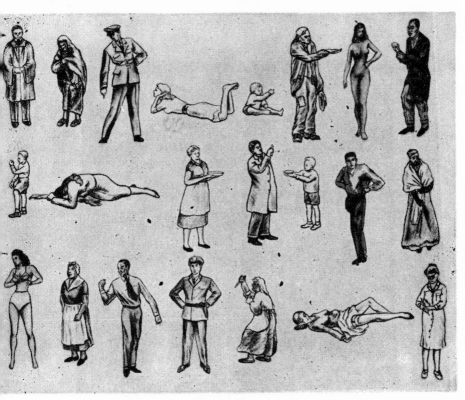

FIGURE 2. ARRAY 2: FIGURES USED IN SORTING TASKS.

Aggressive scenes

Picture 1. A young adult is choking a young adult of the same sex.

Picture 2. A young adult is punching a young adult of the same sex.

Picture 13. A young adult has hands above head and is holding a plate which (he) (she) is about to throw at an older woman who is cowering.

Picture 14. A young adult has hands raised to the face of an older man as if to slap the older man.

Dependency scenes

Picture 3. A young adult is on a stool with head bowed and arms around waist of an adult of the opposite sex who is standing in back of the central figure.

Picture 4. A young adult is standing with hands out as if pleading with an adult of the same sex who is standing in the background with back to the central figure.

Picture 5. A young adult is on knees in front of an adult of the opposite sex. The adult on knees is looking up to the standing adult as if imploring the latter.

Sexuality scenes

Picture 6. A couple is in bathing suits on a beach. The man is over the woman and is kissing her.

Picture 7. A standing couple is embracing and kissing. For these two romantic scenes the same pictures were used for both sexes.

Physical harm scenes

Picture 8. A young adult is falling backward in mid air.

Picture 9. A dog is attacking a young adult who is recoiling from the charging animal.

Control scenes

Picture 10. A young man and woman are standing together looking up at a picture.

Picture 11. Two men are standing while one lights the cigarette of the second one.

Picture 12. Two women are standing together; one is handing a cup and saucer to the second one. The control stimuli were the same for each sex.

Figure 3 illustrates the 14 stimuli.

Figure sorting task: Array 3

Each subject was shown a third array of 22 figures, but the instructions differed from those used with Arrays 1 and 2. This time each adult was required to divide all the figures into two groups on the basis of one concept; and four responses were obtained.

Wechsler-Bellevue Intelligence Scale—Form I

Following the four sorts, part of the Wechsler-Bellevue Intelligence Scale (Form I) was administered. Each subject was administered five

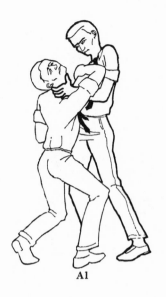
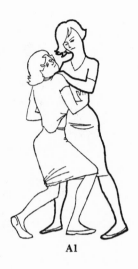

A1   A1

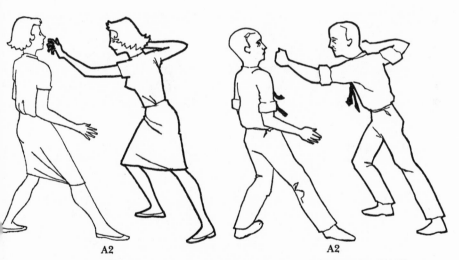

A2   A2

FIGURE 3. STIMULI USED IN TACHISTOSCOPIC PERCEPTION TASK.

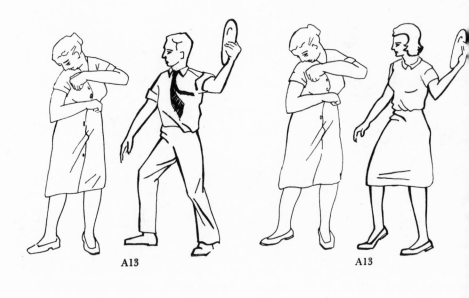

A13 A13

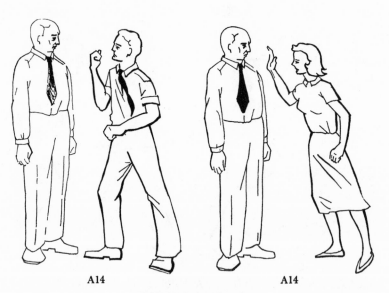

A14 A14

FIGURE 3 (continued)

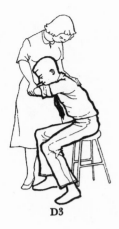

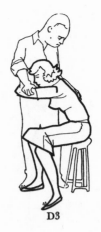

D3   D3

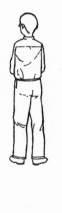

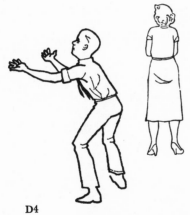

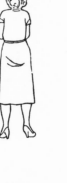

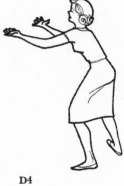

D4   D4

FIGURE 3 (continued)

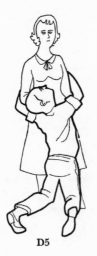

D5

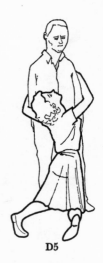

D5

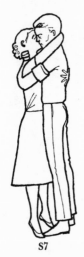

S7

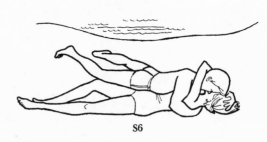

S6

FIGURE 3 (continued)

44

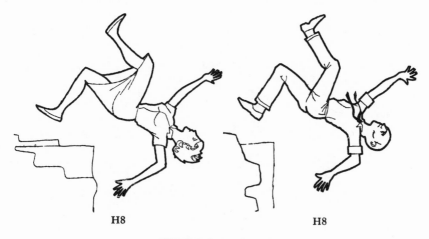

H8   H8

FIGURE 3 (continued)

verbal scale subtests and three performance scales in the following
order: information, comprehension, similarities, arithmetic, digit sub-
stitution, block design, picture completion, and vocabulary.

Hanfmann-Kasanin Concept Formation test

Each subject was administered the Hanfmann-Kasanin Concept
test (1936).

Figure sorting task: Repeat with Array 1

Each subject was again presented with the figures from Array 1 and
asked to produce six additional conceptual groupings.

Figure sorting task: Restricted procedure

All of the figures in Arrays 1 and 2 were pooled into a larger array
of 44 figures. Each subject was then given the following instructions:

Now let us consider this large group of figures as one array. I am going to
select one figure from the array, hand it to you, and ask you to *point* to all

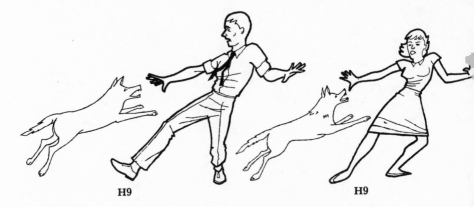

H9   H9

FIGURE 3 (continued)

the figures you would classify with the one I gave you on some common basis. You may use any basis you wish in classifying the figures and you may point to one or more figures. Please tell me the basis of your classification before you begin to point.

Each subject produced 10 additional sorts to 10 different stimulus figures.

Recall of tachistoscopic scenes

The last task in this continuous test session was a recall of the 14 pictures shown in the tachistoscopic recognition task. In most cases, about 90 minutes had elapsed between the completion of the recognition task and the recall. The majority of the subjects recalled at least 12 of the 14 pictures.

Autonomic measurements

Of the group of 35 males who went through both the interview and testing procedures, 30 men returned the morning after the previous test session for an assessment of autonomic reactivity (palmar resistance and heart rate) during conditions of rest and under different

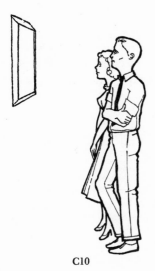

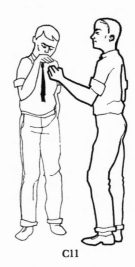

C10   C11

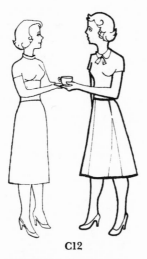

C12

FIGURE 3 (continued)

types of stimulation. Only 15 of the women were able to attend this
session, and their data were not subjected to analysis. The autonomic
information on these 30 males was related to the interview and longitudinal ratings and their performance on the various tests. A detailed
description of this procedure appears in Chapter 8.

In summary, the adult assessment data consisted of the following *independent* sources of information: (a) interview ratings, (b) interpretations of ink blot and picture stimuli, (c) a self rating inventory, (d) tests of conceptualization, (e) tachistoscopic recognition thresholds for conflictful scenes, (f) intellectual ability, and (g) autonomic reactivity.

Footnotes

1. The phrase "longitudinal material" refers to (a) the behavioral observations made in the home, the nursery school and day camp, and the public school, (b) interviews with child, mother, and teacher, and (c) the ratings made on the Parent Behavior Rating Scale and Child Behavior Rating Scale. The Fels Parent and Child Behavior Rating Scales were not consistently available for all of these subjects and, for that reason, Moss gave a greater weight to the narrative summaries. In practice, he first read the narrative material and arrived at a tentative rating. He then checked the Parent and Child Behavior ratings if they were available. When the Behavior Rating Scales confirmed his tentative rating, as was usually the case, he used the former. When the Behavior Rating Scales disagreed with his tentative rating, he would restudy the material and then arrive at a final rating.

2. Most of the variables that failed to yield satisfactory inter-rater agreement required a high degree of inference on the part of the rater (e.g., anxiety in the interview, dependency on the interviewer, projection of aggression).

CHAPTER THREE

The Stability of Behavior: I
Passivity and Dependency

The next four chapters describe the pattern of developmental continuity for a group of behaviors that were assessed during both childhood and adulthood. The areas are passivity, dependency, aggression, competitiveness, achievement, recognition, heterosexuality, sex-role identification, social interaction, fear of physical harm, nurturance, compulsivity, and hyperkinesis. The primary data for each area consist of two sets of correlations. The stability of these behaviors over the first 14 years is expressed by the correlations among the four sets of longitudinal ratings made by Howard Moss. The predictive validity of these childhood ratings for adult behavior is expressed by the correlations between the childhood ratings and the ratings for comparable variables made after the adult interview. The interview and longitudinal ratings are completely independent. *Each of the authors made their ratings without any knowledge of the protocols studied by the other.*

However, the ratings for each of the four developmental periods were all made by Howard Moss, and the reader may question the independence of these assessments. It will be recalled that the rater first read all the material for one age period for each child before proceeding to the next age period. A span of 6 to 8 months typically intervened between the evaluation of the data for any one child for contiguous periods. The amount of material studied, the number of ratings made (approximately 4500), and the interval of time between the evaluation of a specific child for two successive periods was sufficiently large to guarantee a high degree of retroactive inhibition. Furthermore, independent ratings of the material produced satisfactory interrater reliabilities (see Appendix 1).

Two additional sources of information support the assumption of relative independence of the longitudinal ratings. First, the stability coefficients between age periods were not uniform. A significant degree of stability was obtained only for certain variables and, on occasion, for one sex and not for the other. Some of the relationships that occurred could not be anticipated by any of the implicit theories of the rater. Some hypotheses that were reasonable, a priori, were not verified. For example, low negative correlations were obtained between ratings of mastery behavior for Period I and mastery behavior for subsequent age periods. This was due to the fact that the Period I ratings were measuring lack of satiation with simple sensory-motor tasks. The ratings for older age periods emphasized competence in symbolic skills.

Finally, the assumption of independence of ratings among the four age periods was buttressed by the total pattern of relationships between the longitudinal variables and external criteria, such as the adult test scores and interview variables. Despite these considerations, however, halo effects within the four sets of ratings are possible. For this reason we plan to emphasize the relationships between the child and adult ratings, for these data are completely independent.

For a variable rated for all four age periods, the correlations between Periods I and II, I and III, I and IV, II and III, II and IV, and III and IV were computed. The correlations were computed for males, females, and for the total sample.

As noted in Chapter Two, selected variables were not rated for all periods because they were only appropriate for a certain age. A few variables (e.g., withdrawal from tasks) were rated for only one period, precluding the possibility of evaluating the childhood stability of that trait. Ratings were only made when the rater felt that the data were sufficient to make a confident evaluation. Stability correlations are not presented where the sample of boys or girls fell below 10 (as sometimes happened for Period IV correlations).

For each of the behavior clusters, interview ratings were correlated with corresponding longitudinal variables for each age period. These coefficients provide a profile of the predictive power of childhood behavior for different developmental periods.[1]

PASSIVE AND DEPENDENT BEHAVIOR

The childhood cluster consisted of six variables, which are briefly defined below.

Variable 13: Passive reaction to frustration

This variable was rated for all four periods. It assessed the degree to which the child acquiesced or withdrew in the face of attack or frustrating situations, in contrast to an active attempt to overcome and deal with environmental frustrations.

During the early years passivity was manifested through behaviors such as: (a) retreat when dominated by sibling, (b) no reaction when goal object is lost, (c) withdrawal when blocked from goal by environmental obstacle, and (d) withdrawal from mildly noxious or potentially dangerous situations. During the school years, the passivity rating was based primarily on (a) withdrawal to attack or social rejection and (b) withdrawal from difficult and frustrating task situations.

Variables 14, 91, 92: Dependence on female adults

Variable 14 was rated for Periods I and II and was an assessment of general dependent tendencies toward female adults (primarily the mother). The rating was based on seeking of affection, requests for instrumental aid, and reluctance to be separated from the adult.

Variables 91 and 92 were rated for Periods III and IV and were a refinement of the general dependency variable. Affectional dependence (Variable 91) emphasized seeking of affection, acceptance, and emotional reassurance from adults. Instrumental dependence (Variable 92) emphasized the seeking of assistance in problem situations.

Variable 77: Independence

This variable was rated for Periods II, III, and IV and evaluated the occurrence of independent behaviors in threatening and problem-solving situations. Independence and dependence were rated on separate scales because of evidence suggesting that these two variables are only moderately related (Beller, 1955, 1957, 1959).

Variable 16: Anxiety over loss of nurturance

This variable, rated for Periods I, II, and III, evaluated behavioral signs of anxiety (e.g., crying, protest, emotional upset) when a source of nurturance was withdrawn or when the child anticipated loss of love or support from parent or parent figures.

STABILITY OF LONGITUDINAL VARIABLES

The stability coefficients for these variables are presented in Table 1 for males, females, and the pooled sample.

Passivity

A passive, in contrast to a retaliatory, reaction to frustration was highly stable for boys and girls during the first 10 years of life. For the pooled sample, many of the stability correlations exceeded the .001 confidence limit. The greatest degree of stability occurred, as might be expected, for contiguous age periods (Periods I to II, II to III, III to IV). Although there was a definite trend for the stability coefficients to be higher for females, the differences between the coefficients for boys and girls were not significant.

The zero-order correlations for boys between Periods I to IV and II to IV suggest that some of the boys who were passive during the first six years shifted to a more active and retaliatory attitude after school entrance. This shift was less marked for the girls.

Dependence on adults

Dependent behavior also showed a moderate degree of stability over the first 10 years. However, the magnitude of these correlations was not as high as those found for passivity. Moreover, dependence during Period II was not as predictive of Period IV dependence as the corresponding correlation for passivity. As with passivity, dependent behavior was most stable between contiguous age periods. The differentiation of affectional from instrumental dependence did not appreciably alter the degree of stability for these behaviors between Periods III and IV.

Independence

This variable showed marked stability for females over the 11-year span from 3 to 14, whereas, for males, only the Period III to IV correlation was significant. Moreover, the Period II to IV correlation for boys was negative ($r = -.33$). The difference between this negative correlation and the comparable, positive one for females ($r = +.64$)

Variable	I–II	I–III	I–IV	II–III	II–IV	III–IV
13. Passivity						
Boy	.67****	.50**	.00	.75****	.24	.60****
Girl	.58****	.66****	.44*	.79****	.51***	.76****
Total	.59****	.59****	.36**	.73****	.39***	.69****
14. Dependency						
Boy	.58****					
Girl	.64****					
Total	.60****					
14–91. Dependency Affectional						
Boy		.36*	.66**	.33*	—.03	
Girl		.33*	.17	.29*	.26	
Total		.33**	.33*	.29**	.07	
14–92. Dependency Instrumental						
Boy		.45**	.04	.24	—.13	
Girl		.36**	.23	.54****	.24	
Total		.38***	.26	.39****	.14	
91. Affectional dependency						
Boy						.41*
Girl						.34*
Total						.35**
92. Instrumental dependency						
Boy						.56***
Girl						.34*
Total						.45***
77. Independence						
Boy				.28	—.33	.52**
Girl				.55****	.64****	.65****
Total				.43****	.21	.62****
16. Anxiety loss of nurturance						
Boy	.25	.24		.08		
Girl	.30	.29		.36*		
Total	.28*	.33*		.30*		

* $p < .10$; two tails   *** $p < .01$; two tails
** $p < .05$; two tails   **** $p < .001$; two tails

was statistically significant ($p < .01$). It will be recalled that dependence for Period II was also negatively associated with Period IV dependence in boys.

This sex difference is probably the result of the differential cultural expectations for independence in males and females, and this hypothesis will be pursued in detail in a later section. Briefly, it is suggested that the culture maintains a more permissive attitude toward independence or dependence in females. Young girls are often rewarded for being passive and dependent but not consistently punished for acts of independence. It is reasonable to expect that a pattern of independent or dependent behavior would remain relatively constant (in the absence of unusual trauma) for females. For boys, on the other hand, independence is intimately linked with the traditional masculine prototype for the American middle class. These expectations for independence are usually enforced when the child enters school. At that time parents, teachers, and peers encourage behaviors that are consistent with the idealized conceptualization of the male role. The potential for conflict over dependent behavior is, therefore, greater for males than for females, for if the boy does not exhibit independence of action, he is subject to social punishment and guilt.

It might be anticipated that some boys who were dependent during the preschool years would shift toward greater independence when they reached school age. This shift would reduce the stability of this behavior. This interpretation is supported by analysis of the sex differences obtained when the childhood ratings for passive and dependent behavior were correlated with adult interview material.

The following series of verbatim excerpts from the observations on one boy illustrate this shift from early dependence to school age independence.

Subject 855

As a young child S showed an excessively dependent tie to his mother, and at 2 years of age exhibited a demanding request for help in a score of minor stress situations.

At 2 years of age the nursery-school observer noted:

"S had the habit of crying over very minor accidents. He cried less whenever just the teachers were around, but he still wept about a little tumble in the grass as if his mother were around."

When S and the mother visited the Institute:

"S accompanied his mother to the interview. He accompanied her upstairs and did not want mother to leave him, although he had left her willingly to go for his mental test. He cried for several minutes but finally quieted down. According to the mother, S seems to like nursery school and does not object to going. He cried only once when mother left him, and he insists that she accompany him inside."

At 3 years of age, a baby brother was born, and S showed some regressive behavior. At $3\frac{1}{2}$ years the home visitor wrote:

"S had a period of serious regression for a couple of months that was obviously related to his jealousy of the new baby, though he showed no aggression toward him. S relapsed into baby talk, refused to dress himself (which he could do completely before), wet the bed two or three times a week, and even made the statement, 'I don't want to be a big boy like ——, I want to be a baby like——.'"

By age 5 S began to show signs of suppression of dependent behavior. This shift was accompanied by the mother's relaxation of her protective attitude toward him. The mother told the Fels visitor:

"For the first few years I am terribly close and intimate with my children, then I want them to become emancipated and independent, and the transition is probably too abrupt."

When S started school there were wide swings from dependent to independent behavior as if he were attempting to resolve these opposed needs. The home visitor noted that he fluctuated between moods in which he was a rough, tough, swaggering little boy and moods in which he demanded a great deal of physical affection.

By age 8 the conflict had been resolved in favor of independence. He became a leader with his peers, began demanding more freedom of action, and actively rejected a physically close relation to his mother. At $8\frac{1}{2}$, the home visitor wrote:

"The 5 or 10 minutes that S spent in the house were irksome to him. He was completely engrossed in his desire to get back outdoors and play. The mother commented that S had shown a sudden surge of independence this year in his Christmas planning. Formerly he would go over his list with her, seeking suggestions and help in planning. This year he brushed her aside."

This marked shift from dependence to self-sufficiency was less frequent among the girls and is due, in part, to the differences in sex-role standards regarding independent behavior.

Anxiety over loss of nurturance

Ratings of this variable showed minimal stability during the childhood years. Although the pooled correlations were positive, none attained a high degree of statistical significance. Two factors may have contributed to the low stability of this variable: the emergence of defenses against blatant signs of anxiety and the highly inferential nature of this variable.

Anxiety over loss of nurturance is likely to elicit defensive maneuvers that mask evidence of this anxiety in overt behavior. Moreover, the amount of inference involved in assessing this variable was greater than that required for most of the other variables. These considerations may explain why this behavior yielded low stability coefficients.

PASSIVE AND DEPENDENT BEHAVIOR IN ADULTHOOD

In order to assess the continuity of these behaviors into adulthood, each of the six child variables was related to six interview variables describing facets of adult passivity and dependency. Four of these adult variables differentiated among various figures to whom the adult might turn for gratification of dependency motives. The adult variables were dependency on love object, dependency on parents, dependency on parent substitute figures and friends, withdrawal from stressful situations, conflict over dependency, and seeking dependent gratifications in vocational choice.

Interview Variable 5: Dependency on love object

This variable assessed the degree to which the individual viewed his spouse or sweetheart as a reliable source of support and advice and the frequency with which he (or she) turned to a love object for instrumental help with problems or emotional reassurance. Major sources of evidence for this rating included (a) reluctance to make decisions without consulting love objects, (b) perception of love object as wiser and more stable than the subject, and (c) a feeling that the subject relied on the love object for reassurance and guidance in crisis situations. Approximately half of the sample were married, and, except for two subjects who had not established any heterosexual relationships (and were not rated on this variable), all the adults had developed one or more close relations with love objects.

Table 2 presents the correlations between passivity and dependency in childhood and adult dependency on love object.[2]

The major finding is that girls who were highly dependent on female adults during Period III established a passive and dependent re-

TABLE 2. RELATION BETWEEN CHILDHOOD BEHAVIOR AND ADULT
DEPENDENCY ON LOVE OBJECT

Child Variable	Age	Males	Females	Total
Passivity	0–3	.47**	.26	.34**
	3–6	.16	.20	.17
	6–10	.25	.33*	.31***
	10–14	.26	.23	.33**
General dependency	0–3	.03	.35*	.23
	3–6	.09	.10	.08
Affectional dependency	6–10	.12	.35**	.26**
	10–14	.25	.24	.22
Instrumental dependency	6–10	.08	.39**	.27**
	10–14	.09	.25	.33**
Independence	3–6	.00	−.13	−.05
	6–10	−.02	−.35**	−.22*
	10–14	−.25	−.41**	−.41***
Anxiety loss of nurturance	0–3	−.02	.07	.04
	3–6	−.07	−.39*	−.21
	6–10	−.18	.01	−.05

* $p < .10$; two tails
** $p < .05$; two tails
*** $p < .01$; two tails
**** $p < .001$; two tails

lationship with their husband or boy friend during early adulthood.

For the men, the correlations were in the expected direction but much lower in magnitude and not statistically significant. For adult males, a dependent relationship with a love object is not a likely consequent of a passive and dependent attitude during the early school years. The ratings prior to age 6 were generally less predictive of adult behavior than those made for Periods III and IV. For the men, the only significant correlation involved passivity during the first three years ($r = .47$; $p < .05$). Since dependency during Period I did not predict adult dependency on love object, it appears that early passivity may be a predisposition of special significance. Discussion of this point is reserved for a later section.

How can we account for the greater stability of dependency for the females? It will be recalled from Table 1 that passivity and dependence showed decreasing stability for boys over the first four age periods. For example, the correlations for passivity went from .67 for Periods

I–II to .00 for Periods I to IV. It is suggested that during the period from preschool to preadolescence, several sets of forces oppose the temporal continuity of a passive and dependent predisposition.

The primary reason for this lack of continuity in males is the development of conflict over passive and dependent behavior. A passive orientation to problems is inappropriate for the male role. As boys approach school age, the important figures in their lives begin to manipulate rewards and punishments in an attempt to encourage independence and autonomy in stressful and problem situations. Moreover, the boy begins to model his behavior after heroes who symbolize dominance, retaliation, and independence, and who regard passivity as synonymous with infancy, senility, and femininity. Some boys therefore, become conflicted over a passive orientation. This conflict, which does not swell to such strong proportions in middle-class girls, leads to minimal continuity between childhood and adult dependency for males.

In our discussion of the stability of dependency, the assumption of greater dependence conflict for men will be used as an integrating principle to explain many of the results to be reported. Each of the adult dependency variables showed greater stability for women than for men.

Independent support for the hypothesis that dependent behavior is less acceptable to men than to women came from the subjects' performance on the tachistoscopic task. One measure of dependency conflict was each subject's recognition threshold for the dependency scenes. A complete description of the relationship between performance on the tachistoscopic task and other variables appears in Chapter Eight. However, the burden of our argument is eased if we mention here that men had much greater difficulty recognizing the dependent scenes than the women (the sex differences were statistically significant). See Table 1, Chapter Eight. For the aggression pictures, on the other hand, the women had significantly higher thresholds. There were no sex differences for the neutral scenes. Moreover, those men who were rated as highly dependent on love object recognized the dependent scenes *earlier* than the men who avoided a dependent relationship with wife or sweetheart (see Appendix 23).

Thus the men had greater difficulty than the women in recognizing dependent action, and, behaviorally, independent men had greater difficulty than dependent men. This supplementary information suggests that dependent behavior is less acceptable to males than to adult females and adds validity to the *ad hoc* explanation we have imposed on the sex differences in the stability correlations.

The following excerpts from the material on two women illustrate the relationship between degree of passive and dependent behavior during childhood and the strength of a dependent attitude toward love objects.

Subject 2280

As both child and adult S adopted a dependent role with others. During Periods II and III, she was passive in her reaction to peer attack and problem situations, and she often sought out adults for help in time of stress. At 5 years of age the nursery-school observer wrote:

"When another child used force against her, S gave very little resistance. She not only yielded quickly but she showed very little emotional upset, often smiling as a child snatched a toy from her. . . . On a few occasions of rather violent teasing by the other children, S sought the protection of an adult, but more often she merely withdrew from the situation."

When S was 7 years of age, the home visitor wrote:

"She presents the picture of a sensitive, delicate child who is both timid and nervous."

At 7½ years of age, she was interviewed at the Institute.

"This child seems to be rather infantile in her interests, ability, and alertness. She seems very well adjusted but she gives the impression of a rather restricted child with babylike interests."

The day-camp observer described S at 8½ years of age:

"S is the most easy-going member of the group. She had a short period of shyness, but after that she was one of the girls. She liked being with the other children, had excellent relationships with them, and was amiable in almost any situation."

When S was nine, the mother was interviewed at the Institute and reported:

"S is very easily discouraged, not only with regard to school work, but with regard to other things. She hates to fail at anything."

At 9½ years she was characterized as follows:

"S appeared at day camp as a simple, pleasant girl without any striking motivation. She is socially outgoing and was anxious to conform. She likes to please adults and children very much. She was accepted by the other children although she was not popular in the sense of being sought out particularly. She was very ready to admire other people. This characteristic gave her charm and made her acceptable in social situations. She seemed quite unconcerned about problems over dominance and submission."

During the school years, S was consistently described as a passive child who withdrew from anxiety-arousing situations and displayed strong needs for affection from both adults and playmates.

During the adult interview she indicated a strong dependent relation to her husband.

E: "Do you feel that your husband leans on you for support?"

S: "No, I don't think he does (S laughs)—In fact, I'm quite sure of it. He didn't tell me about this new job he took."

E: "How are the responsibilities divided up in your family right now? Would you like them to be changed in any way; would you like to assume more responsibility for the running of the household; would you like him to assume more, or do you think it's perfect just the way it is?"

S: "Well, it seems like I've got all the responsibility of the kids all of the time. I would like for him to kind of help too, I think that's only right because the kids, well, I think things are going to change now since he'll be on this new job. He'll be home for supper and, at the most, a couple of nights a week, and he'll be there more—and—you know, I think that is right. . . . After all, they are his responsibility too—he should—course, I know he has lots—a lot to do, too—but I think he should be—ah—there to help me—a little bit (S laughs)."

E: "Some women lean on their husbands for support, advice, or ideas, but aren't comfortable about this; they wish they didn't."

S: "I don't feel bad about it."

E: "You don't feel bad about it?"

S: "Oh, no—I, I, I just have to have somebody to say—'Yes, go ahead and do that'—the I'm all for it now—but I don't like to do it on my own."

She preferred to let her husband manage the financial negotiations of the family because "he knows more than me about these things." She viewed her husband as she viewed her parents—omniscient and reliable, and these figures were perceived as sources of nurturance to whom she frequently turned for counsel and support.

In the tachistoscopic situation, this woman recognized the dependency scenes early. On the second exposure of the scene of the "woman on her knees in front of a man," she reported:

"A male and a female—the male is standing—the female was on her knees and it looked like she was begging forgiveness—or something."

To the picture of a woman imploring an older woman in the background, she replied:

"There's a female on the right about seventeen—she had her arms out trying to tell somebody—or beg forgiveness for something—maybe it was her mother."

Subject 1173

S is a 21-year-old unmarried woman who was in her senior year in college and one of the most independent women in the sample. As an adult, she had a strong need for recognition by others, combined with a striving for achievement-related goals. She liked to nurture others and often sought out situations in which she could give advice, support, and encouragement to peers. She was trying to sever any semblance of a dependent relation with her mother and derogated the latter because the mother seemed to be dependent upon her for companionship. Her relationship with men was consistent with the above pattern. She avoided men who attempted to place her in a passive role and she was having difficulty establishing a satisfactory heterosexual relationship.

The following verbatim excerpts are from the longitudinal observations on this woman.

AGE 3 YEARS, 4 MONTHS: SUMMARY OF
FELS NURSERY SCHOOL OBSERVATIONS

"S seems to be able to control and channel her behavior so that she got done just what she wanted to get done. In this activity she was very independent and capable. She was very social but also had a streak of aloof self-sufficiency, and she always made her individuality felt. She was what might be called a strong personality; often very intense, quite stubborn. . . . Her most outstanding characteristic was her consistent independence and integrity. In spite of the fact that she imitated and followed certain boys, she seemed to do this very much from her own choice and never lost the flavor of her individuality. She was capable of being social and seemed to enjoy contacts, but at all times she was her own master. She would often withdraw from play and go on in her own direction at any time that she wished. . . . She was independent with adults and, at times, negativistic just to be devilish. She seemed somewhat self-conscious and had some cute little tricks. . . . In all, she could be characterized best by being called 'tough minded.' She shows determination and will, originality and spark, curiosity and interest in factual detail. She likes to quibble and argue, to verbalize, to construct, to accomplish. She is an individualist, independent and stubborn."

AGE 5 YEARS, 4 MONTHS:

FELS NURSERY SCHOOL OBSERVATION

"S seems to be a vigorous, ruthless, competitive, highly sensual young woman, but one felt quite often that antagonism toward others was simply a direct response to their behavior. . . . She has grown far more social and also popular with an increasingly large crowd of special friends in a gang. She could be, when she chose, quite a successful leader, forging ahead and organizing a group on a hike, directing them and arranging things, and particularly keeping order in a fair sharing of the tools in the carpentry shop. . . . Many of S's conflicts with the adult world seemed a direct imitation of a certain boy. She needed a chance to grumble, would scornfully refuse any adult suggestions or orders, would usually go officially ahead to carry them out. She was quite demanding, often shouting an order to an assistant. . . . With her other work the same drive for strong achievement was also evident, sticking to anything until it was finished, whatever the group stimuli."

AGE 7 YEARS: OBSERVATION IN FELS DAY CAMP

"S came accompanied by one friend. S did not seem overwhelmed by the large proportion of adults around, but in her sturdy self-sufficient manner went ahead with her own activities. Her friend was at first rather shy and withdrawn, and S, with her usual confident bullying and bossing of the adults, tended to take the girl under her wing and make sure she had a good time. S remains an exceptionally eager, imperturbable young woman. On a number of small issues she did insist on her own way, on just how long she would stay in the gym and play before lunch, but was quite reasonable about making compromises. She chose a rather difficult necklace to make and got quite mad when it didn't work out well. She kept doggedly with it, very self-sufficient and continuing all on her own after getting some initial advice. . . . Her major effort was put on self-appointed tasks, to be able to master jumping over the horse at the gym where she took numerous tumbles until she succeeded. In spite of her distractability and preference for the apparatus, she did set to learning the new skills required there."

AGE 9 YEARS: REPORT FROM TEACHER

"S is one of the most responsible children in the group. . . . She is self-reliant, independent, and knows how to plan her time well. She enters all games with enthusiasm, is very well coordinated. She is full of personality and 'joie de vivre.'"

As an adolescent S was self-sufficient and sought roles that allowed her to nurture peers and have power over them. An independent approach to problems characterized much of her behavior, and this predisposition was as clear at age 3 as it was in young adulthood.

Interview variable 6: Dependency on parents

A second resource for dependent gratifications is the family. For married females, love objects were usually regarded as more appropriate sources of nurturance, and the married women relied on their husbands more than their family. However, some adults retained a dependent tie to their family during the early adult years. Parents were used as sources of advice, financial support, and encouragement. Dependency on the family was manifested in the form of frequent visits, phone calls, requests for advice on choice of career, choice of college, or major purchases, and a reluctance to move away from the parents.

Table 3 presents the correlations between childhood behavior and adult dependency on parents.

The results resemble those found for dependency on love object. The women who had been highly passive and dependent during Periods III and IV were likely to behave dependently with their family. The stability coefficients for the men were even lower than those found for love-object dependency. The slightly positive relation for men between childhood passivity and love-object dependence dropped to zero for this variable. For young men, a close and dependent relationship with wife or sweetheart was viewed as more appropriate and, therefore, more acceptable than dependence on mother or father. A dependent orientation toward the family was viewed as a regressive and threatening motive. To confide in one's wife, on the other hand, is somewhat more congruent with standards for adult behavior. It would appear that, for men, the relation with a love object may be a more sensitive index of the strength of dependent motives than the character of the relationship with the family.

TABLE 3. RELATION BETWEEN CHILDHOOD BEHAVIOR AND
ADULT DEPENDENCY ON PARENTS

Child Variable	Age	Males	Females	Total
Passivity	0–3	—.32	.17	—.08
	3–6	—.28	.05	—.11
	6–10	—.18	.29*	.00
	10–14	.01	.47**	.16
General dependency	0–3	—.16	.21	.05
	3–6	—.04	—.08	—.03
Affectional dependency	6–10	.00	.30*	.10
	10–14	.03	.47**	.25
Instrumental dependency	6–10	.02	.12	.06
	10–14	.17	.46**	.23
Independence	3–6	.18	—.19	—.02
	6–10	—.04	—.29**	—.16
	10–14	.10	—.39**	—.11
Anxiety loss of nurturance	0–3	.18	.12	.15
	3–6	.24	—.15	.09
	6–10	—.09	.16	.03

* $p < .10$; two tails
** $p < .05$; two tails
*** $p < .01$; two tails
**** $p < .001$; two tails

One of our men verbalized the anxiety over seeking nurturance from the family.

Subject 303

S was an active, aggressive, and independent man for whom dependency was a source of strong conflict. He said he did not like to go to anyone for help because it made him feel uncomfortable.

E: "Are there any people at all that you would go to when you have a problem and want advice?"
S: "I don't like to go to people at all."
E: "Do you have any idea why? Why don't you tend to do this?"
S: "Well—because I—ah—feel that—if I were to go to anybody I would go to my buddies—and—well—I think my buddies don't know anything more about it than me."
E: "I see—you know as much as they do—well, how about your parents? Do

you feel that on most problems they wouldn't be able to give you advice that you could use?"

S: "They could probably give me advice—but—ah—it's just the fact that I wouldn't take it."

E: "You wouldn't take it?"

S: "I doubt it."

On the first tachistoscopic exposure of the scene with the "man with his arms imploring a second man," S replied:

"Two boys playing catch—about 9 or 10 years old."

S also distorted the scene of a "man on his knees in front of a woman." On the first trial he said:

"That was a lady and a little child—I'll say she's about 45—and I believe the child was a little girl about 9 years old—they're crying and the mother was holding her."

At the third exposure:

"There's a mother and it looks like a little boy—she's holding him and it looks like he's crying—he's about 8—or 9—or maybe even younger."

On the last exposure, at one second, S was confused by the stimulus:

"That still looks like a little kid down there—whoever drew that picture is crazy and it looks like she's holding him up—she's got her arms wrapped about him and he's—sorta leaning up against her—I'd say he's about 12 years old."

Variable 55: Dependence on friends

Friends and extrafamilial authority figures are a third resource for advice and encouragement. However, there is often a qualitative difference between the nature of the dependent tie to friends in contrast to the bond to love object or parents. Typically, a less intimate and less emotionally charged relation is developed with peers and older authority figures, and the nurturance sought usually takes the form of advice rather than a request for affection and emotional support.

The seeking of advice from teachers, coaches, college pals, bridge partners, and neighbors usually arises in a context that requires realistic, problem-solving decisions. It is generally less regressive than an emotionally laden request for reassurance from mother or spouse.

Table 4 presents the correlations between childhood behavior and adult dependency on friends.

In general these correlations are neither as high nor as consistent as those found for the previous two variables. It is important to note, however, that the correlations reversed their directions for the females.

TABLE 4. RELATION BETWEEN CHILDHOOD BEHAVIOR AND ADULT
DEPENDENCY ON FRIENDS

Child Variable	Age	Males	Females	Total
Passivity	0–3	.05	.28	.16
	3–6	—.01	.15	.07
	6–10	—.03	.07	.00
	10–14	.02	—.44**	—.18
General dependency	0–3	.00	.22	.16
	3–6	.07	—.08	.03
Affectional dependency	6–10	—.01	—.04	—.05
	10–14	.52**	—.26	.07
Instrumental dependency	6–10	.14	—.16	—.03
	10–14	.25	—.55**	—.23
Independence	3–6	.00	—.07	—.12
	6–10	—.08	.16	.05
	10–14	—.13	.47**	.24
Anxiety loss of nurturance	0–3	.17	.27	.25*
	3–6	.10	.02	.10
	6–10	—.12	.24	.13

  * $p < .10$; two tails
 ** $p < .05$; two tails
*** $p < .01$; two tails
**** $p < .001$; two tails

The *independent* school-age girls were *dependent* on friends in adulthood. For the males, on the other hand, Period IV dependency was
positively associated with adult dependent behavior. This was the first
instance in which adult dependency for men showed a significant association with childhood dependency during the school years.

The pattern of correlations for the females suggests that there is a
psychological difference between dependence on friends, on the one
hand, and or husband or family on the other. The girls who were unusually dependent on adults during ages 10 to 14 avoided an overly
dependent posture with friends, but established an emotionally dependent bond with their families.

When these women required nurturance they sought out this more
reliable and more gratifying source of support. It is as though a dependent tie to family figures precluded the establishment of an emotionally dependent attachment to extrafamilial figures. The girls who
were independent of their families during preadolescence remained

independent of them as adults. They gratified any needs for nurturance through the less intimate relationship with teachers and friends.

It appears that excessive dependence on parents during preadolescence is prognostic of a strong, continuing need for an emotionally supporting relationship with family in adult women. Relative independence from the family is a sign that the childhood tie to parents is being severed. As adults these women sought advice from extrafamilial figures.

Only one of the correlations for the men reached significance, and it is dangerous to attach too much significance to the positive relation between emotional dependence during age 10 to 14 and adult dependence on friends. At a speculative level, it is suggested that the men were highly conflicted over seeking support from love objects or parents and displaced these motives to more acceptable and less regressive sources of nurturance. Mother and wife were viewed by many adult males as symbolic of childhood sources of nurturance and, in flight from this regressive orientation, the men chose figures outside the family orbit. Moreover, the men probably viewed their dependence on friends as problem solving in character rather than as a need for affective reassurance.

A desire for nurturance was present in all of our subjects, but the culture dictated the routes by which this need would find gratification. For the women who were unusually dependent as children, family and husband served this role. The less dependent girls sought out friends and parent substitutes. Many of the men were forced either to displace this response to friends or to completely inhibit its expression. Two men rejected a dependent relationship with all three sources of support. These men were anxious over a passive or dependent posture with any person. One was an aggressive farmer whose façade of belligerence and cynicism buried any expression of dependent needs. The second sought power over others through intellectual accomplishment, and this power precluded his becoming dependent on anyone. Both men were unable to describe accurately the picture of the man on his knees in front of a woman, even at the last exposure at one second. At this exposure the majority of the sample were able to describe accurately the content of the picture, but the aggressive farmer reported:

"Woman on the left, man on the right proposing to her."

The independent intellectual distorted the scene to a greater degree.

"A woman and a boy age 10. . . . she has her arms around him— she's sort of upset by the whole thing and she's comforting him."

These interpretations contrast with the response of a man who was extremely dependent on parents, friends, and teachers. On the first exposure (at 0.01 second) he reported:

"A male and a female about 25—he's done something wrong and he's begging his wife to forgive him—he's down on his knees."

The dramatic difference in the pattern of correlations for women involving dependency on family versus friends suggests the importance of differentiating dependent behavior *with respect to the goal object from whom the nurturance is sought*. If we had attempted to assess over-all dependent behavior, without regard for the goal object, many of the correlations would have been negligible, and we would have concluded that dependent behavior was not stable. The specification of the goal object in motive-related behaviors adds a vital dimension to a description of the response.

Variable 46: Withdrawal from stressful situations

When an individual encounters problem situations he has three alternatives: to deal with the problem independently, to seek help from others, or to withdraw. The variable of withdrawal evaluated the adult's tendency to retreat from situations that were viewed as tests of competence or from situations in which the subject expected task failure or social rejection. Some common examples included the avoidance of positions of responsibility, postponing difficult tasks or decisions, changing major area of study in college because of anticipated failure, and reluctance to interact with strangers. One of our subjects left college in her first year because of an exaggerated feeling of inadequacy. One of the men wanted to teach at a college, but doubted his ability, and finally took a position in an elementary school system in order to avoid the possibility of failure in the more desirable but more challenging role.

It is reasonable to assume that the tendency to withdraw in the face of anxiety is an acquired reaction that develops, in part, from a series of failure experiences. Why should it be related to a young child's dependency on adults? The exaggerated anticipation of failure is often nourished by extreme passivity and dependency during the first six or seven years of life. If the child is consistently passive and dependent in the face of difficult problems, he is likely to acquire the belief that he is helpless when confronted with difficult problems. If the child fails to learn that he can effectively solve problems autonomously, he will expect failure when crises arise. Withdrawal is one probable reaction to a conviction that failure is the most likely outcome. Childhood passivity and dependency, therefore, might be prognostic of the adult tendency to withdraw from failure situations. Table 5 illustrates the relationships between childhood dependency and adult withdrawal.

The results are similar to those found for dependency on love object and parents and clearly indicate that *passivity during Periods III and IV is a reliable predictor of withdrawal in adult women.* The correlation between Period IV passivity and adult withdrawal ($r = +.67$) was the highest coefficient in this entire series. It will be recalled that childhood passivity was based primarily on incidence of withdrawal to frustration. Thus a tendency to withdraw from potential failure experiences was stable from preadolescence through adulthood.

For men, passivity for age 10 to 14 showed only a suggestive relationship with adult withdrawal. The differential stability for the sexes could be a product, once again, of the greater conflict over withdrawal behavior in adult men. Flight from threat or challenge violates one of the defining characteristics of traditional masculine behavior. The

TABLE 5. RELATION BETWEEN CHILDHOOD BEHAVIOR AND ADULT WITHDRAWAL FROM STRESS

Child Variable	Age	Males	Females	Total
Passivity	0–3	−.06	.22	.07
	3–6	.06	.26	.15
	6–10	.27	.48***	.35***
	10–14	.36*	.67****	.50****
General dependency	0–3	−.04	.17	.07
	3–6	.08	.05	.04
Affectional dependency	6–10	.19	.32*	.26**
	10–14	−.24	.18	.00
Instrumental dependency	6–10	.00	.23	.11
	10–14	−.17	.43*	.20
Independence	3–6	−.05	−.29	−.12
	6–10	−.31*	−.35**	−.33***
	10–14	−.25	−.57***	−.46***
Anxiety loss of nurturance	0–3	.16	−.38*	−.16
	3–6	−.08	−.18	−.12
	6–10	−.09	−.05	−.08

 * $p < .10$; two tails
 ** $p < .05$; two tails
 *** $p < .01$; two tails
 **** $p < .001$; two tails

internal standards incorporated by some of our men instructed them to attack problems and to be counterphobic in the face of threat. This inner directive would lead to suppression of withdrawal and attenuate the continuity of this behavioral reaction.

Variable 7: Conflict over dependency

This interview variable was highly related to the preceding ones. The rating was based on derogatory statements about dependent people, a refusal to be dependent or passive with another person, and an unwillingness to admit to dependent motivation. The subjects who were very dependent with parents or love objects typically received a low score for dependency conflict. This variable allowed the rater to be somewhat more inferential, to go beyond the overt behaviors, and to integrate a wide variety of data. Table 6 presents the correlations for this variable.

TABLE 6. RELATION BETWEEN CHILDHOOD BEHAVIOR AND ADULT CONFLICT OVER DEPENDENCY

Child Variable	Age	Males	Females	Total
Passivity	0–3	—.05	—.21	—.12
	3–6	—.02	.00	—.01
	6–10	—.15	—.45**	—.33***
	10–14	—.30	—.39**	—.39***
General dependency	0–3	.07	—.15	—.07
	3–6	.12	.03	.10
Affectional dependency	6–10	—.04	—.17	—.13
	10–14	—.01	—.36	—.19
Instrumental dependency	6–10	—.02	—.12	—.09
	10–14	—.16	—.35	—.41***
Independence	3–6	—.12	.06˙	—.05
	6–10	.15	.31*	.25**
	10–14	.49**	.33	.44***
Anxiety loss of nurturance	0–3	—.09	.00	—.02
	3–6	—.04	.38*	.15
	6–10	.24	.00	.11

* $p < .10$; two tails
** $p < .05$; two tails
*** $p < .01$; two tails
**** $p < .001$; two tails

The relationships were not as striking as those reported for the more behavioral variables. The major result, as might be anticipated, was that passive girls had minimal conflict over dependency as adults. The results are in the same direction for the males but not as significant.

Variable 4: Dependency and vocational choice

At a more speculative level, it was assumed that strong dependent needs might also find expression in an emphasis on financial security in vocational preference. Concern with financial security and avoidance of risk in occupational choice are often regarded as a derived form of dependency motivation, and childhood dependence might be associated with this form of security seeking. Table 7 presents the correlations between childhood behavior and an emphasis on the financial security of a job in adulthood.

TABLE 7. RELATION BETWEEN CHILDHOOD BEHAVIOR AND ADULT DEPENDENCY IN VOCATIONAL CHOICE

Child Variable	Age	Males	Females	Total
Passivity	0–3	.00	.25	.10
	3–6	−.03	.24	.07
	6–10	.05	.55****	.22*
	10–14	.22	.54***	.30**
General dependency	0–3	−.04	.02	.03
	3–6	.00	.16	.08
Affectional dependency	6–10	.16	.04	.09
	10–14	.08	.13	.11
Instrumental dependency	6–10	.13	.20	.13
	10–14	.07	.30	.07
Independence	3–6	.00	−.38**	−.24*
	6–10	−.03	−.40**	−.23*
	10–14	−.28	−.48**	−.31**
Anxiety loss of nurturance	0–3	.16	−.19	−.01
	3–6	.08	−.18	.01
	6–10	−.18	.00	−.03

* $p < .10$; two tails
** $p < .05$; two tails
*** $p < .01$; two tails
**** $p < .001$; two tails

Passivity and lack of independence in girls was clearly associated with a concern for job security. In most cases this concern was reflected in the woman's preference that her husband remain in a financially secure position rather than seek greater remuneration at the price of greater risk. For the men, the correlations were negligible.

EVALUATIVE DISCUSSION

Passivity and a dependent orientation to adults during childhood showed a remarkable degree of developmental continuity among girls. Period I passivity predicted passivity during Period IV ($r = .44$). Period IV passivity predicted both adult withdrawal ($r = .67$), and adult dependency on parents ($r = .47$). There was, therefore, a small group of girls whose preference for passive withdrawal in adulthood had its roots in the preschool and early school years. On the other hand, there was also a group of girls who characteristically acted upon problems with autonomy and independence.[3]

This behavior showed moderate stability for boys over the first 10 years, but predictability of adult responses was generally poor. For some of the males, a shift from a passive-dependent posture to an independent and counterphobic one occurred during the school years. These men tended to come from families that viewed independence and self-sufficiency as a requisite for maturity.

Subject 2313

One of the boys who showed a marked shift from dependence to independence had a father who placed unusually high values on autonomy of action for himself and his sons. As the boy approached preadolescence he experienced direct familial pressures for independence. The change in his behavior is apparent in the following excerpts.

At $2\frac{1}{2}$ years of age he was described as unusually passive and cautious.

"S spent an unhappy week at nursery school. He cried a great deal and looked ready to cry even when he was not actually doing it. He drew away when other children approached him, and he seemed afraid of them. Usually he stood around and looked lost."

At $4\frac{1}{2}$ years of age passivity was still a prepotent response.

"S was one of the group's most isolated members. He was noncompetitive, unassertive, and sedentary. He shrank from actual physical contact with others and his relationships with peers were mild, long-distance verbal ones. S was petrified at rough handling. When he was verbally rebuffed or teased he smiled weakly and put his hands behind his back. S was the most eclipsed member of the group because of his apprehension, shyness, and inhibition."

By age 8 some shift toward independent behavior had occurred. There was a forced independence and swagger, and S had learned to use his intellectual skills as a weapon of power over others. He lectured and bragged to his peers, and the fear and apprehension that were manifest at age 4 were more disguised. S became less dependent on his family and more committed to an intellectual life.

As a late adolescent, the conflict associated with withdrawal from stress had swelled in intensity. S's internal standards did not permit retreat from potential failure situations. At age 16, for example, he realized that he was still afraid of dating girls and decided that there was only one effective way to conquer this fear. He invited to a dance the most popular girl in the school even though he had never been with her before. The primary reason for inviting her was to test his ability to conquer his fears.

As an adult he derogated dependent behavior and dependent people.

E: "Did you ever go to your family for advice with any problems?"
S: "My father was not approachable, and I didn't go to him for advice—in fact—he used to tell me to solve my own problems by myself, and I felt uneasy about going to him for help—ah—my mother—she wouldn't know what to tell me anyway."

His conflict was revealed in his perceptual interpretation of the picture of the man on his knees. On the first exposure, he reported:
"A woman in her thirties—holding a boy 8 or 9—she was comforting him."
On the second exposure:
"A woman in her early thirties with a little boy—she was cheering him up—comforting him or something—perhaps comforting him because something happened to him."
On the third exposure he said:
"A relatively young woman—the man in the foreground has been badly hurt and she was leaning over him—she was trying to pick him up—to get some kind of medical attention."
On the fourth exposure he retreated to his earlier perception and replied:
"A woman in her middle twenties in front of a younger boy—13 or

14—she's trying to pat him on the head—and that's figuratively and not literally—to cheer him up—or something."

Subject 2943

S was as passive as the boy described above during childhood. However, the father of this boy was a weak and frightened man who was completely subordinate to his wife. The mother protected the boy and accepted his fragile reactions to stress. Passivity was acceptable to both parents and excessive independence or autonomy was met with parental disapproval. As both child and adult S was one of the most dependent subjects in the sample. The interviewer questioned him about dependency in adulthood.

E: "What do you tend to do when there are problems or decisions that you have to make?"

S: "Like the job—the new job I went to—I heard about it and I talked to my teacher—then when I had the chance I talked to my parents about it—and then I decided to take it."

E: "Now when you say 'I talked to my parents,' did you talk to them as if you were really interested in what their views were or because it was appropriate to do so?"

S: "Well—I wanted to know—what they—if they thought it would be good for me—or not."

E: "And you are interested in their opinion?"

S: "Yes, I wanted to know what they thought."

E: "As to your parents—did you talk to both of them—or just Mom—or Dad?"

S: "Both."

E: "Both—well, when you do have problems, are you more apt to go to one than to the other?"

S: "No—I don't think so."

E: "When you are faced with a problem—are you apt to talk it over with them?"

S: "Yes—uh-huh—I try to if I have the chance—if I'm home and if the decision doesn't have to be reached right then—I will talk it over with them."

E: "Can you give me some more things you have talked over with them—in the last year—or year and a half?"

S: "Well—like going to school—I talked it over with them and the—and a teacher at high school too, I talked with him about it—and then I arrived at the decision to go."

E: "Do you feel close to your folks?"

S: "Well—I mean I still like to look to them for decisions—and help—I mean I don't want to rely on them—entirely—I like to make my own decision in the end—but I like their help on it."

E: "Some adults do and some adults do not feel a certain bond of closeness to their parents. Do you feel a bond?"

S: "Well—in a sense—yes—I want to see them—that is, I just don't want to be shut off from them—entirely."

S's minimal conflict over dependency was evidenced in his early recognition of the scenes illustrating a man on his knees in front of a woman. On the first exposure, *S* reported:

"A male and a female—they look like they are about 25—it looks like the man has done something wrong and he's begging his wife to forgive him—he's down on his knees."

SOCIAL CLASS AND DEPENDENCY

The best estimate of social-class position for this sample was the amount of formal education achieved by the parents. Occupation was often misleading, for many of the farmers in the group had college degrees and middle-class values. Housing and neighborhood were also poor indices of class in this semirural area. Each parent was assigned a score (1–6) based on amount of formal schooling, and these values were correlated with the longitudinal and adult interview variables.

The educational level of the child's parents was not consistently associated with passivity or dependency in early childhood. Correlations between education of each of the parents and passivity for Period I or II were all close to zero (range of .00 to .13). Dependence during Periods III and IV also failed to show a statistically significant association with parental education.

However, adult dependency showed some complex association with the educational level of each of the parents (see Table 8).

For the men, the only significant association was between maternal education and dependency on love object. For women, the results were quite the reverse. Maternal education was not highly related to love-object dependency, but paternal educational level was inversely related to love-object dependency.

The men with well-educated mothers were more dependent on sweetheart or wife than the men with poorly educated mothers. The women with well-educated fathers avoided a dependent relationship with love objects. It is tempting to speculate on these correlations.

The boy with the well-educated mother may develop a respect for the knowledge and competence of a woman. In marriage he may

TABLE 8. RELATION BETWEEN EDUCATIONAL LEVEL OF PARENTS AND
ADULT DEPENDENT BEHAVIOR

	Men		Women	
Adult Variable	*Father*	*Mother*	*Father*	*Mother*
Dependency on love object	.18	.42**	−.34**	−.17
Dependency on parents	.01	.09	−.27	−.15
Dependency parent substitute	.06	.24	.25	.33**
Dependency conflict	.19	.01	.50***	.32**
Withdrawal	−.06	.04	−.27	−.31
Dependency vocation	−.10	.01	−.18	−.11

** $p < .05$; two tails
*** $p < .01$; two tails

generalize this attitude to his wife. Why then did the girls behave in
the opposite manner? The women with well-educated fathers were
more conflicted over dependency and reluctant to assume a passive
role with men. These women came from homes where the traditional
sex-role characteristic of passivity with men was not encouraged. Independence of action and career choices were valued, and this freedom
from the restrictive pressures of traditional sex typing may have led
to a reluctance to assume a dependent role with men.

A PARTIAL REPLICATION

The significance of the present findings is limited by the omni-
present possibility that this sample was atypical and replication would
fail to confirm the stability of passive behavior. Since the Institute's
longitudinal program is continuous, we had available an independent
group of 90 children who had been observed during the first six years.
These data provided the opportunity for an independent replication
of some of these results.

Initially a group of 45 girls and 45 boys born between 1941 and
1959 was selected, none of whom were members of the present long-
term study. An undergraduate student, who was unfamiliar with any
of the children in the Fels' study, was trained to rate the observational
reports on these children (seven-point scale) for passivity and dependency during the first three years. In order to avoid the psycho-

logical interference associated with making ratings for a large number of variables, only three variables were rated: passivity, dependency, and task mastery. Initially the student rated 12 cases previously rated by HM to assess the reliability of her ratings. The reliability coefficients were .86 and .88 for passivity and dependency, respectively.

Replication 1

Of the 45 girls rated for the first three years, 15 had visited the Fels experimental nursery school during 1959 and 1960 when they were between 3 and 6 years of age. The children came to the nursery school for from one to three sessions, each session lasting 3 weeks, and each session separated by a 6 to 12 month period. The regular Fels nursery-school observer, who had no knowledge of the child's behavior at home or of the student's ratings, rated each child for a variety of variables after the 3-week nursery school period was completed. These ratings were based on a schedule of time-sampled observations in which each child was observed for 10-minute periods once or twice daily for each of 15 days. The reliability of this particular observer's ratings had been ascertained on two separate occasions (1957 and 1959) with two separate individuals, for six variables related to passivity, dependence, and aggression. The average inter-rater reliabilities for the two sessions ranged from .54 to .97, with a median coefficient of .83.

These two independent sets of ratings (the student's ratings for age 0 to 3 and the Fels observer's ratings for age 3 to 6) were then correlated for the 15 girls. The sample size for boys was negligible, and correlations were not computed.

The girls who were passive during age 0 to 3 were, during age 3 to 6, low on dominance with other girls ($r = .54$; $p < .05$) and likely to withdraw from the peer group to solitary play with paints, blocks, and paper ($r = .74$; $p < .001$). The dependency rating for 0 to 3 had similar correlates with preschool behavior. The girls who were dependent for 0 to 3 were rated low on dominance from 3 to 6 ($r = .50$; $p < .05$) and prone to withdraw from the peer group ($r = .47$; $p < .10$). In sum, a passive reaction to frustration during the first three years was predictive of withdrawal from strange peers during the preschool years. These findings parallel the results found with the original and larger group of subjects. The girls who were rated as passive during Period I were, during the preschool years, nondominant with same sex peers and socially withdrawn ($r = .43$; $p < .10$, $r = .44$; $p < .10$, respectively).

The short-term stability of peer dominance and social withdrawal was assessed with a group of 14 girls who had visited the Fels nursery school twice between 3 and 6 years of age. The average time lapse between the two visits was one year. The Fels observer's ratings for these two periods were correlated, and the stability coefficients were .72 ($p < .01$) for dominance of peers and .67 ($p < .01$) for social withdrawal. Thus the tendency to be assertive or passive with same sex peers showed moderately high stability over a 12-month period for this small but independent group of girls.

Replication 2

Most of the 90 children whose behavior had been rated for the first three years of life were between 7 and 17 years of age when the student had made her ratings. The longitudinal files contained observations on their behavior at home and in the nursery school. After eliminating the 15 girls described above (Replication 1), 61 cases remained, each with adequate observational data for 3 to 6 years of age. Adequate data were defined as a minimum of three home visits and two nursery-school reports. Two raters (a graduate student in psychology and one of the authors [JK]), who had no knowledge of the ratings made on these subjects for age 0 to 3 by the undergraduate student, divided the 61 cases equally and rated each child for four variables: (1) passivity in the face of aggressive attack from a peer, (2) social withdrawal, (3) general passivity [i.e., over-all rating that combined (1) and (2)], and (4) dependence on female adults.

TABLE 9. STABILITY OF PASSIVITY AND DEPENDENCE OVER THE FIRST SIX YEARS: REPLICATION SAMPLE

(35 boys; 26 girls)

| | Age 0–3 | | | | | |
| | Passivity | | | Dependence | | |
Age 3–6	Boys	Girls	Pooled	Boys	Girls	Pooled
Passive to attack	.18	.48***	.33***	.35**	.30	.31**
Social withdrawal	.26	.17*	.21	.26	.16	.22
General passivity	.23	.36	.30	.35	.31	.33***
Dependency	.10	.16	.10	.33	.14	.23

* $p < .10$; two tails
** $p < .05$; two tails
*** $p < .01$; two tails

Table 9 presents the correlations between passivity and dependence for 0 to 3 (as rated by the student) and each of the four variables rated for age 3 to 6.

The girls who were passive during 0 to 3 continued to be passive during the preschool years ($r = .48$; $p < .01$). For boys, the rating of early dependency was the better predictor of preschool passivity and dependency ($r = .35$; $p < .05$).

The results from these analyses of independent samples of children lend strong support to the conclusion that a passive orientation to attack and a tendency to withdraw from novel social situations are moderately stable characteristics during the childhood years, and perhaps longer.

THE SIGNIFICANCE OF EARLY PASSIVITY

The stability of passive behavior during the childhood years was striking. Intensive study of the observations on the school-age children who fell at the behavioral extremes of this dimension suggested that the tendency toward passivity during preadolescence was already apparent during the first two years of life. Passivity during the first three years was significantly associated with a consistent cluster of school-age behaviors (ages 6 to 10): avoidance of dangerous activity, absence of physical and verbal aggression, conformity to parents, and timidity in social situations (see Chapter Six for details). Moreover, the boys who were passive during Period I avoided sports and other traditional masculine activities during the preadolescent and adolescent years. The four boys who were rated as most passive during the first six years chose intellectual careers as adults (music, physics, biology, psychology). The four least passive boys chose more traditional masculine vocations (football coach, salesman, and two engineers).

There are, therefore, tentative bits of evidence that link early passivity with direct forms of passivity during late childhood or with derivative behaviors, such as failure to adopt masculine interests (in boys), conformity, nonaggression, and social withdrawal during the school years. This cluster of behaviors has a theoretically meaningful consistency that invites systematic attention to the significance of passivity during the early developmental years.

An independent team of investigators has also concluded that early passivity is a stable characteristic of the child (Thomas et al., 1960). This group studied 74 children during the first two years of life; the primary data consisting of detailed interviews with the mother (six interviews during the first two years). These interviews were scored for factual statements about the child's behavior. Analysis of the interviews suggested that a passive approach to new situations was relatively stable over this period. The authors wrote:

Qualitative examination of the data also permits the delineation of another characteristic of individuality which is of special psychiatric interest. This concerns the character of the child's reactions to a new situation, whether it be the bath or the introduction of solid food in early infancy, vaccinations or the first awareness of strangers, the attempt to enforce the prohibition of dangerous activities or the initiation of toilet training at two years, or the first contact with nursery school at three years. In each instance, there is striking consistency in the pattern of the individual child's reaction to the new situation. This pattern is actually compounded from elements involving certain of the nine categories defined in the quantitative analysis, namely activity level, approach or withdrawal, intensity, mood, adaptability, attention span and persistence. *Some children respond quietly and placidly to a new situation, approach it at once and adapt quickly and smoothly. At the other extreme are those children who withdraw sharply and violently from a new situation, persist tenaciously in their old behavior, and adapt irregularly and slowly* (italics ours).

The initial reaction to social situations may affect the responses of other people involved and influence the whole character of interpersonal interaction (Thomas, Chess, Birch, and Hertzig, 1960, p. 109).

It is perhaps no coincidence that a dimension of assertiveness versus nonassertiveness has always been popular in descriptions of human behavior. Inventories and rating scales used with children and adults repeatedly include a continuum of social assertiveness in contrast to passive withdrawal.

Moreover, a recent study of 34 pairs of identical and 34 pairs of fraternal twins (same sex) suggested that a dimension of social withdrawal versus social extraversion may have a genetic component (Gottesman, 1960). Each of the adolescent subjects was administered the *Minnesota Multiphasic Personality Inventory* and Cattell's *High School Personality Questionnaire,* and intraclass correlations were computed for each of the scales in the two tests. The scales that showed a significantly greater degree of similarity between identical rather than between fraternal twins were closely related to a social withdrawal dimension (Gottesman, 1960).

This last finding on twin similarities, together with the evidence suggesting the early age at which a passive predisposition emerges, tempt speculation on possible constitutional correlates of a passive approach to environmental stresses. There are some highly tentative, but tantalizing, data that support this possibility.

CONSTITUTIONAL CORRELATES OF PASSIVITY

Passivity was more stable for females than for males, and investigators typically find that passive and dependent behaviors are more frequent among girls and women than among boys and men. We generally assume that this difference is largely a product of training. However, Bell (1960) and Knop (1946) suggest that neonatal girls are more likely than boys to display motoric passivity. Furthermore, Harlow (1962) has found that infant male macaques are more likely to make threatening gestures and less likely to withdraw in the face of attack than infant females. Thus there is some beginning evidence suggesting that the constitutional differences between males and females may be associated with a passive-active behavioral continuum.

A second source of evidence involves the autonomic reactivity of our adult male subjects. For the adult men who were rated as passive during the first three years of life showed nonvariable cardiac activity at rest. It will be recalled that 30 of the adult males were seen for a session in which heart rate and palmar resistance variability were assessed under different conditions (see Chapter Eight for details). The index of resting cardiac arrhythmia was obtained by measuring the trough to peak changes in the cardiac cycle in a 10-minute rest period, casting these into a frequency distribution, and choosing the third quartile value as the measure of cardiac arrhythmia. Of the 30 males for whom cardiac arrhythmia measures were available, 14 were rated on passivity during the first three years of life. The 6 boys who were below the median on early passivity were all above the median on degree of heart rate arrhythmia in adulthood. Of the 8 most passive boys, 6 were below the median on cardiac variability in adulthood ($p < .05$). Thus passivity in childhood was associated with a minimal degree of spontaneous cardiac arrhythmia in adulthood. The adult men who were rated as highly dependent on love objects also had lower arrhythmia scores. Thus early passivity was indirectly linked to the degree of spontaneous arrhythmia of the cardiac cycle. Moreover, the Laceys (Lacey and Lacey, 1958 [a]) have found that college males with low cardiac arrhythmia scores were less able to sustain a set to react quickly in a simple, motor-reaction time situation. One is tempted to add that they were more passive during this laboratory task.

Thus far we have presented possible relationships between biological variables and passivity that are without a theoretical context.

There is, however, one type of constitutional variable that might be implicated in male passivity, for which a reasonable rationale can be constructed. This variable involves the child's physique.

Several studies indicate that an individual's bony chest diameter (e.g., width at the tenth rib) is an excellent index of his fat-free body mass—an anatomical characteristic that appears to be genetic in origin (Behnke, 1959). Children born to two large-chested parents, in contrast to those born to two small-chested parents, are taller and heavier during the growing period (Garn, Clark, Landkof and Newell, 1960). Moreover, these larger children have higher mental test scores on the Merrill-Palmer Scale at 2 years of age and on the Stanford-Binet at 3 years of age. By school age these differences have vanished (Kagan and Garn, in press).

Unfortunately, only a small group of our children with ratings on passivity for age 0 to 3 were the products of matings of two large- or two small-chested parents (16 children born to large-chested parents and 11 to small-chested parents). The children of two small-chested parents were more likely to be rated as passive during the early years than the children of large-chested parents. Although this difference was not statistically significant, it suggests that muscle mass and behavioral passivity may be associated.

Let us assume that a boy with low muscle mass is predisposed initially to adopt a passive orientation to the environment. It would be reasonable to argue that the child's future encounters with the social environment might exaggerate these initial tendencies. That is, if the boy entered the preschool period with a prepotent tendency to withdraw from physical attack, from strange social situations, and from vigorous gross motor games, subsequent social learning experiences would strengthen this withdrawal habit until it became a stable part of his behavioral repertoire. As mentioned earlier, passivity in boys during the first six years predicted social anxiety, avoidance of sex, and nonmasculine interests in adulthood (see Chapter Six).

A young boy is expected to be skilled with gross motor games and able to defend himself physically. The child who fails to develop these habits is likely to encounter peer rejection, which, in turn, will result in feelings of inadequacy and social anxiety. Such feelings should lead to even more persistent withdrawal behavior.

It is reasonable to suppose that boys with low muscle mass might have more difficulty perfecting those masculine skills that lead to peer acceptance. Furthermore, the public media's stereotype of the ideal male portrays an individual who is tall, broad, and muscular. The preadolescent boy who perceives a major discrepancy between his body image and his conception of the cultural ideal is likely to develop an expectancy of rejection and subsequent anxiety. A boy's physical characteristics, therefore, make him susceptible to the acquisition of an anxiety-arousing self-concept and anticipation of social rejection, because of the association between an expectancy of peer rejection (by both boys and girls) and the absence of sex-appropriate physical attributes. The work of Mussen and Jones (1957, 1958) on early and late maturing boys and the early research of Sanford et al. (1943) support this line of reasoning. Boys who are late maturing, and, therefore, deviate from the culture's ideal body build, tend to be less popular and reveal greater feelings of inadequacy than early maturing boys.

Thus one rationale for a relation between behavioral passivity and constitution is based, in part, on a link between passivity and muscle mass during the early years of life, followed by an incorporation of the culture's attitude toward males who are small and frail and who, therefore, are likely to be deficient in those physical attributes that define the male ideal. Learning experiences, therefore, strengthen an initial, unlearned disposition toward passivity.[4]

In sum, although the data from the present study and those of other investigations must be regarded as highly tentative, they suggest two hypotheses that merit attention: (1) a predisposition to passivity is a function, in part, of biological variables and (2) the foundation for extreme degrees of passivity, or its derivatives, in late childhood, adolescence and adulthood are established during the first six years of life.

Footnotes

1. We chose this strategy (i.e., correlating clusters of childhood variables with phenotypically similar adult variables) over a factor analytic procedure, in part, because the sample size for each sex was relatively small and not constant for all coefficients.

As the reader studies the coefficients relating child and adult behavior he should bear in mind that the child or adult variables in any one cluster (e.g., dependency or aggression) are not completely independent of each other. The complete sets of intercorrelations among the longitudinal or interview variables appear in Appendixes 32 and 33 and the interested reader should study them.

2. In an earlier paper (Kagan and Moss, 1960a) preliminary correlations were presented between child and adult passive-dependent behavior. These earlier correlations were based on data from 54 subjects rather than on the complete group of 71 subjects.

3. Anxiety over loss of nurturance showed minimal stability during childhood and negligible links to adult behavior. It has been suggested that it is difficult to assess this variable from descriptions of overt behavior. The three borderline correlations all occurred for women and suggested that signs of anxiety over loss of love during the preschool years were predictive of a reluctance to become dependent on love objects and high conflict over dependency. It is possible that the girl who anticipates rejection might begin to defend against a dependent attitude toward people, since she does not expect gratification of these needs. Rather than become vulnerable to rejection and the anxiety attendant upon an unsatisfying reliance on others, the individual might inhibit dependent overtures.

4. Dr. Irving Gottesman recently informed the authors of an unpublished study on 43 adolescent males in which he found a positive relation between ponderal index (ratio of height to cube root of weight) and the social introversion scale of the MMPI ($r = .36$) and a negative relation between ponderal index and the dominance scale of the MMPI ($r = -.31$). Thus tall, thin adolescent boys tended to be socially withdrawn and nondominant with peers. The corresponding correlations for adolescent girls were not significantly different from zero.

CHAPTER FOUR

The Stability of Behavior: II
Aggression

Aggression is a second behavior system that begins its growth during the first five years. Traditionally a response was labeled aggressive if the goal of the behavior was assumed to be psychological or physical injury to a person or person surrogate. We have adhered to this definition. As with dependency, the display of aggressive acts is a regular concomitant of development. The slapping or pushing of an age mate, the destruction of a sibling's new fort, and the stinging verbal attack are regularly observed in the behavior of many children.

Aggression, like dependency, is subject to socialization pressures, for the child does not have complete license to unleash his anger when he chooses. In addition, as with dependency, the occurrence of overt aggression is a function of both the threshold for motive arousal and the intensity of anxiety associated with direct expression of this behavior.

In contrast to dependency, however, the potential for conflict over aggression is greater for females than for males. The pattern of social rewards and traditional sex-role standards act in concert to discourage the direct expression of aggression in girls and women. It might be anticipated, therefore, that aspects of aggression would be more stable for males than for females. This is precisely what occurred, for overt aggression to mother and frequent tantrums during childhood predicted adult aggressivity for men but not for women.

This chapter contains a detailed description of the pattern of stability for different aggressive behaviors. The format follows that of the previous chapter. A cluster of seven aggressive variables was rated for part or all of the four childhood periods, and abridged definitions of these variables follow.

Variable 1: Aggression to mother

This variable, rated for all four age periods, assessed behavioral manifestations of direct hostility toward the mother, for example, striking the mother, flagrant disobedience, verbal attacks, chronic resistance to maternal requests.

Variable 2: Physical aggression to peers

This variable was only rated for the first three periods because of its infrequent occurrence for ages 10 to 14. The rating was based on the occurrence of unprovoked, physical attacks on same sex peers.

Variable 3: Indirect aggression to peers

This variable was rated for all four periods and assessed occurrence of unprovoked, nonphysical aggression toward same sex peers, for example, verbal threats or taunts, teasing, destruction or seizure of a peer's property.

Variable 12: Behavioral disorganization

This variable was rated for all four periods and evaluated the degree of behavioral disorganization displayed by the child when he encountered frustration or attack. Evidence of disorganization during the early years included violent crying and tantrums. During the school years the rating was based on uncontrolled destructive activity, rages, and tantrums. One might view this rating as an index of the child's tolerance for frustration.

Variable 28: Conformity to adults

This variable, rated for all four age periods, evaluated the degree to which the child accepted, and practiced, the rules, standards, and requests of adult authorities, primarily parents and teachers. The rating was based on degree of obedience to parents and teachers and the tendency to enforce adult rules with other children.

Variable 82: Dominance of peers

This variable was rated for Periods II, III, and IV and assessed the child's attempts to direct and control the behavior of other children.

Variable 83: Competitiveness

This variable was included in the aggression cluster because of the potential aggressive gratifications involved in attempting to defeat a peer in a game or task situation. This form of aggression is socially approved and, therefore, differs from the previously defined behaviors. Competitiveness, rated for Periods II, III, and IV, evaluated the degree to which the child became involved in games or tasks that were tests of relative superiority and assessed his tendency to structure inter-personal relations in terms of competition for superiority.

STABILITY OF LONGITUDINAL VARIABLES

The stability coefficients for these seven aggressive variables over ages 0 to 14 are presented in Table 1.

Aggression to mother

Expression of hostility to the mother showed moderate stability only for the contiguous age Periods II to III and III to IV. *Aggression to mother during the first three years was not highly predictive of behavior during later childhood.* The minimal stability for Periods I to III and II to IV indicates that the tendency to express aggression toward the mother underwent a major change in some children during the first 14 years.

Physical aggression to peers

In contrast to aggression to mother, this class of behavior was highly stable over the first 10 years of life. All of the stability coefficients for the pooled sample exceeded the .01 level of confidence. The greater stability for peer-directed, in contrast to mother-directed, aggression could be due to the fact that the mother is less tolerant of open expressions of hostility toward herself than she is of peer-directed aggression. This possibility is consonant with the recent work of Sears, Maccoby, and Levin (1957). Since peer-directed aggression is less subject to punishment and conflict-induced suppression, it is more likely to exhibit long-term stability. Further, aggression with peers can have secondary gains, for it is sometimes instrumental in attaining power positions with peers. The attainment of these social rewards nourishes the developmental continuity of this behavior.

TABLE 1. STABILITY OF AGGRESSION FOR CHILDHOOD PERIODS I TO IV

Variable	I–II	I–III	I–IV	II–III	II–IV	III–IV
1. Aggression to mother						
Boy	.24	.22	−.19	.61****	.23	.56***
Girl	.26	.08	.36*	.59****	−.02	.49***
Total	.24*	.16	.14	.61****	.11	.53****
2. Physical aggression to peers						
Boy	.86***	.30		.48**		
Girl	.82****	.69***		.70****		
Total	.89****	.56***		.59****		
3. Indirect aggression to peers						
Boy	.59***	.49**		.67****	.64**	.71****
Girl	.44**	.48**	.53*	.61****	.56***	.60****
Total	.52***	.49***		.64****	.51****	.67****
12. Behavioral disorganization						
Boy	.11	.08	.35	.57****	.52***	.67****
Girl	.14	.12	−.02	.48***	−.03	.25
Total	.13	.11	.12	.55****	.23*	.47****
28. Conformity						
Boy	.53***	.29	.27	.76****	.16	.53***
Girl	.06	.05	−.24	.47***	.35*	.68****
Total	.32**	.21*	.01	.60****	.34**	.66****
82. Dominance						
Boy				.78****	.72**	.84****
Girl				.73****	.59***	.56***
Total				.73****	.53***	.66****
83. Competitiveness						
Boy				.61**		.75****
Girl				.61***	.73***	.64***
Total				.61****		.67****

* p < .10; two tails *** p < .01; two tails
** p < .05; two tails **** p < .001; two tails

Indirect aggression to peers

This variable also manifested moderately high stability over the childhood years. Even the Period II to IV comparison was significant. The boys' correlation for Period I to IV was not presented because it was based on less than 10 cases. Thus peer-directed aggression, in the form of fighting or verbal attack, showed impressive stability from the preschool years through early adolescence.

Behavioral disorganization

This variable showed a rather unusual stability pattern. The occurrence of tantrums, irritable crying, or rage reactions during the first three years had no relationship with apparently similar behavior during the subsequent 11 years. Furthermore, for Periods II, III, and IV, this reaction to frustration was more stable for boys than for girls. The coefficients for Periods II to IV and III to IV were significantly greater for boys than for girls ($p < .05$; two tails).

The lack of continuity for Period I disorganization could be due to the fact that irritability and long crying episodes during the early years are diffuse reactions to frustration that are not always directed at a specific social object and are not as effective in overcoming frustrations as the more organized aggressive response of the preschool years. Aggression to peers, on the other hand, is an organized, and often effective, act directed at a specific target. A child who is irritable and easily upset during the first two to three years of life is not necessarily the child who will display uncontrolled rages or tantrums during the school years.

The following verbatim excerpts furnish a concrete illustration of the lack of relation between irritability during Period I and behavioral disorganization during the school years.

Subject 006

During the first half year S was an unusually irritable baby who cried for long periods of time. Novel situations with strange adults elicited long periods of energetic wails. At 8 months of age the home visitor wrote:

"This family is tied down both by S and the farm. It is growing more difficult to leave S at the home of the grandparents while the parents go to a movie. S cries continuously while they are gone and occasionally starts so early that they do not go. She is highly dependent upon her mother and whimpers when she goes out of the room."

"The observer thought that the mother was feeding S too rapidly and jabbing the spoon into her mouth too roughly. In any case S started to cry, got very red, and could not be distracted. Mother turned in desperation to the home visitor and said: 'What shall I do? She does this all the time.' S is not yet bowel-trained and has irregular movements. S is less easily startled now than she was as a baby, but she still can be characterized as nervous. According to the mother, 'S has a terrible temper.'"

Several weeks later S and the mother were seen at the Institute.

"When mother and S were ready to leave, mother put on S's outdoor clothing. S began to cry and continued to do so all during the dressing process. According to the mother, S has a will of her own, and, when she is determined, she makes it known by crying lustily."

One month later the mother was interviewed.

"The mother was very willing to talk and, as usual, was very much interested in S and tried to recall any incident that might be interesting. She is a little worried about S's temper. S has a strict routine, and she becomes angry, crys, and grows red all over when the routine is upset in any way. S has a definite idea about what she wants and when she wants it, and she objects if not satisfied. The mother remarked that she supposed that S had inherited her temper from someone in the family."

During the second year S resisted toilet training and would cry violently when placed on the pot. She continued to use her crying spells as a way of manipulating the mother.

At 2 years, 3 months the home visitor wrote:

"Mother said that S was so determined that she usually 'won out' in any conflict between the two. Her behavior depends almost entirely on her state of health and the amount of sleep she has had. Some days, tractable and pleasant; other days she is in tears most of the time. Mother said she disciplined S by spanking her or sitting her on a chair. She admitted that her disciplinary techniques usually failed; however, any attempt to make S do something she didn't want to do usually makes her behavior worse than it was before. The mother remarked, 'it is best to let her alone; gradually she will tire of what she is doing; then it is possible to distract her.'"

Toward the end of the third year S still showed a low-frustration tolerance and a diffuse and disorganized reaction to attack.

The nursery-school summary at 2 years, 8 months read:

"S was independent, willful, slow moving and deliberate. S was prob-

ably most interesting because of what might be called her 'temperament.' She had a definite personality and individuality which characterized her more accurately than an actual record of her moment-to-
moment behavior. Much of her behavior seemed to have an emotional
basis. She was highly independent, and she fought and resisted when
attempts were made to suggest other actions for her. She liked to do
things by and for herself and often jerked away or grew emotional
when frustrated. She was rather irritable, more so on some days than
others. She would frown, complain, or fuss at small annoyances such
as being crowded, touched, or having a toy upset. She was quite willful, wanted to have things her own way and wanted to be allowed to
do as she pleased. If she were coerced sharply, she could display a
violent temper in which she wept, howled, and stamped her feet. She
turned this off and on rather quickly."

"These outbursts, mild or serious, were always the result of some
kind of interference or blocking. When she was uninterrupted and
allowed to go her own way, she was very peaceful and often quietly
happy."

During the fourth year there was a gradual change in the ease with
which her temper could be aroused, and disorganized outbursts became less frequent. When S was 3½ years old, the nursery-school observer wrote:

"S wasn't ready to take all the rough-housing and actual hostility that
went on, and, when directly attacked or accidently pushed, she would
turn to a young boy in the nursery school for protection, defense, and
comfort. It is hard to say how much of this reaction is due to lack of
social dominance and how much is relative disinterest in the materials.
She was easily dispossessed of toys and seldom acquired toys from
others."

"In relation to this boy, the things that stood out were mutual
warmth and shared play and his protection of her against the aggression of others and frustration from objects."

"S was seldom interruptive in free play as she wasn't aggressive or
destructive, and she seldom objected when stopped from sucking an
object; she simply waited and substituted something else."

The shift toward docility was more apparent in the report written
when S was 4½ years old.

"The most startling change was S's behavior with adults. Last year,
in spite of the fact that the staff was fond of her, they all considered her
as one of the most difficult kids to get along with. They never knew
what word or gesture would strike her the wrong way and provoke a
burst of anger. This year she was not only friendly but actually warm,

in initiating either joking, affectionate or physical contact with adults. There is a great deal of gayety and responsiveness to adults as individual people, and during story hour her enjoyment seemed to be divided between the fun of listening and the chance to sit on an adult lap."

"Last year S had been outstanding for her refusals. This year she was not only willing to be examined but also showed some enjoyment over it."

In an interview with her mother when S was 6 years old, the mother reported that:

"S is responsive to suffering or weakness in others. The mother described a scene that took place when her husband brought home a lamb born with bad eyes. He intended to work on the lamb right in front of the children. S broke in and told him, 'I love that little lamb, I don't want Daddy to hurt him.' "

S was interviewed when she was 6 years, 3 months.

"S attended the winter interview with two boys and seemed very pleased to have the chance to be with some other children. In her contacts with them S showed a great deal of just plain inexperience of how to deal with other children, talking to them in an ultrasweet voice. She commented to one of the adults, 'Those are cute little boys,' and addressing them, 'Come here, boys.' Somewhere she seems to have been thoroughly indoctrinated with the idea of a sex stereotype. In the sandbox she gave a long lecture on the different kinds of fun had by boys. S was unable to enter into the dramatic play of the boys and seemed really puzzled by it. When the boys in the swing were doing dive-bombing and strafing, they pretended to shoot at her. She came to an adult and asked in a thoroughly puzzled tone, 'They're just joking, aren't they?' "

When S was 8 years, 3 months, the home visitor noted:

"The difference between S and her younger sister is quite striking. S, who is the older, is quiet, passive, and cautious. The younger, only 4 years old, is the initiator; active and reckless. This younger sister resents it if S orders her around. On the other hand, S seems perfectly willing to follow the younger sister's demands and requests. These two little girls are the best of friends and seem to get along together unusually well."

When S was 9 years old, the home visitor wrote that:

"S seems to be such a conforming little girl, eager to do what is expected of her."

This series of descriptions captures the shift from extreme irritability at 2 years to the docility and conformity present at 8 years of age. It is not implied, however, that irritability and low frustration tolerance during the first few years are of no psychological significance. The particular girl described above developed into one of the two most psychologically disturbed women in our sample. As an adult she displayed shallowness of affect, and disturbed and incoherent communications. Thus extreme irritability in this girl was prognostic of a variety of significant derivative behaviors. But it was not a precursor of the violent rage or tantrum behaviors that are displayed by some school-age children.

The selective stability of behavioral disorganization for boys could be due to the existence of differential permissiveness for rage reactions in school-age boys and girls. The uncontrolled, and sometimes violent, motor discharge characteristic of a rage reaction are ill-suited to the role prescription for a middle-class girl. Females can be aggressive, but the cultural pressures dictate that its expression be verbal and controlled. Moreover, violent outbursts are more frequently ascribed to the male than to the female in the public media's dramatizations of sex-role behavior. Thus parents are less apt to expect this behavior in girls, more anxious when it occurs, and more prone to suppress it. There are, of course, alternative interpretations of this finding. For example, unknown constitutional processes may favor a low threshold for rage behavior in boys. Regardless of the cause, however, this class of behavior was more stable for boys than for girls.

Conformity to authority

Adoption of an acquiescent posture with parents and teachers was very stable for Periods II to III and III to IV, but of minimal stability over the longer span from 3 to 14 years of age. Although conformity during the first three years predicted conformity for age 3 to 6 in boys, it was not highly related to conformity for ages 6 to 10 or 10 to 14. *Thus aggression to mother, behavioral disorganization, and conformity during the first three years of life were not sensitive indicators of analogous behaviors during the school years.*

Dominance

Dominance of peers was stable for both sexes over the span 3 to 14 years of age. Even the Period II to IV coefficient was moderately high ($r = .53$, $p < .01$; two tails). The stability of this variable parallels the stability of indirect aggression to peers, and these variables are highly correlated with each other (correlations in the nineties for Period II and in the eighties for Periods III and IV). Attempts to dominate, control, or verbally attack peers are not punished consistently and are usually effective in attaining power and leadership positions with peers. This combination of minimal or inconsistent punishment together with the secondary gains are likely to facilitate the stability of those classes of responses.

Competitiveness

As with dominance, a competitive attitude with peers was highly stable for Periods II, III, and IV. The boys' correlation for Period II to IV was omitted because of the small number of subjects. A competitive attitude facilitates the acquisition of peer-approved skills, and most of the parents and teachers in the sample regard competitiveness as a healthy orientation. The appearance of this disposition during the preschool years is prognostic of competitive behavior during the elementary and high school period.

In the previous chapter we described an analysis of the short-term stability of selected preschool behaviors for a group of 14 girls who were observed for two nursery-school sessions (about one year apart) during the period 3 to 6 years of age. The stability coefficients for three aggressive variables for this small group were as high or higher than those reported for this larger sample. The coefficients were .92 ($p < .001$) for physical aggression, .72 ($p < .01$) for dominance, and .65 ($p < .01$) for indirect aggression. This limited replication on an independent sample adds validity to the findings for the larger group.

AGGRESSIVE BEHAVIOR IN ADULTHOOD

The relation between child and adult aggression is expressed by the correlations between each of these seven longitudinal variables and the seven interview variables related to aggressive behavior, motivation, and conflict.

Interview Variable 15: Aggressive retaliation

This variable assessed the individual's tendency to retaliate with direct verbal aggression or blatant resistance when attacked, teased, frustrated, or restricted by the social environment. The open refusal to cooperate with the request of an employer and outburst of verbal aggression to a spouse, parent, friend, or stranger were the most frequent sources of evidence used in rating this variable. Occurrence of physical aggression in this group of middle-class adults was rare, and the rating necessarily reflected the frequency of verbal attacks or direct resistance to others. It is not difficult to assess this variable in an interview, but its theoretical significance is ambiguous.

The predisposition to aggressive behavior is influenced both by the ease with which anger is aroused and the degree of conflict and anxiety associated with such behavior. A low threshold for anger, coupled with high-aggression anxiety, might not always result in frequent display of aggressive behavior. Aggressive retaliation is most likely to occur when an individual has both a low threshold for anger arousal and low conflict over aggression. Table 2 presents the correlations between the longitudinal aggressive variables and the rating of retaliation.

In contrast to dependency, for which stability was more striking for women, the developmental consistency for aggression was noticeably greater for males. Aggression to mother, behavioral disorganization, and dominance for Periods III and IV predicted adult retaliation for the men but not for the women. The sex differences for the correlations between behavioral disorganization for Periods III or IV and adult retaliation were of borderline significance.

The following excerpts from the case material on Subject 2610 illustrate the association between low-frustration tolerance and aggressive outbursts during the school years and retaliatory tendencies in adulthood. At 7½ years of age the day-camp observer described this boy as:

"An impetuous, irresponsible child with lack of judgment and often purposely mean and malicious. He likes to bust up constructive activities of others with destructive and violent acts. He was noisy most of the time and, in any group, would disrupt its organization. He was rather infantile in these destructive activities. He cried easily, was easily frustrated, and would kick up a crying tantrum when he didn't get his way."

The mother felt that S was much too aggressive, and he was unpopular with his peers because of this behavior. On the other hand, she was somewhat fatalistic and remarked, "S is much like his father, nervous and a fighter. All the _____ are fighters."

After a visit to the Institute when S was 10 years old, the observer wrote:

"S came in with his customary whoop. He dashed cars across the bridge, knocking down portions of it, building it up again with much noise and thumping. During the course of the morning, he managed

TABLE 2. RELATION BETWEEN CHILDHOOD BEHAVIOR AND ADULT
AGGRESSIVE RETALIATION

Child Variable	Age	Males	Females	Total
Aggression to mother	0–3	.19	.11	.14
	3–6	.25	.00	.15
	6–10	.32*	.09	.24*
	10–14	.47**	.13	.31**
Physical aggression to peers	0–3	−.06	−.57**	−.27
	3–6	.15	−.51**	−.06
	6–10	.02	.23	.10
Indirect aggression to peers	0–3	.44	−.10	.11
	3–6	.30	.00	.16
	6–10	.27	.27	.26**
	10–14	.31	.15	.28*
Behavioral disorganization	0–3	.28	−.21	.03
	3–6	.12	.05	.13
	6–10	.37**	.03	.22*
	10–14	.51***	.09	.34**
Conformity	0–3	−.29	.01	−.15
	3–6	−.11	.05	−.04
	6–10	−.26	−.11	−.20*
	10–14	−.24	.02	−.13
Dominance	3–6	.30	−.10	.06
	6–10	.44***	.29*	.37***
	10–14	.48**	.17	.37**
Competitiveness	3–6	.17	−.37	−.11
	6–10	.33*	−.12	.11
	10–14	.34	−.24	.10

* $p < .10$; two tails
** $p < .05$; two tails
*** $p < .01$; two tails
**** $p < .001$; two tails

to demolish the bridge with much pleasure. He bombed the Tinker-
Toy parts, and, in all, his play was quite destructive. He painted several
muddy-brown pictures, one of a girl and one of three faces, Japanese,
German, and one unidentified, with bombs bursting around them,
torpedoes exploding, and a rather colorful battleship under full steam.
Later in the afternoon he raced around in the snow with Mary. He
evidently teased her, since she came in very indignantly. Left alone, S
amused himself by throwing snowballs at passing college students. . . ."

"At the Institute, S ransacked the house while he was looking for the underground railway passage that presumably had been under the house. He was uncontrolled and heedless of property or person in his play. He had to be coaxed to endure the test session, and this response seemed to be a hostile reaction to adult authority. His moods were changeable. Happy one minute, sullen the next, and these moods were rather unpredictable as to their occurrence."

An excerpt from a report of a visit to S's school when he was 10 years old was similar in tone.

"S clumped loudly whenever he walked and needled the teacher a great deal in annoying ways. Whenever she spoke to him for talking out loud, his reply was a blank stare and a 'What?' S was almost insolent in his manner to the teacher. During the spelling test he drew airplanes on the blackboard. He erased them at the teacher's request, but wrote his spelling downhill. The teacher reproved him, and he erased it and did the same thing all over again. He made flip remarks to the class and was generally a nuisance throughout the morning. S was rather smug and sarcastic. One girl sighed at the arithmetic test and said, 'It was very hard.' S replied, 'It's easy as pie, just use your brain—what brain?' During the visit he disturbed the whole room twice by noisy trips to the pencil sharpener in a defiant, sullen, cross, and cocky attitude."

At 11 years old, the following summary was written after an annual day-camp session.

"S's play was of a blustering, aggressive sort with little quiet persistence in it. He liked active games, easy activities with quick success, lots of noise and action. He appeared to like 'baiting' the adults; he liked daring authorities by a slim balance more than the actual end product. He liked to run wild in the yard and did this most of the time with an abandoned sort of violent physical effort. S has a loud voice, which he likes to throw around a lot. He loved strange and anal-sounding grunts and groans and sings at the top of his voice. He has no real group cooperative play. He showed off, clowned a lot, and initiated a lot of aggressive play with other boys."

During the adult interview, when S was 27, he indicated a low threshold for anger and frequent retaliations to personal attack.

E: "Can you remember the last time you were mildly irritated at anyone?"
S: "I get irritated at drivers everyday. I'm driving in traffic—there's usually some idiot that wants to pull out in front of you or something like that. I'm inclined to get too upset about things like that and be criticized for blowing-up like that."
E: "Do you tend to blow-up if somebody makes an error?"

S: "Yeh—I swear sometimes. Let's see, this morning or last night some character pulled out of the filling station right in the path of a gasoline truck,
and he came swerving over into my lane, wasn't very close, but I said a few
things under my breath. I get kinda excited about a lot of things. I blow
off a lot of steam verbally, and don't do much else—."

E: "What do you tend to do if you come home at night and your wife is
irritated with you?"

S: "Well—that depends on the mood I'm in. Sometimes I'll blow-up. Generally, I get too obnoxious and get to feeling guilty and try to smooth
things over."

E: "Is there any issue that tends to cause most friction between you and your
wife?"

S: "Nothing in particular; well, she criticizes my sloppy habits, like saying I
should hang up my coat or something."

E: "And what do you say to this?"

S: "Well, I don't remember exactly. I think I got angry the other night; it
wasn't so much. I mean I realize I should have hung my coat up; it was
the way she said it. I forget just how it was."

E: "What do you tend to do when someone insults you?"

S: "If somebody gets to insulting me, I insult them right back."

The failure of peer-directed aggression to predict retaliation in adult
men may be due, in part, to the fact that the verbal barbs, rough-
housing, wrestling, and fighting that occur among school-age boys
reflect attempts to practice behaviors that define the traditional male
role. The poking or shoving of a peer is just as often the acting out of
a fantasy in which the boy is a soldier or detective hero as it is the
expression of strong resentment. The forces determining aggressive
retaliation in adulthood are more closely linked to low-frustration
tolerance and low-aggression anxiety than to the need to maintain one's
sex-role identity. Thus, peer-directed aggression should be less predictive of adult aggressivity than behavioral disorganization or aggression
to mother. The latter responses are less appropriate behavioral supports for a masculine identification and, hence, more likely to be a
reflection of aggressive motivation.

For women, there was a negative relationship between peer aggression and adult behavior. The girls who were physically assaultive with
peers during the first six years were least likely to be retaliatory as
adults. Moreover, aggression to the mother and behavioral disorganization, which were prognostic of adult behavior for men, showed zero-
order correlations for the women.

The absence of stability for the females appears to be a result of
more intense aggressive conflict. Direct attacks on the mother, fighting,
and rage behavior violate the community's conception of a "well-

mannered young lady." These tendencies are more consistently punished in girls than in boys (Sears, Maccoby, and Levin, 1957). Moreover, the ego ideal of the typical adolescent girl is not likely to include explosive aggression as a desired attribute. A girl is apt to develop stronger inhibitions and more intense conflict over aggressive behavior than a boy during the preadolescent and adolescent years. The establishment of these inhibitions will dilute the continuity of this behavior from adolescence through adulthood.

In essence, the same argument that was used to rationalize the differential stability of dependency is called into service again to interpret the differential stability of aggression. The adults' performance on the tachistoscopic tasks supports the assumption of greater aggressive conflict for women. The four aggressive scenes illustrated aggression to peers and older adults. For three of the four scenes (a young adult in a belligerent posture toward an older man, a young adult striking at a peer, and a young adult choking a peer), the women produced more distortions and had higher recognition thresholds than the men ($p < .01$) and showed delayed recall of these scenes ($p < .05$). See Chapter Eight for details.

Moreover, the women who were rated as highly anxious over aggressive behavior, in contrast to those with low anxiety, had greater difficulty recognizing the scenes in which a woman was slapping at a peer or an older man ($p < .10$).

To illustrate, a woman who rarely expressed aggression as an adult and was docile and nonaggressive as a child had difficulty interpreting the scene of the woman shaking her finger at an older man. On the first exposure (0.01 second), she replied:

"The figure on the left is a male and the female is on the right; I don't know what they're doing."

On the second exposure (0.02 second), she reported:

"Male on the left and teenage female on the right; she's showing him something."

A second woman who showed low anxiety over the expression of aggression accurately described this scene on the first exposure.

"Woman on the right, man on the left; they were arguing. She was pointing her finger at him and laying down the law."

In sum, the tachistoscopic data supported the assumption that conflict over aggression was more pronounced in women than in men.

The negative relation between physical aggression during Period III and retaliation in adult women finds support in a longitudinal study (Sears, 1961). These investigators initially interviewed a large group of mothers of 5-year-old children and assessed, among other things, the child's overt aggressive tendencies. When these children were 12 years old, they were administered a set of scales designed to measure aggressive behavior and aggression anxiety. For 84 boys, severity of conscience at age 5 was positively related to aggression anxiety at age 12 ($r = .30$; $p < .01$). The corresponding relation for 76 girls was negative ($r = -.24$; $p < .05$). Similarly, the relation between overt aggressive behavior at age 5 and aggression anxiety at age 12 was positive for girls but negative for boys. Thus girls showed a shift in degree of aggressive conflict over this seven-year period.

These independent data are supportive of the hypothesis that preschool aggression in girls is met with more punishment than similar behavior in boys. This punishment leads to strong conflict over aggressive behavior in adolescence and adulthood and suggests why preschool aggression is not a good predictor of adolescent or adult aggression in females.

The patterns of intercorrelations among the child behaviors (see Appendix 32) indicate that aggressive behavior to peers during Periods II and III was highly correlated with a cluster of behaviors that are traditionally associated with masculinity (e.g., status striving, interest in mechanical activity and athletics, hyperkinesis, competitiveness, and dominance). Aggressive behavior with peers is one of a cluster of traits that is congruent with the culture's conception of masculine behavior. Most of the above behaviors were also associated with peer-directed physical aggression for girls (e.g., a nonpassive approach to frustration, masculine interests, nonconformity to parents, hyperkinesis, competitiveness, and dominance). These responses in girls are apt to meet with strong opposition from friends, teachers, and the wider social community. The resulting conflict is likely to produce inhibition of aggressive behavior in order to attenuate the anxiety over alienation from the social environment as well as a discrepancy between a girl's behavior and her schema of the ideal female personality.

Interview Variable 16: Ease of anger arousal

This variable was more inferential than the rating of retaliation. The interviewer evaluated the individual's threshold for anger, the ease with which mild frustrations led to irritability and anger. Ease of anger arousal did not take into account the frequency of overt aggression, and this variable might be regarded as an estimate of aggressive motivation. Table 3 contains the relevant correlations between childhood behavior and adult anger threshold.

TABLE 3. RELATION BETWEEN CHILDHOOD BEHAVIOR AND ADULT
ANGER AROUSAL

Child Variable	Age	Males	Females	Pooled
Aggression to mother	0–3	−.02	.19	.02
	3–6	.39**	.10	.27**
	6–10	.37**	.23	.32**
	10–14	.77****	.24	.51****
Physical aggression to peers	0–3	−.16	−.18	−.20
	3–6	.06	.02	.06
	6–10	−.03	.36*	.07
Indirect aggression to peers	0–3	.23	.11	.13
	3–6	.17	.24	.21
	6–10	.26	.45***	.35***
	10–14	.16	.24	.22
Behavioral disorganization	0–3	.35	.04	.20
	3–6	.30*	−.06	.12
	6–10	.42**	.12	.29**
	10–14	.52***	.08	.37***
Conformity	0–3	−.12	.05	−.05
	3–6	−.10	.05	−.03
	6–10	−.09	−.04	−.07
	10–14	−.26	−.08	−.19
Dominance	3–6	.10	.18	.15
	6–10	.25	.26	.25**
	10–14	.47**	.09	.35**
Competitiveness	3–6	−.25	.05	−.08
	6–10	.34*	.27	.30**
	10–14	.25	−.08	.12

* $p < .10$; two tails
** $p < .05$; two tails
*** $p < .01$; two tails
**** $p < .001$; two tails

The results are similar to those found for aggressive retaliation. *Aggression to mother and behavioral disorganization during ages 6 to 14 were highly related to adult anger arousal for men, but not for women.* The coefficients for the males were typically higher than those for the females; the sex differences for the correlations involving aggression to mother and disorganization for Period IV were statistically significant ($p < .05, < .10$, respectively).

It appears that the anger-arousal variable (Variable 16) was a more sensitive index of potential for adult aggression than the rating of retaliation (Variable 15). For example, childhood aggression to mother among boys showed a stronger relation with adult anger arousal than it did with adult retaliation. For girls, indirect aggression to peers during age 6 to 10 showed a significant association with adult anger arousal, but a minimal association with retaliation. Finally, for males, aggression to mother and behavioral disorganization *during the pre-school years* showed a significant association with anger arousal, but not with retaliation. Ease of anger arousal was apparently a more sensitive index of enduring aggressive predispositions than the rating of verbal retaliation to attack.

Subject 1650 provides one of the best illustrations of the relationship between maternal-directed aggression and behavioral disorganization during childhood, and a low threshold for anger in adult men.

At 3½ years of age, during a visit to the Institute for an examination, S had a rather extreme rage reaction.

"S sat on my lap and then left me. When I picked him up, he had an uncontrolled spell. I held him until he stopped and then laid him down. Later, when I tried to measure him, he woke up and screamed and started to hold his breath."

During the early school year S was unusually destructive, and in the nursery-school and day-camp setting he was irritable and violent. When S was 7 years old, a visit to the home yielded the following observation:

"The mother reported that there had been no recurrence of his breath-holding behavior lately. When S is particularly tired or thwarted, he will stiffen and say, 'I won't.' *This reaction is directed only to his mother.* His mother avoids telling him he must do things, thus staying within his tolerance."

"The mother is afraid that S will be unable to adjust to other people when he grows older unless he masters his temper. When he is thwarted, opposed, or annoyed in any way, his face grows white with anger."

During a visit to the home one year later, the observer noted:

"S was plowing several rows of cabbages and persisted at the task although it was very warm. After three quarters of an hour, he left his work to get a handful of sparrows from the barn. They had just been hatched. He threw them about, squeezed them unmercifully, stretched their necks, and generally tortured them. In the end, he finally left them to die on the ground."

When S was 9 years of age, the mother told the Fels interviewer that she was troubled by S's temper outbursts. The mother described situations in which S had a rage reaction when he is asked to do anything, regardless of the reasonableness of the request.

As a preadolescent S was interviewed at Fels and was noticeably resistant.

"S was rather uncommunicative during this interview. He simply says, 'He doesn't know' when you ask him questions about anything, and he is very noncommittal. I have the impression of a boy with a terrific need of inviolacy, a boy who seems to resent any intrusion into his life. It seems that he has a mental set against coming to the Institute because the Institute represents intrusion."

At 12 years of age, following a day-camp experience, the observer wrote:

"S is really good-looking; rather ruddy under his darkness, with a well-built frame. He has a hang-dog sort of growl and a sullen, glowering expression on his face. He makes a distinction between adults and other children. With other children he raced hard and displayed a rough-house quality of play with boys. He certainly did not seem to like adults or the things that adults suggested for him to do. On many tests there was open resentment and rebellion shown, and he would say, 'I can't do it. I can't do these things. Why do we have to do them?' S seems to have a grudge against the world."

As an adult, the inviolacy and suspicion noted during childhood were still apparent. During the interview and testing sessions, S was hostile, suspicious, and resistant. His answers were short, brief, and, at times, spoken with fury. He harbored strong feelings of hostility and derogation toward anyone with status or authority. At one point in the interview he stopped, looked directly at the interviewer, and with clenched jaw said, 'I only like common folk.' He was easily angered by any frustration, and he verbally attacked his wife, his child, his landlord, and strangers.

In the interview S was asked:

E: "When was the last time you were provoked?"
S: "It usually happens with the landlord, and I tell him what I think. I told him off and everything else. He is the kind of a guy, it's like water shedding off a duck's back."
E: "Let me name some circumstances that happen to most people. I would like to know what you would do in these situations. Suppose your wife has had a hard day and when you come home she is irritable with you. What would you do in that situation?"
S: "I'm . . . irritable too, just like she is. Why . . . you know, that's just one of those days."
E: "What are you like if your boy gets pesty with you?"

S: "He better leave me alone; he knows enough to leave me alone."
E: "What would you do if someone was rude to you?"
S: "I'd say what I think and that's it. If they don't like it, they don't have to."

Under direct questioning S said that he believed that hate and power strivings were basic qualities of human nature. He felt that if you were not tough and aggressive, "You would not get anyplace in this world."

As might be expected, he recognized the aggressive scenes early. On the second exposure of the illustration of two boys fighting, S reported:

"Fellow on the left, man on the right, he is going to poke him one."

To the picture of the man about to strike a woman, S replied:

"Woman on the left in her fifties, man on the right. He is going to hit her."

On the second exposure illustrating the man with fists clenched in front of an older man, S reported:

"Middle-aged man on the left, boy on the right; he is going to poke him one."

Interview Variable 14: Competitive behavior

Open retaliation, irritability, and low-anger thresholds often lead to social rejection and interpersonal friction. Competitiveness, on the other hand, is a socially more effective method of expressing hostility. Competitiveness is generally approved by both peers and adults; it leads to socially valued rewards, and it facilitates the development of selected skills. The aggressive element in competitive behavior resides in the implicit set to defeat another person; the attempt to overpower an adversary and to gain psychological superiority. The hostile intent in a competitive attitude is supported by clinical descriptions of capable people who repeatedly fail in academic or vocational situations. These individuals equate competitiveness with hostility and are troubled by the fact that in order to obtain a high grade or a desirable job assignment they must defeat a peer. The anxiety that accompanies this conflict can lead to inhibition of productivity.

Some of our subjects expressed the anxiety that is often associated with defeating a peer in a game. One talented and insightful young woman, who was in a highly competitive graduate program, withdrew from school because she became tense and uncomfortable in this intellectually aggressive setting. She recognized that in order to succeed she would also have to become intellectually aggressive with her peers. She felt that this competitiveness was incompatible with her concep-

tion of herself as nonaggressive and threatening to her sex-role identification. The anxiety over the aggressive component in intellectual competition was strong enough to drive her from a potentially productive
career.

Two of our subjects verbalized the conflict implicit in a competitive
situation. One young woman replied to the interviewer's query:

E: "Do you tend to play hard and try to win in various recreational games,
like tennis, for example?"
S: "Yes, I do think that the concentration and the effort—this is something
that I really put into it—I want to win. There are some instances in which
I want to win more than others—some I don't care about—but in some
instances I even feel uncomfortable winning. If a fellow had asked me to
play tennis and had never seen me play tennis before—then went out on
the courts and then he wasn't very good, I would feel uncomfortable by
beating him—I—ah—."
E: "You would sort of let up on him?"
S: "I'd tell myself not too—but I'd find that I would probably play on his
level—anyway—or the same with a close girl friend of mine—who—as—is
kind of unaware—."
E: "As to how good you are?"
S: "Yeh—in my tennis skills—and has asked me to play—I would feel uncomfortable being really aggressive and really beating her—ah—although
there are other instances in which the person I'm playing against is very
aggressive or is—in my estimation—not being fair—or—if somebody I
don't really care about has jokingly said that they are going to beat me,
this you know can tend to—."
E: "Make you more competitive?"
S: "Yes—and I think I would be more competitive in this situation."

The comments of one of the men also revealed a conflict over competitiveness.

E: "Do you try to win when you play ping-pong?"
S: "Depends on who I'm playing. Sometimes I just, when I'm not sure I'm
going to win, I don't try real hard."
E: "When you feel that a guy's too good for you?"
S: "Possibly too good for me, I'll just play along and make it a fair score,
but I. . . ."
E: "You don't try real hard?"
S: "Yeh—but even sometimes when I think I can beat him, even if he is real
good, I don't try real hard."
E: "Why not?"
S: "I don't know. I like to win. I feel pretty good. . . . I feel pretty proud of
myself when I win, you know. And when I know I can beat 'em, a lot of
times I'll play 'em later on and I'd let 'em beat me."
E: "Why do you think?"

S: "I'm not too sure though. I know some of them after they've . . . well, yeah, cause some of them, they beat me, you know and then all of a sudden I up and . . . stomp 'em; they don't like that at all, boy; they don't like that. They make some pretty rough comments about me—daggone, you know. And I guess I've construed it that they don't like me because I beat them that way."

In our population, athletics, related recreational skills, or intellectuality were the most frequent sources of competitive strivings among the men. Although there were a few women who chose physical skills as an arena for competitive gratifications, most of them viewed intellectual activity as the channel for their competitive energies.

Table 4 contains the correlations between childhood behavior and adult competitiveness.

For the men, the pattern of correlations differed somewhat from those found with aggressive retaliation and anger. *Both indirect and physical aggression to peers for age 6 to 10, in addition to aggression to mother and disorganization, showed a significant association with adult competitiveness.* It will be recalled that peer-directed aggression had negligible associations with adult retaliation or anger arousal. Similarly, conformity toward adults for Periods II, III, and IV was negatively associated with adult competitiveness, but minimally related to retaliation or anger threshold. Thus, when competitiveness was the adult criterion for men, childhood aggression with both peers and adults as well as behavioral disorganization were prognostic of this class of aggressive behaviors.

It was suggested earlier that peer aggression in boys was motivated in part by the need to practice behaviors that defined the male sex-role. Peer aggression failed to predict retaliation or anger arousal in adulthood because it may have been only tangentially related to aggressive motivation. A competitive attitude in adult men is part of the traditional masculine role prescription. In sum, we are assuming that some of our men were competitive because this behavior supported the idealized masculine conception they held for themselves and because it was a method of gratifying hostile feelings toward others. Adult competitiveness serves multiple motives, and it is not unreasonable to assume that both peer-directed aggression as well as behavioral disorganization would be associated with this predisposition.

For girls, the results were more equivocal. Aggression to mother during age 3 to 6 and disorganization during age 10 to 14 were negatively associated with adult competitiveness. The differences between the male and female correlations for these two variables were significant ($p < .01$). *However, competitiveness for age 6 to 10 predicted*

TABLE 4. RELATION BETWEEN CHILDHOOD BEHAVIOR AND ADULT
COMPET·ITIVENESS

Child Variable	Age	Males	Females	Pooled
Aggression to mother	0–3	.00	.08	.08
	3–6	.37**	−.57***	−.02
	6–10	.36**	−.09	.20
	10–14	.28	−.07	.20
Physical aggression to peers	0–3	.11	.02	.06
	3–6	.34	.29	.36**
	6–10	.46**	.08	.44***
Indirect aggression to peers	0–3	.31	.22	.26
	3–6	.56***	.18	.37***
	6–10	.51***	.07	.33***
	10–14	.45**	−.03	.39***
Behavioral disorganization	0–3	.13	.00	.08
	3–6	.11	.11	.18
	6–10	.34**	.15	.33***
	10–14	.59***	−.39**	.25*
Conformity	0–3	−.34	−.23	−.29**
	3–6	−.40**	.00	−.21*
	6–10	−.48***	−.09	−.37***
	10–14	−.54***	.15	−.33**
Dominance	3–6	.28	.01	.07
	6–10	.59****	.29*	.44****
	10–14	.36	.00	.30*
Competitiveness	3–6	.39	.14	.26
	6–10	.51***	.52***	.47****
	10–14	.39*	.08	.28*

  * $p < .10$; two tails
 ** $p < .05$; two tails
*** $p < .01$; two tails
**** $p < .001$; two tails

*adult competitive behavior ($r = .52$, $p < .01$). Unlike the boys, the
girls who were overtly aggressive with peers or mothers did not become competitive adults.*
   It will be recalled that behavioral disorganization and competitiveness in boys were stable from 3 to 14 years of age. For girls, only competitiveness showed continuity over this 11-year period. There seems
to be a differentiation of uncontrolled aggression from competitiveness
during the girls' childhood years. For boys, these two dimensions re-

main more closely associated, suggesting some degree of similarity in dynamics.

The intercorrelations among the various aggressive variables for Period III support this statement (see Appendix 32). For boys, competitiveness was highly related to aggression to mother, physical aggression to peers, behavioral disorganization, and nonconformity. For girls, competitiveness showed no significant associations with any of the above four variables.

Intellectuality was the major area of competitive activity in the adult women, and these competitive females came from homes where both parents were well educated. The correlations between educational level of mother and father and adult competition in women were .36 and .43 ($p < .05$). For males, the corresponding coefficients were only .13 and .19. Thus competitiveness in the adult woman was associated with a family atmosphere that valued intellectual superiority. It is possible that intellectual competitiveness in women is more a reflection of a need for intellectual mastery than a sensitive index of aggressive motivation.

Interview Variables 17 and 38: Aggressive conflict

In addition to estimates of aggressive predispositions, the interviewer attempted to assess anxiety over expression of aggressive behavior and the degree of repression imposed on angry thoughts and feelings. Two related variables were used. *Aggression anxiety* evaluated the person's reluctance to express overt aggression due to fear of disapproval, rejection, or guilt. The second variable, *repression of aggressive thoughts,* assessed the degree to which the subject was unaware of angry feelings or thoughts and denied these ideas, especially in situations where such motivation was appropriate. The individuals who were given a high rating on this variable rarely criticized anyone; they denied resentment or irritation toward other people, and they pushed from consciousness, awareness of aggressive motives. If these adults behaved aggressively, and occasionally they did, they were unaware of the hostile intent of their behavior. Table 5 presents the correlations between childhood behavior and adult anxiety and repression.

The pattern of correlations was similar for both variables. *Absence of aggression to mother and a high degree of conformity during age 6 to 10 were prognostic of adult aggression anxiety for both men and women. Behavioral disorganization during Periods III and IV was nega-*

TABLE 5. RELATION BETWEEN CHILDHOOD BEHAVIOR AND ADULT ANXIETY
AND CONFLICT OVER AGGRESSION

Child Variable	Age	Aggression Anxiety			Repression Aggression		
		Males	Females	Pooled	Males	Females	Pooled
Aggression							
to mother	0–3	.02	−.34	−.08	.22	−.12	.08
	3–6	−.12	−.02	−.08	−.05	−.04	−.05
	6–10	−.44***	−.42**	−.43****	−.41**	−.30	−.36***
	10–14	−.42**	−.36*	−.36**	−.56***	−.02	−.28**
Physical aggression							
to peers	0–3	.03	−.19	−.04	.11	−.44*	−.10
	3–6	−.21	−.19	−.18	−.01	−.40*	−.18
	6–10	−.13	−.22	−.14	−.14	−.20	−.17
Indirect aggression							
to peers	0–3	−.02	−.31	−.07	.16	−.43*	−.06
	3–6	−.17	−.17	−.17	.02	−.29	−.12
	6–10	−.22	−.29*	−.25**	−.18	−.17	−.17
	10–14	−.01	−.05	−.05	−.11	−.04	−.08
Behavioral disorganization	0–3	−.22	−.06	−.13	−.45**	−.09	−.27*
	3–6	−.12	−.02	−.08	−.17	−.02	−.11
	6–10	−.39**	−.18	−.27**	−.38**	−.13	−.26**
	10–14	−.34*	−.14	−.23*	−.54***	−.07	−.34**
Conformity	0–3	.08	−.02	.03	−.10	−.10	−.10
	3–6	.25	.16	.21*	.06	.06	.06
	6–10	.44***	.35**	.36***	.31*	.22	.26**
	10–14	.25	.11	.17	.20	−.02	.09
Dominance	3–6	−.30	.16	−.04	−.20	.00	−.08
	6–10	−.28	−.13	−.21*	−.23	−.04	−.14
	10–14	−.16	−.12	−.14	−.58***	−.27	−.42***
Competitiveness	3–6	−.10	−.04	−.07	.07	−.27	−.08
	6–10	−.33*	−.02	−.17	−.39***	−.14	−.29**
	10–14	−.01	.33	.12	−.32	.15	−.10

* $p < .10$; two tails
** $p < .05$; two tails
*** $p < .01$; two tails
**** $p < .001$; two tails

tively related to adult anxiety and repression, but only for the men.
Childhood aggression to peers showed no strong relationship with
aggression anxiety in adult men. We have argued previously that peer-
directed aggression in boys fulfills sex-role requirements and, therefore, is not as closely related to aggressive motivation as mother-
directed aggression or behavioral disorganization. The lack of relationship between childhood teasing and fighting in boys and later
aggression anxiety or motivation supports this argument. Moreover,
absence of competitive behavior in childhood was more closely associated with repression of aggression in adult men than in adult
women. This finding is congruent with the previous suggestion that
competitiveness is more closely linked with aggressive motives in men
than in women. For the men, an extremely competitive attitude seems
to require an acceptance of the hostile intent of competitive en-
deavors.

In summary, a conforming and nonaggressive attitude toward the
mother and other adults during the early school years is associated
with a repression of anger and an inhibition of aggression that remain
with the individual through adolescence and early adulthood.

Interview Variables 12 and 13: Criticism of parents

The previous variables have been concerned with aggressive behavior, motivation, or conflict. The final two interview variables in
this cluster were of a different character. They dealt with the adult's
criticism of his mother or father in response to the interviewer's direct
probes for this material. The tendency to criticize one's parents is not
necessarily related to overt aggression toward them. These variables
measured the degree to which the individual entertained conscious
attitudes of disappointment or resentment toward the values, behavior, or personality of his parents, and his willingness to disclose
this material. This rating should be regarded as a measure of conscious hostility toward the parent.

One of the primary reasons for including these variables was to
assess the relationship between childhood aggression toward the
mother and adult criticism of her. Psychotherapists often infer the
character of the early mother-child interaction from the patient's
adult attitudes, and it would be of interest to know if a critical attitude toward the mother is indeed a derivative of earlier aggression
toward her. Table 6 contains the correlations between childhood behavior and adult criticism of each of the parents.

TABLE 6. RELATION BETWEEN CHILDHOOD BEHAVIOR AND ADULT CRITICISM
OF PARENTS

Child Variable	Age	Criticism Father			Criticism Mother		
		Males	Females	Total	Males	Females	Total
Aggression to mother	0–3	−.19	.39*	.07	−.04	−.20	−.16
	3–6	−.01	.41**	.16	−.03	−.06	−.05
	6–10	.04	.06	.05	−.07	.20	.03
	10–14	.40*	.00	.18	.00	.01	−.03
Physical aggression to peers	0–3	.11	−.05	−.03	−.05	.26	.00
	3–6	.00	.03	−.01	−.29	.34	−.03
	6–10	−.14	.07	−.06	.01	.36*	.09
Indirect aggression to peers	0–3	−.10	.03	−.09	.00	.16	−.06
	3–6	−.01	.04	.01	−.22	.11	−.04
	6–10	−.30*	.13	−.08	−.04	.29	.10
	10–14	−.25	.11	−.07	.29	.15	.06
Behavioral disorgan- ization	0–3	.00	.41**	.21	.17	−.35*	−.10
	3–6	.12	.03	.05	−.01	−.10	−.09
	6–10	−.05	−.10	−.07	.13	.03	.03
	10–14	−.09	.11	.00	.11	−.31	−.08
Conformity	0–3	.05	−.12	−.02	−.28	.11	−.06
	3–6	−.01	−.12	−.06	.10	.00	.04
	6–10	.18	−.13	.01	.00	.08	.08
	10–14	−.14	−.04	−.08	.09	.00	.09
Dominance	3–6	−.08	.19	.09	−.23	.02	−.04
	6–10	−.27	−.05	−.15	−.03	.10	.03
	10–14	−.14	.16	.00	.37	.21	.19
Competitiveness	3–6	−.45	.10	−.11	−.41	.35	.07
	6–10	.10	.00	.05	−.03	.29	.13
	10–14	−.26	−.02	−.14	.31	.30	.25

* $p < .10$; two tails
** $p < .05$; two tails

There was no relationship between childhood aggression or conformity to the mother and criticism of her during the interview. Indeed, none of the childhood aggression variables showed a strong and
consistent association with criticism of either parent.

EVALUATIVE DISCUSSION

Aggressive behavior toward the mother and frequent episodes of behavioral disorganization in the 10-year-old boy were moderately good predictors of retaliatory behavior and ease of anger arousal in adult men. Although indirect aggression to peers was highly stable over the years 3 through 14, this class of behaviors was not prognostic of the more direct manifestations of adult aggression.

It was difficult to predict adult aggressive behavior or anger arousal for women from their childhood behavior. We have suggested that this is because young girls are subjected to more severe socialization of aggression than are boys. Excessive aggressivity in a school-age girl is gradually brought under control through the action of two sets of forces. The patterns of rewards and punishments issued by parents, teachers, and friends act in concert to suppress both open forms of aggression and angry feelings. The content of the culture's definition of the ideal female also influences the girl's fantasied conception of how she should behave. As a result of these processes (i.e., identification with nonaggressive models and direct punishment for hostility), a conflict is established. One effect of this conflict is the inhibition of aggression and attenuation of the long-term stability of this behavior.

One of the women in the sample provides a good example of the discontinuity between childhood and adult aggressive behavior.

Subject 121

S was aggressive and destructive as a child, but as adolescence approached, she began to suppress this behavior. As an adult there was a reluctance to display her hostile feelings or behavior because they violated the sex-role standards she established.

At 2 years of age S's nursery-school behavior was often punctuated with aggressive outbursts.

"S seldom talks or shows any outward sign of emotion. She is by far the most physically bold child, doing much jumping and climbing. She often reacts to other children destructively, pushing them down, pulling out hair, and absconding with toys."

At home her behavior was similar to that shown in the nursery school. The home observer wrote:

"S often treats her younger sister roughly, pinching and pushing her. The mother thinks it is more a matter of curiosity than of meanness or resentment of the baby's presence. S is the same way with other people, adults and children, attacking them and pushing them over, and then standing back to see the effect."

Two years later, at 4 years of age, S's nursery-school behavior was clearly competitive and aggressive.

"S was habitually aggressive, but she was not a successful leader. She was very competitive and seized every opportunity to equal or excel the feats of the other children. She liked to tease, and she had great sport with Mary and Peter, both of whom would yell or whine when she plagued them. Occasionally she played cooperatively with others, but more often she put herself in the role of a rival. S complied with adult requests at times, but at other times resisted with all her might. She needed to be reminded to take turns and to respect property rights. It was not because she did not know about these nursery-school principles, but rather because she could get such a rise out of other children by pushing in front of them or by snatching at their toys."

When S visited day camp at $6\frac{1}{2}$, the predisposition toward unprovoked aggression was still clearly present.

"S was somewhat shy and wary in social situations and made few social advances. She was almost eager in her response when others made advances to her. She seemed to expect that she might not be accepted and was surprised and pleased when other children were nice to her. S was very easy to have around when she was busy. Sometimes in free moments she went a little wild. The other children complained that she pushed them, knocked their sand constructions down, or poked her finger in their clay work. These outbursts were over in a flash. She needed no provocation other than idleness to start her off. She never made excuses for her behavior or even admitted anything about it. S was out for her own advancement and was sort of a lone wolf. She seemed to feel no deep identification with the group or with any of its members."

During the early school years S was independent, and verbally rebellious and attacking. She was competitive with peers and began to gain some peer respect because of her daring, verbal skills and athletic prowess. By age 10 a dramatic shift occurred in her behavior. She became interested in her attractiveness to boys, and this new motive was accompanied by a sharp decrease in overt aggression. At age 10 the day-camp observer wrote:

"There has been a good deal of change in S's appearance: straightened posture, hair washed clean with French braids, and frilly, nice clothes. The big thing seems to be the big shift in S herself. She no longer needs to express her hostility and alienation toward the world. She has the possibilities of becoming a very attractive little girl. Socially S has loosened up a great deal. Though no one in this group was congenial with her, she was much more outgoing than in previous years. At the races she got to the tomboy state, loudly boasting and jeering at one girl for being so awkward. *Most of the time she had a quiet, almost demure, air about her, listening to what others had to say and smiling in a friendly fashion."*

At 10½ S was interviewed at the Institute and reported a dream sequence that disclosed the essence of her conflict. She has a strong need for power over others, but wanted to retain a feminine identification. Thus blatant forms of aggression were replaced with more subtle methods. The psychologist's notes of the interview follow:

"S is having a number of dreams. They do not seem to be of the nightmare variety, but are obsessional, and she wakes up with a heavy sense of despondency. Last night she had a wish-fulfillment dream in which she was so beautiful that every man fell immediately in love with her and she could have whatever she wanted. The emphasis in the dream seemed to be on the sense of power that this physical attractiveness gave her. A policeman tried to arrest her, and she seduced him into letting her go. She went up to the store with expensive goods and got the manager to give them to her. As S related this dream, she began acting it out, half laughing at herself as she did so."

"Later in the talk, as we got on to S's plans for the future, she said, 'I'd like to be a housewife and a pianist.' Asked what she would do if she were a man, she said, 'She would still play piano and have kids,' and then she suddenly burst out with the wish that she were a boy. Men have so much more fun, they play soccer and baseball, and do not have to be dainty. S hates daintiness, high heels, and having to daintily trip-along. If she were a boy, she could have her hair cut in a crew-cut, never have to bother about it. She says her younger sister also wishes she were a boy and that her mother puts no pressure on them to be dainty. *It is just the outside world that does.* Her mother doesn't care about appearances at all herself, and as a girl, she was one of the best fighters in the neighborhood.

The perception of a cultural pressure to adopt traditional feminine traits is clearly verbalized by this insightful girl. We have repeatedly referred to this process in order to explain many of our results. The cultural prescription of sex-appropriate behaviors forms a limiting wall that the child finds difficult to scale. These cultural rules set definite limits on the external form of every child's overt behavior pattern.

By 12½ years this girl had adopted more completely the traditional feminine-role behaviors. The home visitor wrote:

"S has passed conspicuously into adolescence. Since the last time I saw her, her breasts have developed noticeably, and she has a very pretty figure and is becoming quite attractive. The mother told me privately that S had bought a new bathing suit, a one-piece affair, and when she tried it on for the family, her older brother gave a long, low whistle, which embarrassed her terribly. Mother shows considerable interest in S's appearance and in helping her to become attractive. She mentioned today that before school starts, she plans to take S to a hair stylist for a special cut. She also remarked that S says she wants to grow up and marry and have children, 'so that's what we're getting ready for'."

S did very well academically in high school and college and decided to go to graduate school. On first impression S appeared quiet, reserved, and neither competitive nor aggressive. She became conflicted over an intellectual career because the required competition in graduate school threatened the self-image she was trying so hard to retain. She was sufficiently insecure about her conception of herself as a woman that intense involvement in an intellectually aggressive atmosphere made her uncomfortable. During the adult interview she tried to explain why she withdrew from graduate school.

S: "I have the feeling that if you're going to do something so weird and peculiar, you at least have to feel thoroughly right about it."
E: "And you didn't feel right about it?"
S: "No. Everything didn't quite fit somehow. I mean, a woman who really has a good motivation in her field and—and is also secure in her own values and relationships, feels pretty much at home there (in graduate school) I think."
E: "What kind of woman do you feel would have felt secure in that situation?"
S: "What kind of woman would have?"
E: "Yes."
S: "Well, like there were one or two people there, they had either a real— well, one of them worked and she knew that—ah—that she wanted to be an engineer, and she wanted a degree, and she was very happily married. I had the feeling she—felt secure in her personal life, and secure in what she was doing, and she was pretty. She knew that there were discriminations against her. She didn't have the feeling 'Do I really belong here,' and that kind of thing."
E: "But you did have these thoughts?"
S: "You're never—it was sort of a lonely position, in a way, because—you can't go with them—I mean, men are more groupy and women are more groupy, and it's sort of hard for one woman to be a part of a men's group.

You know, eating lunch together and that kind of thing. They were very—the guys were nice. They were understanding and friendly, by and large, but I never quite felt as though you really were a part of things, such as in a really mixed group."

E: "So, in part, you felt that this was primarily a masculine situation, and this was a threat to your concept of yourself as a woman?"

S: "Yes, I think so, 'Are you really a woman or are you a man' type?"

E: "That could have been involved then?"

S: "Yes. I think it was. Quite definitely. The feeling of not—of wanting to establish myself as a person rather than—if you realized that the pressure was going to be like that, you could go to a school, at least, like—well, the University of _____, which I think has more fraternities and sororities. But when you don't even take that into consideration as a factor, well, then you're stuck with it. There you are—and it hits you."

E: "You had no idea this would happen?"

S: "No. Most people don't though. They say, 'Oh, boy—what fun! All those men! It doesn't work that way. It is nice in a way; it's just not enough."

When the interviewer asked about S's reaction to frustrating situations, she indicated a reluctance to retaliate, even though she might have felt angry.

E: "When you are annoyed, what do you do?"

S: "What do I do? Nothing. Just keep a straight face. One time I was so concentrated on controlling myself that I could hardly move. The girl said, 'Do you have a stiff neck?' I was just so rigid. When I'm annoyed, it's usually not what they're doing that I'm annoyed at as much as the position it puts me in. If someone does something, and I'm mad, that is, completely at cross-purposes with what I happen to want to do in the situation, it doesn't annoy me unless it throws me out of kilter. I always figure rather than get annoyed and start that whole thing up, so that they realize I'm annoyed, I might as well do what I have to do to make what I want out of the situation, so I won't be annoyed anymore."

E: "You're only annoyed when the behavior of another person, in some way, interferes with what you want to do?"

S: "Interferes and when I can't—umm—when I haven't made peace with that interference somehow, you know. It doesn't matter if it interferes, you know, if I want to plan something, and somebody comes in and says, 'Will you do something else,' or if I—you know, I think, 'Well, that's my job.' You know."

E: "Besides your boss, who else, as you think of it, is more apt to annoy you and irritate you by the things they do?"

S: "My boss and the two people that give me work—that I'm not sure is necessary, sometimes."

E: "Are these men or women?"

S: "One of them is a woman and one is a man. I get annoyed sometimes—

let's see—there's one guy that, whenever I go anywhere and he's there, he's sort of a nice guy, but he really does annoy me. He's just sort of a hang-dog type of guy. And, gee whiz, I guess it's because, to a certain extent I react against it because—being lonely, you know, not having a decent relationship built, it's a temptation to sort of take him up on the implied offer. I suppose it's partly rationale that I don't just sort of move away and forget it, you know."

E: "In general, when at the moment you are deeply angry at someone, a friend, boy or girl friend, are you more likely to express it verbally at the time or not say anything?"

S: "Do nothing."

E: "Not say anything? Because you don't want to alienate them?"

S: "Yes, I suppose that's it. I don't know why I don't. The only person that I've ever gotten in the hang of really expressing what I felt was my roommate last year. She was brilliant, temperamental, and a strong-minded person and I finally—we would just flare up at each other—just because it was so murderous not to. With her I would get so mad that I just couldn't—just go off and cool down. I'd stay mad at her."

E: "What kind of thing did she do?"

S: "Oh, the precipitating things were—were not very simple, I suppose. We had different ways of life. She had no concern with neatness and order at all. I didn't mind our room, I didn't mind doing her laundry, I didn't mind emptying the trash all the time—most of the time. But sometimes, you know, it's her turn to wash the dishes, and two days later, they're still not washed, you get mad. I don't think that would have bothered me if we had had a basic understanding, but I guess—umm—there was some antagonism between us that I've never really pinned down. Partly, I guess, on my part. I realized this fall when I was listening to some music that we used to play last year and the feeling came back to me, all of a sudden, of this enviousness of her freedom. She would do what she felt like doing. All the time she was buying the food that she felt like eating. It didn't matter how expensive. She could afford it. She was on a Woodrow-Wilson scholarship, which helped. She would study till all hours and sleep till all hours. Her room was in a constant chaos—piles of books. And it just hit me then—how I envied her—her freedom."

E: "Would you say, in general, that you are easily irritated or not?"

S: "I would say sort of medium."

E: "Medium?"

S: "Yes."

E: "When you're in an argument with someone and they start getting very excited and there is a note of anger present, are you apt to persist in your argument or not?"

S: "I like to try to get out of it, I guess. Because I can get involved too. And I know that when I do that, the first thing it indicates is how insecure I feel about what I'm saying. The only time I used to really get into this was when I went with a certain guy last year. The feeling that he was just as right as I was was what really threw me for a loop or that I had nothing to take hold of to say why I felt the way I did. *So, in general, I just try to back out of it if people get me angry or if I think I'm going to get angry."*

S's preference for withdrawal from situations where she might be tempted into aggression was in sharp contrast to the destruction and aggression that characterized her childhood behavior.

Suppression of aggression in order to maintain a feminine sex-role identification was probably one of the major reasons for the minimal continuity of overt aggression in the present sample of women.

Educational level of family and aggressive behavior

Aggressive behavior in boys during the childhood years showed no consistent relation to the educational level of either parent. However, the girls with well-educated parents were more verbally aggressive with peers and less conforming with adults during age 10 to 14 than girls from poorly educated families. The better educated parents were more tolerant of deviation from sex-role standards and, therefore, of aggressive behavior in their daughters. Table 7 presents the correlations between educational level and the seven adult interview variables.

TABLE 7. RELATION BETWEEN EDUCATIONAL LEVEL OF PARENTS AND ADULT AGGRESSIVE BEHAVIOR

Adult Variable	Men		Women	
	Father	Mother	Father	Mother
Retaliation	−.03	−.14	−.17	−.16
Anger arousal	−.06	−.13	.05	−.02
Competitiveness	.19	.13	.43***	.36**
Anxiety	.33**	.26	.07	.13
Repression	.17	.12	.04	.11
Criticism of Father	−.34**	−.32**	−.08	−.12
Criticism of Mother	.10	.02	.26	.06

** $p < .05$; two tails
*** $p < .01$; two tails

The adult women who were competitive came from well-educated families, whereas competition in men was not a function of parental social class. There was no relationship between parental education and either aggressive retaliation or anger arousal.

Culture, constitution, and aggression

The data summarized in this and the preceding chapter indicate that aggressive behavior showed greater stability for men, while dependency showed greater stability for women. These are the facts. Several interpretations suggest themselves. We have stressed the role of differential conflict as the result of the culture's definition of appropriate sex-role behaviors. The tachistoscopic data support this interpretation. Developmental continuity for aggression or dependency appears to be facilitated by congruence with the cultural prescription for sex-appropriate traits. However, these findings can be used as grist for those who wish to assume constitutional determinants for these response tendencies. Males of all ages have a higher proportion of muscle tissue than girls (Garn, 1957; Garn, 1958), and some recent data tentatively suggest that infant girls may have greater pain sensitivity than infant boys (Lipsitt and Levy, 1959). Finally, aggressive and destructive play in very young children is typically much more frequent among boys than among girls, and Harlow (1962) has found that infant-male macaques show more threatening behavior in the face of attack than infant-female macaques. The early emergence of these sex differences (in monkey and man) tempts one to speculate on the possible relevance of constitutional factors for passive and aggressive behavior dispositions. It is possible that the differential stability of dependency and aggression for males and females is the product of a complex interaction in which constitutional variables find support in the behavioral rules promoted by the child's culture.

CHAPTER FIVE

Stability of Behavior: III
Achievement and Recognition

The previous two chapters have dealt with behaviors that are moderately conflictful. Conflict over passivity, dependency, and aggression is learned during the first 10 years, and if the conflict is strong, major changes can occur in the behavioral expression of these motives. These conflict-induced changes reduce the stability of overt manifestation of these behaviors.

Achievement and recognition behaviors, on the other hand, are socially valued responses for both boys and girls. These behaviors are not subject to differential sex-role standards in most middle-class families and, therefore, do not elicit the anxiety that is associated with practice of the socially censored acts of passivity and dependency by boys and aggression by girls. Although failure to achieve can be a source of anxiety, striving for gratification of these motives among our middle-class children gained general support from the social milieu. It might be anticipated, therefore, that the stability of achievement and recognition behavior would be generally high for both males and females, in contrast to the pattern found for the previous two response clusters. This expectation was verified in the data to be presented.

Achievement and recognition are considered together because the overt behaviors that gratify these motives overlap to a large degree. Achievement is defined, after McClelland et al. (1953), as behavior aimed at satisfaction of an internal standard of excellence. The goal of achievement behavior is self-approval for performing tasks at a level of competence that an individual had previously established as satisfying. In recognition behavior, the goal is some positive reaction from other people—a social acknowledgment of the individual's skills. For the present sample, the areas of competence that were most highly prized were intellectual, athletic, mechanical, and artistic abilities. Although competence in these areas brought feelings of self-satisfaction, acquisition of these skills also resulted in social recognition. Family, peers, and teachers awarded praise and prizes for academic, athletic, or artistic achievements. Hence it is extremely difficult to differentiate achievement and recognition motives. Involvement in school work or long hours of baseball practice can indicate strong achievement or recognition motives, or both. The data to be presented reveal a high, positive correlation between these two variables. This could mean either that our methods were not sufficiently sensitive to separate these two motives or that it is impossible to measure the desire to improve at a skill, independent of the person's desire for social recognition for this improvement.

The achievement cluster included nine variables rated for all or part of the four longitudinal periods. As noted earlier, HM had no knowledge of the child's intelligence test scores when he made the ratings. The achievement variables are briefly defined below.

Variable 25: General achievement—mastery behavior

This variable was rated for Periods I, II, and III and was a global assessment of achievement-oriented behavior without differentiating the specific content of the behavior. The rating was based on the child's persistence with challenging tasks, games, and problems and his involvement in activities in which a standard of excellence was applicable. For Period I, emphasis was given to persistence with perceptual motor activities (e.g., building block towers, stringing beads, coloring, and drawing). For Periods II and III, the greatest weight was given to interest in and persistence with intellectual, mechanical, and athletic activities.

For Period IV, achievement behavior was rated for three more delimited areas: intellectual, mechanical, and athletic tasks.

Variable 98: Intellectual achievement

This variable evaluated the child's attempt to master language and numerical skills, his motivation to perform well in the school situation, his involvement in knowledge acquisition, amount of time spent in reading, and interest in scientific projects.

Variable 99: Mechanical achievement

This variable assessed the child's attempts to master mechanical skills, for example, carpentry, mechanical toys, motors, and arts and crafts.

Variable 100: Athletic achievement

This variable assessed the degree to which the child showed involvement in physical skills and the time spent in athletic activities.

Variable 19: Recognition behavior

This variable, rated for Periods III and IV, evaluated the child's desire for status goals and social recognition and the intensity of his behavioral efforts to obtain these goals. The common goals sought included: academic recognition, leadership positions with peers, athletic honors.

Variable 83: Competitiveness

This variable, assessed for Periods II through IV, was defined in Chapter Four. It evaluated the degree to which the child competed with peers for superiority on any task. Major areas of competition were the school situation and athletics.

The six variables described above deal with behaviors directed at attainment of achievement or recognition goals. However, fear of failure is intimately associated with achievement behavior. If the child anticipates failure in a task situation, he may withdraw from the task even though his motivation is high. The following three variables deal with fear of failure and withdrawal from task situations.

Variable 88: Expectancy of task failure

This variable was rated for Periods III and IV and assessed the degree to which the child anticipated failure in challenging task situations. Evidence included statements of inadequacy to parents and interviewer and signs of avoidance of achievement-related situations.

Variable 84: General withdrawal

This variable was rated for Periods II and III and assessed the degree to which the child avoided situations in which he anticipated task failure or social rejection.

Variable 101: Withdrawal from task situations

This variable was rated only for Period IV and dealt with withdrawal from task situations in which the child anticipated failure.

STABILITY OF LONGITUDINAL VARIABLES

Table 1 presents the stability coefficients for these nine variables.

Variable 25: Achievement behavior

Involvement in task mastery during Period II was associated with mastery during Period III and with high levels of intellectual achievement behavior during age 10 to 14 for both sexes. The correlations with Period IV mechanical achievement were lower, and concern with athletic prowess among boys age 10 to 14 was *negatively* associated with early achievement behavior. The stability coefficients for Periods III to IV or II to III were generally higher than comparable coefficients obtained for dependency and aggression.

Achievement behavior during the first three years was unrelated to mastery behavior for Periods II, III, or IV. Indeed, the Period I rating showed a slight negative relationship with subsequent mastery. This finding has some important implications.

The behavioral evidence used in making the Period I rating differed from that used to assess mastery for the older age periods. Since the 2-year-old child did not initiate complex intellectual, mechanical, or athletic strivings, persistence with simple perceptual motor tasks (stringing beads, coloring, building towers) seemed a plausible basis for an early rating of mastery. However, these behaviors can also be viewed as reflecting a high threshold for satiation with simple stimulus materials. Achievement behavior at the older ages involved symbolic problem-solving activities that were more similar in form to adult mastery behavior. It could be argued, therefore, that mastery during Period I reflected a dynamically different process than achievement strivings during the school years.

The data suggest that persistence with sensory motor tasks is not predictive of future achievement strivings. The 2-year-old boy who patiently builds block towers, strings beads on a shoelace, or sits for 30 minutes sticking pegs into holes is neither the third grade's scholar nor the eighth grade's creative scientist.

After the fact, it is reasonable to assume that perseverative manipulation of simple objects is not a necessary precursor of intellectual curiosity or mastery motivation with symbolic material. Kounin (1941) has suggested that brighter children satiate more rapidly on simple

TABLE 1. STABILITY OF ACHIEVEMENT AND RECOGNITION BEHAVIOR FOR CHILDHOOD PERIODS I TO IV

Variable	I–II	I–III	I–IV	II–III	II–IV	III–IV
25. Achievement behavior						
Boy	−.28	.06		.27*		
Girl	−.14	−.07		.56****		
Total	−.20	−.03		.45****		
25–98. Intellectual achievement						
Boy			−.19		.39*	.81****
Girl			−.18		.68****	.76****
Total			−.19		.54****	.78****
25–99. Mechanical achievement						
Boy			−.16		.23	.40**
Girl			−.40		.49**	.45**
Total			−.01		.21	.27**
25–100. Athletic achievement						
Boy			.27		−.41*	−.26
Girl			.15		.16	.30*
Total			.25		−.16	−.02
19. Recognition behavior						
Boy						.77****
Girl						.47****
Total						.61****
83. Competitiveness						
Boy				.61**		.75****
Girl				.61***	.73***	.64***
Total				.61****		.67****
88. Expectancy of failure						
Boy						.58***
Girl						.66****
Total						.70***
84. Withdrawal						
Boy				.56***		
Girl				.09		
Total				.30**		

TABLE 1. (CONTINUED)

Variable	I–II	I–III	I–IV	II–III	II–IV	III–IV
84–101. Withdrawal tasks						
Boy					−.41	−.06
Girl					−.16	.56***
Total					−.19	.22

* $p < .10$; two tails
** $p < .05$; two tails
*** $p < .01$; two tails
**** $p < .001$; two tails

sensory motor tasks. Furthermore, infant intelligence scales, which mainly tap sensory motor development, are poorly related to intelligence and achievement test results obtained during the school years.

The hypothesis that Period I mastery is qualitatively different from later achievement gains support from the negative correlation between the Period I mastery rating and Stanford-Binet IQ at age 6 ($r = −.34$ and $−.11$ for boys and girls, respectively). The correlations between Period II mastery and child's IQ at age 6 jumped to $+.53$ and $+.80$ for boys and girls ($p < .01$). The dramatic difference between these pairs of correlations, together with the assumption that the Stanford-Binet score measures level of conceptual development, indicate the independence of early persistence in sensory motor coordinations from the mastery of academic skills.

In describing the course of intellectual development, Piaget differentiates two major eras of mental functioning: the sensory motor and conceptual stages (Piaget, 1952). The former covers the first two years of life and involves the acquisition of basic perceptual motor coordinations. Symbolic activity is minimal during this time. Conceptual thought is characterized by the use of language, symbols, and imagery in the child's intellective adaptation to his environment. Piaget's distinction between sensory motor and conceptual processes is somewhat analogous to the differences between Period I and Period II mastery behaviors.

There is no theoretical scaffold to support a hypothesis of continuity between the desire to spend a long period of time piling blocks into high towers and the motivation to acquire language and numerical skills. Some psychologists and many parents have implicitly assumed this association because it is intuitively more appealing to postulate continuity rather than discontinuity in mental functioning.

Longitudinal observations on two boys provide a dramatic illustration of the discontinuity between early persistence with simple materials and mastery behavior during the school years.

Subject 2313

S was a highly motivated and excellent student in elementary and high school. He received a scholarship to college, graduated valedictorian of his college class, and won a competitive fellowship to graduate school. When interviewed as an adult, he expressed a strong motivation for achievement and recognition, and he looked forward with confidence to an intellectually creative career.

However, at age 2½ S was distractible and gave no clue to his future achievements.

"S spent an unhappy first week at nursery school. He cried a great deal and looked ready to cry even when he was not actually doing it. He drew away when other children approached him as if he were afraid of them. He required much adult attention to get him to do anything. He stood around, did nothing, and looked rather lost. After the first week, he became happier and played primitively in the sand out-of-doors. He did some climbing on ladders and slid alone. *In the room, his activity was not constructive. He did a lot of wandering from room to room, and he liked to throw things: balls, colored cubes, or tin dishes.* He watched the other children a great deal, identifying himself with the play of others by laughing when they did. Despite S's lively coloring he was not a lively, dramatic child. In fact, the teachers remarked that when they were tallying up the children to see who was there, they were always most likely to forget S's presence."

Let us contrast this summary at 2½ with a nursery-school report three years later, at 5½ years of age.

"S was one of the most adult-centered children in the group. The particular quality of his relationship is hard to describe. It was on a very verbal level. He came to tell you things, show you things, act things out, and explain things. S has a very active play life. There was a constant stream of verbal descriptions, and an observer would know every minute of the time what S was doing, what technique he was using, and why he was doing it. *S seemed to have a very strong calvinist sense of needing to get things done and not wasting time.* He would say, 'In a few minutes I will be through with this.' Although he was still ineffectual in holding on to things, he had really become more skilled."

"By choosing the less coveted objects and getting into an obscure corner in which to work, he had a chance of carrying his projects through. S seemed really happy just to be making things. There was a great emphasis on the detail without an over-all pattern. The Christmas tree gave him a very good goal to work toward, and he did more than his share of hanging materials. At the end of the session S was one of the most jubilant in wrapping up his booty to take home."

"In his scrutiny of the books and the retelling of the stories there was an emphasis on every tiny detail; every part coming in its right sequence. S often asked questions to find out where parts fit in; how this different world of nursery school was supposed to run; what peoples' ideas about things were. Once told, he would store the knowledge away for the future. S was a great storyteller; long lectures on how things worked and on events at home. S's exceedingly high standards and an inability to relate to the world are his most salient features."

At 16½ years of age he was interviewed at the Institute.

E: "Would you tell me some of the things you are interested in?"
S: "Oh—my grade standards, various forms of amateur scientific research— I like to play around with. Like down at school, every once in a while I read about something interesting that someone has done, and if facilities permit, I like to try it out."
E: "Anything else you are interested in?"
S: "Well—I read a good bit—my main format of reading is in the science fiction class. I kind of enjoy learning. Of course, I may be rather conceited, but I don't think, except in a few classes, I actually learn anything. However, it excites my interest toward discovering things for myself."
E: "Are grades important to you?"
S: "Oh, I like to have them—I figure I should get along with a B just as well as an A, but then I don't have to work much harder to get an A, so I might as well have it."

This developmental sequence contrasts sharply with the pattern shown by Subject 2253. At 2½ years of age S appeared highly motivated to master simple skills.

"S was mild and quiet on his entering day at nursery school. He interested himself in playing with beads and remained relatively mild during the whole day. He learned to stick up for his rights. S was one of the busiest and most tenacious children in the group. His attention span was long for a child of his age. Sometimes he changed play equipment only twice in an hour. Outside he played on the slide and in the sandbox. He rode a small tricycle very well. He was tense whenever he was faced with learning a new physical stunt like climbing or jumping from a board but gained confidence rapidly and performed very creditably. Inside the room, he was interested in all kinds of equipment. He played with clay for long periods of time, used beads, pounding boards, and the small cars. He built better things and built much more often than the other children. He understood well what adults asked of him and usually cooperated nicely. He learned to feed himself better and ate more food and more varieties of food than the other children."

At 3 years of age he was still mastery oriented.

"S liked to ride bicycles and he spent most of his time in that activity. In the house, he proved to be an excellent builder. He used to make roofed garages and train sheds and run the cars and trains in and out of them. He liked to play with clay a lot. He was silent and talked neither to adults nor to children. He defended his property rights vigorously and physically. He did not seem to be enthusiastic nor particularly happy about being in nursery school but found the toys interesting and was busy doing something all the time. He was usually intent on his work and not distractible."

However, by 5½ years of age the persistence and mastery present at age 3 had disappeared.

"S's continued lack of speech isolated him from successful social contacts and skewed his behavior toward the physical, emotional side. During the first few days S refused to speak at all; during the last sessions he broke out into a few impulsive words when excited. He speaks rapidly and almost undistinguishably in a high, thin voice. S held to his sphinxlike silence under very trying circumstances. S whizzed about hard and fast on a bicycle and tried all the apparatus with no apprehension. He was wiry and strong and could fight scrappily. *Indoors his play was functional and quite simple.* He liked to construct with blocks and pushed trains over the floor in low-order play. *In general, he did little that was original or creative.* He did not paint; his play work was primitive and simple; his ideas were not well developed nor of long duration. He did catch on well to what others were doing, and when he was given a social role, he carried it out satisfactorily. He gave no overt evidence of fantasy play, and it was impossible to say what he was thinking." Most of S's attention and effort were centered on the other children. He was apprehensive and shy. Most of the time he would get some toy, do some simple manipulations of it, and keep an eye out for others."

At 6 years of age S was observed in his public-school setting.

"S was one of the most restless children in the group, playing with string and giggling. He kept his eye out for the teacher but felt no compulsion to study. On a test of reading, S scored the lowest of all the children in the group. His voice was weak, and his attention wandered a good deal. Throughout the morning he gave very little attention to the business at hand and was immature with his classmates. He picked his nose a great deal, watched the others, and did a lot of whispering. He seemed to have no idea of working alone. On the playground he was a nuisance, calling attention to himself in socially undesirable ways."

During high school S did poorly in academic subjects and was involved neither in athletics nor in extracurricular activities. As an adult S was working as an unskilled laborer in a metal shop. He was dependent on his family and showed little concern with task mastery in any area. His only interests were in driving his car and watching stock-car races.

This pair of admittedly extreme cases clearly illustrates the discontinuity between persistence with simple motor tasks during the first three years and mastery motivation in late childhood and adolescence.

Variable 98: Intellectual achievement for Period IV

The ratings for Periods II and III were weighted with intellectual activities because this area of competence was highly valued by most of the parents of these children. Thus achievement during ages 3 to 10 was most highly related to intellectual, rather than athletic or mechanical, achievement during ages 10 to 14.

The correlation between Period II achievement and intellectual mastery during ages 10 to 14 was higher for girls than for boys, suggesting that stable intellectual strivings may emerge earlier in the girl than in the boy.

The correlation between Period III achievement and Period IV athletic achievement was significantly higher for females than for males ($p < .05$). Recognition-seeking behavior showed considerable stability over the years 6 through 14, and the coefficient for the males was higher than that found for the females ($p < .05$).

Variable 83: Competitiveness

Competitive behavior was related to both achievement and aggressive motives, for it involved *striving for excellence* in order to *defeat* a peer. The main arenas for competitiveness were the school and playgrounds, since academic and athletic activities invite the development of competitive attitudes. As noted in the previous chapter, this response was moderately stable during childhood.

Variables 88, 84, 101: Expectancy of failure and withdrawal

Fear of failure showed remarkable consistency over the years 6 through 14. The pooled correlation of +.70 was one of the highest coefficients in this series. However, *withdrawal* from potential failure situations over this same age interval was only stable for girls. This sex difference could be related to our often repeated assumption of greater conflict over withdrawal behavior in the boy. The young male adolescent was more likely to attempt mastery of tasks despite the possibility of failure, whereas the adolescent girl who was anxious over failure was more likely to withdraw. During the years 6 to 10 many boys learn to resist the temptation to withdraw from difficult problem situations. The shift from a phobic to a counterphobic attitude during this time would decrease the stability of this defensive maneuver.

ACHIEVEMENT AND RECOGNITION BEHAVIOR IN ADULTHOOD

The relevant adult interview variables were achievement and recognition behavior, competitiveness, expectancy of failure, and predisposition to withdraw from potential failure situations.

Variable 19: Achievement behavior

The interviewer attempted to assess behavioral strivings for task mastery as well as the subject's desire for competence in various skill areas (i.e., achievement motivation). In evaluating achievement motivation, the rater attempted to infer the individual's desire for task mastery apart from his behavioral efforts. The subject who appeared to have strong needs for mastery, but limited opportunity for gratification or a crippling fear of failure, received a higher rating on the motive than on the behavioral variable. These two variables were highly correlated ($r = .98$), and the size and pattern of the correlations with the childhood variables were very similar. For this reason we shall only consider the overt behavioral variable.

The lack of independence for the ratings of achievement behavior and motivation suggests two conclusions. It is possible that achievement motivation and behavior are, in fact, highly correlated, that is, individuals with strong needs for mastery usually engage in achievement activities. It is more reasonable to assume that the interview is ill-suited to assess motive strength when expression of the motive has been suppressed or repressed. Individuals who have a strong need for mastery, but feel that their achievement efforts will end in failure, are apt to inhibit overt goal strivings and deny concern with these goals.

Intellectual competence and knowledge of the environment were the skills most highly valued by this sample. The interviewer approached this section of the interview schedule with an expectation of social-class differences in attitude toward intellectuality. However, almost all of the adult subjects, regardless of educational level, were concerned with this area of mastery. Intellectual power and education were typically regarded as highly desirable goals. The achievement ratings, therefore, were weighted rather heavily with this area of functioning. For the men, mechanical skills and concern with quality of vocational performance were also primary areas of mastery gratification. Athletic proficiency was of minimal importance for most of the sample. Even the men who were still active in sports indicated that this was not their primary achievement area, nor one in which their standards of excellence were very high. For the women, competence in domestic skills and proficiency in artistic hobbies were frequent choices for achievement satisfactions. Table 2 presents the correlations between childhood and adult achievement behavior.

These correlations indicate that degree of achievement behavior at age 10 was a good index of adult achievement behavior for both sexes. Unlike dependency or aggression, achievement behavior was equally stable for both sexes. This is because strivings for accomplishment and proficiency at tasks is appropriate for the behavioral repertoire of both sexes. Achievement strivings do not violate traditional sex-role standards for men or women, and this contributes to the similar degree of stability for both sexes.

As might be anticipated, intellectual achievement for age 10 to 14 showed the highest correlations with adult achievement, whereas involvement in athletics was unrelated to adult achievement.

It should not be surprising that mastery behavior for age 0 to 3 showed no relationship to adult achievement, for Period I mastery was not predictive of achievement during Periods II, III, or IV.

TABLE 2. RELATION BETWEEN CHILDHOOD BEHAVIOR AND ADULT ACHIEVEMENT

Child Variable	Age	Achievement Behavior		
		Male	Female	Pooled
Achievement	0–3	−.12	−.02	−.03
	3–6	−.03	.45**	.24*
	6–10	.46***	.38**	.37***
Achievement				
Intellectual	10–14	.40**	.42**	.36***
Mechanical	10–14	.20	.20	.36**
Athletic	10–14	−.18	.01	−.06
Recognition	6–10	.47***	.40**	.42****
	10–14	.25	.20	.26*
Competitiveness	3–6	.21	.11	.14
	6–10	.30*	.54***	.40***
	10–14	.05	.00	.04
Expect failure	6–10	−.16	−.05	−.07
	10–14	−.34*	−.29	−.32**
Withdrawal	3–6	.00	.07	.05
	6–10	.08	.01	.03
Withdrawal task	10–14	−.08	−.11	−.05

* $p < .10$; two tails
** $p < .05$; two tails
*** $p < .01$; two tails
**** $p < .001$; two tails

Variable 19: Recognition behavior

As with achievement, the interviewer attempted to evaluate the adult's *desire* for status and social recognition independent of his behavioral attempts to obtain these goals. These two variables were highly correlated ($r = .82$ for men and .98 for women), indicating that similar evidence was used in making both ratings. Thus we will only be concerned with the rating of recognition-striving behavior.

The goals that these subjects selected as status-awarding emphasized academic honors, striving for leadership positions in organizations, and vocational choices that had high status characteristics (scientist, doctor, lawyer, artist, composer, economist). These goals and related behaviors were also used to assess achievement strivings. Despite the fact that the interviewer attempted to evaluate the degree to which the incentive was social recognition, in contrast to self-satisfaction, the correlations between recognition and achievement behavior were high ($r = .78$ for men and .85 for women).

Table 3 presents the correlation between the childhood ratings and adult recognition behavior.

The correlations were similar in size and pattern to those found for the adult achievement variables. The only differences, and these were slight, occurred in the relationships involving intellectual achievement and expectancy of failure during age 10 to 14. Low fear of failure during Period IV was a slightly better predictor of adult recognition strivings than of adult achievement behavior. Similarly, intellectual achievement during Period IV was more highly associated with adult recognition striving than with achievement behavior. This latter find-

TABLE 3. RELATION BETWEEN CHILDHOOD BEHAVIOR AND ADULT RECOGNITION STRIVINGS

| Child Variable | Age | Recognition Behavior | | |
		Male	Female	Pooled
Achievement	0–3	.01	−.22	−.07
	3–6	−.11	.49***	.23*
	6–10	.57****	.51***	.51****
Achievement				
Intellectual	10–14	.60****	.56***	.58****
Mechanical	10–14	.46**	.02	.30**
Athletic	10–14	−.17	−.09	−.12
Recognition	6–10	.42**	.48***	.45****
	10–14	.36*	.39**	.36***
Competitiveness	3–6	.06	.09	.08
	6–10	.24	.52***	.37***
	10–14	.27	.06	.21
Expect failure	6–10	−.27	−.20	−.23*
	10–14	−.62***	−.40**	−.55****
Withdrawal	3–6	.05	.06	.07
	6–10	.07	−.06	.00
Withdrawal task	10–14	−.26	−.37*	−.28*

   * $p < .10$; two tails
  ** $p < .05$; two tails
 *** $p < .01$; two tails
**** $p < .001$; two tails

ing suggests that children who strive for high grades and academic honors in secondary school are likely to seek social recognition through intellectual pursuits in adulthood.

The similarities in the pattern of correlations for achievement and recognition behavior are more striking than the differences. This congruence suggests an intimate relationship between behavior aimed at satisfying internal standards of excellence, particularly in intellectual pursuits, and the search for social recognition for this competence.

Interview Variable 35: Concern with intellectual competence

This variable was singled out for special attention because the American middle-class places a unique value on the acquisition and perfection of intellective skills. The family, public media, and the school effectively communicate the attitude that knowledge of the physical environment, a high IQ, facility in speaking and writing, and cultural sophistication are personally satisfying, economically valuable, and status-awarding characteristics. This attitude permeated the value system of most of the subjects in our sample. Even the few lower-class subjects who did not attend high school regretted leaving school and hoped that their children would obtain as much formal education as possible.

The interviewer assessed each adult's concern with intellectual competence (i.e., how important education, cultural sophistication, curiosity, and acquisition of knowledge were in his value system). It is interesting to note that the inter-rater reliability for this interview variable was one of the highest of any rated ($r = .98$), indicating that this trait is a salient characteristic of the individual.

Table 4 contains the correlations between childhood behavior and adult concern with intellectual competence.

Although the pattern of correlations resembles that found for achievement and recognition, several coefficients were somewhat higher. *As might be anticipated, intellectual mastery during age 10 to 14 was highly predictive of the adult counterpart of this variable.* Involvement in intellectual tasks and concern with school performance in childhood were moderately sensitive indexes of concern with academic excellence in college and mastery of intellectual challenges in one's vocation.

On the other hand, athletic mastery for age 10 to 14 was negatively correlated with adult intellectual concern in men ($r = -.47$; $p < .05$). This is the first instance of a significant, inverse relationship between

TABLE 4. RELATION BETWEEN CHILDHOOD BEHAVIOR AND ADULT
CONCERN WITH INTELLECTUAL COMPETENCE

Child Variable	Age	Male	Female	Pooled
Achievement	0–3	−.08	−.02	−.06
	3–6	.13	.44**	.33**
	6–10	.68****	.49***	.57****
Achievement				
Intellectual	10–14	.66****	.49***	.60****
Mechanical	10–14	.47**	.27	.43***
Athletic	10–14	−.47**	.02	−.30**
Recognition	6–10	.37**	.55****	.46****
	10–14	.24	.40**	.36***
Competitiveness	3–6	−.08	.06	.00
	6–10	.25	.50***	.38***
	10–14	.06	.24	.13
Expect failure	6–10	−.29*	.01	−.11
	10–14	−.51***	−.40**	−.48****
Withdrawal	3–6	.26	.17	.20
	6–10	.14	.22	.18
Withdrawal tasks	10–14	−.21	−.23	−.20

* $p < .10$; two tails
** $p < .05$; two tails
*** $p < .01$; two tails
**** $p < .001$; two tails

an aspect of childhood mastery and adult achievement. The boys who became ego-involved in athletics during early adolescence withdrew from tasks that involved intellectual mastery. This phenomenon did not occur among the females.

It is certainly not suggested that all adolescent boys who become involved in athletics avoid mastery of intellectual skills. This particular sample, however, included boys who chose either sports or school as an area of achievement. There were very few boys who chose both. This bifurcation of interests at age 10 to 14 was responsible for the negative correlation between adolescent athletic mastery and adult concern with intellectual competence.

Those boys who emphasized athletics were not academically motivated and had been doing poorly in school. Similarly, the boys who were motivated academically were incompetent in athletics and avoided gross motor games. Each boy made a choice during preadolescence as to his area of primary competence. He took inventory of his assets and liabilities and directed himself toward those activities that maximized the likelihood of success and minimized the possibility of failure.

This schizm between athletic and academic pursuits did not occur for the girls. Involvement in tennis or swimming at age 14 was independent of desire for intellectual competence in adulthood. This independence is partially understood if it is assumed that the athletic skills the girls chose as avocations (e.g., tennis, swimming, golf) were not as intimately associated with the sex-role identity of the girl as baseball, football, and basketball were for the boy. For the adolescent boy competence in the traditional team sports is one of the defining characteristics of masculine behavior. Athletic competence is one of the trio of traits—courage, independence, and athletic prowess—that defines the culture's version of the ideal American male. The boy who is identified with this idealized role tends to reject the passivity and nonpragmatic character associated with the acquisition of knowledge. Thus involvement in athletics for some boys involves a rejection of intellectuality. For girls there is less inconsistency between athletic competence and intellectual motivations. Both are viewed by the adolescent girl as appropriate mastery areas.

Interview Variables 54 and 46: Fear of failure and withdrawal from potential failure situations

The occurrence of achievement behavior is influenced in part, by the individual's expectation of success or failure. The construct of "expectancy of success" assumes pivotal importance in Rotter's (1954) conceptualization of personality as well as in Atkinson's (1957) theorizing about the determinants of achievement behavior. The individual will be tempted to avoid the task situations in which he anticipates failure, despite the presence of strong motivation to excel in that area. Vocational decisions are too often determined by selecting a job that allows the person to maximize the probability of success and minimize the possibility of humiliating failure. The statement, "I like physics, but I'm not sure I can make it—so I decided to major in sociology," is frequent in the office of the vocational counselor. Too often man's decisions are determined more by flight from failure than by the desire to acquire goals that might bring more delight.

The persistent anticipation of failure is the complex product of many historical events. Repeated task failure, identification with an incompetent parent, and communications from significant others im-

STABILITY OF BEHAVIOR: III ACHIEVEMENT AND RECOGNITION

plying inadequate skills can all lead to negative self-evaluations and apprehension in the face of challenging situations. When expectancy of failure is high, the individual is apt to avoid goals and responsibilities that might test his competence. This psychological footwork has one central aim—to prevent the experience of *failure*.

Since failure generally increases and success decreases the gnawing anticipation of failure, we would expect that lack of mastery gratifications during childhood would predispose the adult to a fairly strong fear of failure and the preference for withdrawal from situations that are perceived as tests of adequacy.

The assessment of these two variables (fear of failure and withdrawal) was based on the individual's feelings and reactions in some key problem situations. These situations included feelings about college work, reasons for vocational choices, apprehension about assuming positions of responsibility, confidence in decisions about the family and major purchases, and anxiety in social situations in which the subject felt he might be judged negatively.

Table 5 presents the correlations between the child's behavior and fear of failure and withdrawal in adulthood.

The adult women who were insecure about their intellectual and social competence, and withdrew from situations that were tests of these abilities, behaved similarly as children. They showed minimal attempts at mastery in school, little involvement in intellectual activities, and they withdrew from challenging task situations. *Although the correlation between achievement behavior during Period III and adult fear of failure was negative for both males and females,* the relations between withdrawal in adulthood and achievement, fear of failure, or withdrawal in childhood were generally high for women but negligible for men.

There are two reasons why early achievement anxiety and task avoidance might be *less stable* for men than for women. First, withdrawal is not permitted easy entrance into the list of acceptable traits that define the young boy's ego ideal. Second, the boy feels a distinct pressure to choose a vocation. The 13-year-old girl may avoid making a career choice, but the adolescent boy can not. This external demand for a vocational role pushes some boys with high fear of failure to repress this source of anxiety. They must conquer this fear. In order to be admitted into the world of adult men, a commitment to a vocational skill must be made. The boy, more than the girl, must attempt to conquer anxiety over task mastery. Thus childhood fear of failure might be expected to be less prognostic of adult task withdrawal for men than for women.

TABLE 5. RELATION BETWEEN CHILDHOOD BEHAVIOR AND ADULT FEAR OF FAILURE AND WITHDRAWAL

Child Variable	Age	Fear of Failure			Withdrawal		
		Male	Female	Pooled	Male	Female	Pooled
Achievement	0–3	.02	−.09	−.01	.03	−.08	−.03
	3–6	−.03	−.40**	−.24*	.18	−.48***	−.15
	6–10	−.31*	−.34**	−.34***	−.16	−.40**	−.29
Achievement							
Intellectual	10–14	−.21	−.44**	−.30**	−.15	−.55***	−.30**
Mechanical	10–14	.00	−.05	.00	.11	−.10	−.03
Athletic	10–14	.00	.04	.00	−.21	−.01	−.13
Recognition	6–10	−.36**	−.14	−.26**	−.23	−.32*	−.28**
	10–14	−.22	−.08	−.15	−.16	−.19	−.18
Competitive-ness	3–6	−.18	−.11	−.15	−.27	−.24	−.26
	6–10	−.20	−.23	−.22*	−.28	−.41**	−.35***
	10–14	−.01	−.07	−.04	−.05	−.11	−.09
Expect failure	6–10	.07	.24	.17	.07	.28*	.17
	10–14	.31	.37*	.34**	.26	.50***	.37***
Withdrawal	3–6	.21	.13	.18	.08	.09	.09
	6–10	.13	.35**	.25**	.17	.43**	.31**
Withdrawal task	10–14	.24	.41**	.33**	.40*	.49**	.42***

* $p < .10$; two tails
** $p < .05$; two tails
*** $p < .01$; two tails

Minimal concern with intellectual mastery during Period IV was highly correlated with fear of failure and withdrawal in adult women. The adolescent girls who were the least successful in school became self-doubting adults who usually avoided responsibility, decisions, and avocations requiring effort and skill. These relations did not occur for athletic or mechanical mastery during Period IV. Because intellectual competence was so highly valued by our women, failure to perfect intellectual skills during childhood and adolescence led to serious feelings of inadequacy and a cautious approach to problem situations in adulthood.

Fear of bodily harm and adult intellectuality

The hypothesis that intense involvement in intellective pursuits may be—for the boy—a retreat from the aggressive, active, and competitive atmosphere supported by the dominant peer group is not an original one. The characterization of the poet as "coward" occurs in both story and verse and the presumed causality between these processes has both theoretical and empirical support.

The concept of "maleness" in our society is closely linked with the characteristics of strength, size, daring, aggressivity, instrumental effectiveness, and interpersonal dominance. Both adults and children concur in preferentially ascribing these attributes to men (Jenkins and Russell, 1958; Bennett and Cohen, 1959; Kagan, Hosken, and Watson, 1961). For example, when adolescent boys were asked about wished-for alterations in their physique, increased height and muscle mass were named most frequently (Cobb, 1954; Nash, 1958). It is reasonable to assume that the desire for increased size among boys in our culture reflects the high valuation placed on physical strength, the ability to physically retaliate when attacked, and proficiency at gross motor skills. For this reason, the boy who is afraid of the reciprocal aggression and bodily contact games that characterize the group behavior of school-age boys is likely to suffer peer rejection and to withdraw to more solitary activities. Intellectuality is one area of competence that can provide such a boy with a compensatory sense of adequacy. Thus fear of bodily harm during the childhood years might be associated with the development of an especially strong need for intellectual mastery in those boys who were mentally capable of success in this area. The concept of femaleness is not linked with strength, power, fearlessness, or gross motor skills, and there is no reason to expect this particular sequence to occur among girls.

The longitudinal ratings included assessments of fear of physical harm and avoidance of dangerous activity, and these will be discussed in detail in Chapter Six. The fear-of-harm ratings for Periods I and II were based on avoidance of dangerous play (jungle gym, climbing, wrestling), as well as the presence of irrational fears (the dark, animals). For Period III, intensity of irrational fears and avoidance of potentially dangerous games were evaluated independently. The latter behavior was assessed for Periods III and IV and emphasized reluctance to enter into body-contact games (football, wrestling) or potentially dangerous activities (climbing, hunting, swimming).

Table 6 presents the correlations between fearfulness or avoidance of dangerous activities in childhood and concern with intellectual competence and competitive behavior in adulthood.

The association between childhod fearfulness and intellectual mastery only held for males. The boys who exhibited strong fear of bodily harm during Period II showed the greatest involvement in intellectual pursuits as adults (r = .50; p < .01). This relationship was minimal

TABLE 6. RELATION BETWEEN CHILDHOOD FEAR OF HARM AND ADULT BEHAVIOR

		Competitiveness			Intellectual Concerns		
Child Variable	Age	Male	Female	Pooled	Male	Female	Pooled
Fear of bodily harm	0–3	−.17	−.18	−.14	.18	−.26	−.09
	3–6	−.26	−.03	−.10	.50***	.08	.28**
Phobias	6–10	−.34**	−.17	−.23*	.26	−.01	.12
Avoidance of dangerous activity	6–10	−.37**	−.07	−.24*	.29	.00	.16
	10–14	−.43*	−.34	−.43***	.27	−.63***	−.02

* $p < .10$; two tails
** $p < .05$; two tails
*** $p < .01$; two tails

for girls during the first ten years. However, the girls who were bold and daring during age 10 to 14 became the intellectually oriented adult women. As anticipated, the noncompetitive adult men were fearful and avoided dangerous activities during childhood.

Subject 2313 furnishes a dramatic illustration of the association between fear of injury and intense strivings for intellectual mastery. We have previously described this man as a brilliant student in high school and college (see Chapter 3, p. 72). His major source of gratification, since the early school years, was his intellectual precocity. This area of competence was not only his primary achievement concern but also furnished the foundation of his self-concept.

At 2½ years of age the nursery-school observer wrote:

"S was one of the groups most isolated members. At no time did he ever play an aggressive role in relationship to the other children. He was noncompetitive, nonassertive, and his play was puttering and sedentary. He did make a few approaches to others in which he offered a toy to children, but he usually shrank from actual physical contact with other playmates. His relationships with others were mild, long-distanced, verbal ones. S was petrified at rough handling. If he were verbally rebuffed or teased, he smiled weakly, put his hands behind his back, and verbalized about what he would do or had once done. He quite frequently refused friendly offers from other children, as if he were apprehensive of new experiences. S appears to enjoy himself as long as direct pressure is not brought to bear on him. The most salient thing about S is a binding inhibition and apprehension. He moves tentatively and quaveringly like an old man on an icy day. His whole posture exudes timidity. He is drawn in at the knees and elbows, hunched at the shoulders, his head is poked forward, his hands, often rabbit-fashion, hanging limply from wrists, tucked together at his chest. In any swirl of noise or rough play he becomes terrified and rigid, holding himself away stiffly. In any excitement of his own he constrains himself and draws in tighter and tighter. When excited or afraid he is wound up so rigid that his posture and expression become taut. He had extreme physical fears, and when threatened by falling, precarious situations, or bullying, he was totally unable to control the situation. He was petrified by any physical threat and verbalized this emotion. He had no positive anger to show, and it was almost impossible to rouse him to any aggression."

At 5½ years of age he was similarly described.

"While S's almost total lack of aggression was very striking, it was not at all clear how much of it was because of a deep emotional taboo against aggression and how much he lacked the emotional courage to try it. Several staff members feel that S's fear of being hurt in physical encounters is extreme."

At 8 years of age, fears of harm and feelings of guilt were strong. After an interview at the Institute, the interviewer wrote:

"After we talked for a long time about airplanes and magic, he turned to me and said in a miserable voice, 'My brain is full of too much.' With some urging this 'too much' turned out to be bad words of which he had learned four or five in school but did not want to say them. He says they keep coming up and bothering him. I suggested that perhaps if he wrote them out on a blackboard and erased them, it might help him to get rid of them. He eagerly accepted this technique and, in a straggling hand, printed a few of the more common smutty words on the board. He erased each before printing the next. He breathed hard for a few minutes after this process and carefully wiped all the chalk dust off his hands."

"He also made many references to a fear of being hurt and a concern about colds and germs. He said he wouldn't like to live in a city because of all the noise, which might keep him awake at night. His current ambition is to be a doctor, 'To see the things I want to—like what tonsils look like—and disease.' He seems definitely ambivalent about expressing emotions, but he can't help it at times when, 'Somebody is talking bad to me.' He doesn't show his anger much because, 'The only way you show it is by fighting, and I don't fight.' "

S's fear of bodily harm and expectation of injury from the environment gradually led to strong needs for power over the social and physical environment. *S* sought to obtain this power through intellectual competence. In an interview at 9 years of age *S* expressed these feelings to the staff psychologist.

"*S* is getting along very well in school, making all 'A's' and 'B's' in the fifth grade. He never gets into any fights and says, 'The teacher makes us stay in if there's a fight, so no one wants to fight.' When asked what he wants to do when he grows up, *S* said, 'Well, I want to be a scientist.' I asked him what he liked about science and he said, 'Well I like element study in geology, I have a collection of crystals that I find.' *S* goes to bed at 8:00 P.M. and has a room by himself. He says, 'It takes me about an hour to go to sleep; I think about various things that keep you from getting excited and keep you calm. I try to say the Psalms, but the only one I can remember all the way through is the 23rd Psalm. I also say a few prayers. After a while, my mind gets to scattering, and I think about everything. I think of almost everything: being great, being President, and at other times I think of being a genius, and all kinds of things.' When he said this, I asked, 'Do you think you will be a genius someday?' *S* replied, 'Oh, I suppose so, scientific, of course.' When asked if there were any things that frighten him, he replied, 'Only at night, something, some unexpected noises. I am used to the pitter-patter of mice, but an unexpected noise like hearing a window break scares me a little. I'm not so awfully scared of the dark.' "

S went through elementary and high school with exceptionally high grades and was an outstanding student in college. As a young adult, the desire for intellectual excellence and social recognition was unusually strong. However, the feeling of isolation from peers and fear of attack from the physical environment were still present.

This case, more than any other in our sample, suggests a close link between a strong fear of injury from the environment and the development of a need for retaliatory power through intellectual mastery.

Acquisition of knowledge and intellectual skills can dilute fears of the environment in two ways. A rational understanding of nature gives the child some defense against potential dangers. If he can predict or explain the events that terrify him or rationalize irrational dangers, he has gained some measure of control over these sources of anxiety.

Second, a feeling of intellectual superiority over one's peers can be an effective weapon against feelings of physical impotence and anticipation of attack. Intellectual power often brings status and awe and, as such, is a defense against those who are more physically potent.

Strivings for intellectual competence among the females in our sample were associated with a different set of personality dispositions. The high achieving girls were competitive and rather bold as children. The correlation between Period III competitiveness and adult achievement in women was $+.54$ ($p < .01$); with adult intellectual concerns the correlation was .50 ($p < .01$). The intellectually oriented women showed minimal fear of dangerous games during Period IV ($r = -.63$), in contrast to the fearfulness of the intellectual boy. The achievement-oriented women were confident, counterphobic, and competitive during childhood and adolescence.

Subject 375 was the most achievement-oriented woman in the entire sample. She was single at the time of the interview and in her last year at college. She viewed the world as a source of challenges and was involved in activities that ranged from inventions of kitchen gadgets to guitar playing. She was doing well academically and was entertaining thoughts of becoming a writer on graduation from college. When asked to name the three people she admired most, S listed three former teachers:

"I admired Mrs. _____, for she gave me a sense of values and was a good model for me. I admired Mr. _____. He has wide interests and knows so much about the world; he's a vital man. And Mrs. _____ because she's a thinking person."

A striving for mastery, a counterphobic and confident attitude to problems, and the parental encouragement of these behaviors were all apparent from the earliest observations on this girl.

At one year of age the home visitor noted:

"S is pushed rather vigorously toward developing useful skills and independence by both parents. For example, when the father was given the responsibility of feeding S in the morning, he promptly trained her to feed herself to save him the trouble. The mother is nonchalant and lets S toddle about with minimal protectiveness. The mother fails to bat an eye when S tumbles and crys. S straightens herself out after a perfunctory whimper. S can say half a dozen words and is friendly with all strangers. She is unusually independent and active."

Both of S's parents gave her an unusual degree of autonomy, and she seemed to thrive in this atmosphere. She was active, nonfearful, and curious about her environment. Her speech development was advanced, and her peer interactions had an aggressive flavor. At $4\frac{1}{2}$ years of age, S was described as follows:

"S's body is strong and well coordinated, and there is a great push behind everything she did. She had an exceptionally clear voice, and every word of her amazingly large vocabulary was sharply and distinctly enunciated. Her habitual tone was a bellowing shout, but she could modulate it to fit the particular role she was playing. S was one of the group leaders. Her energy, fund of ideas, and verbal manipulation of the world gave her great skills and dominance of peers. S would occasionally attack others if they stood in the way of an object she wanted. She would vary between a diplomatic explanation of, 'Well I need it' to simply snatching the toy."

"S seemed to seek attention and revel in it. She was as pleased when a crowd was around to witness her battles as when someone admired her art work. S's play always had an element of physical energy. The major part of S's activity was concern with ideas, using her own body and voice for the stage in which she acted out things. She would use dolls as props in her play. Another favorite game was being pregnant. She would wear a doll in her sweater and bring it out with a dramatic pop. S was well aware of her special talent in music and openly compared her superiority with others. For S every relationship was structured in terms of competition, and she was aware of the impact of her behavior on others at all times. S loves to use words, both for show-off value as well as for the pleasure involved in using long words and sentences. S seems to get delight from mouthing sounds and enjoys puns, rhymes, and alliterations for their own sake. S loved aggression. She would often select a dramatic role in which aggression was necessary. She would play the role of an alligator, a dragon, or a bear who was the head of a bear tribe. S would then terrorize the children by telling them what was going to happen to them. Although S always wanted audience attention, her method of trying to acquire knowledge often seemed free of self-consciousness or status drives. Rather, there was a great excitement in wanting to know things. S would give respect to any person if he had a particular art technique which she wanted to learn. She would stand and watch him, even ask him to show her how to do it and work hard until she had mastered it."

This intense need to know and the persistent desire for mastery, which were present as early as 4 years of age, remained a salient aspect of S's personality throughout the school years. At 6 years of age the Fels' observer wrote:

"S has learned to read and vitally enjoys it. She has long, silent periods of concentration and was often enraptured by the story she was reading. She loved trips to the Glen and reveled in the space; sure-footed as a mountain goat and fearless to all danger."

The intellectual challenges provided by the school situation were met and conquered with zeal. She was admired by her peers, for she had a vivid and lively imagination. She enjoyed a battle and adopted a competitive and rivalrous attitude with boys as well as girls.

At 15 years of age her story to Card 17BM of the TAT (picture of a man on a rope) captures her preoccupation with status and mastery goals.

"This is one of the greatest sportsmen of all times, who has broken the record, the speed record for rope climbing. It's the world's record. He is shown going up the rope on one of his latest records that he made."

To Card 14 (silhouette of a person in a window), S verbalized a concern with the acquisition of knowledge.

"This is a high school boy who is interested in studying the stars, but his high school didn't offer the proper education for astronomy, so at night he just stands by the window and wishes with all his might that he could have had the proper education so that he could go on and study things he wanted to study."

S graduated second in her high school class. She was involved in almost all the school activities and devoted special energy to music and athletics.

The competitiveness, confidence, and vitality shown by this girl are in sharp contrast to the apprehension and caution that characterized the boy described previously. Both children were unusually bright and both had unusually strong motivations to master intellective skills. The excerpts from this pair of cases illustrate the significant differences in personality among the high achievement boys and girls in our particular sample.

It is *not* suggested that intellectual achievement in boys is usually a consequent of early childhood fears and withdrawal from the aggressive play of peers. However, when the motivation for intellectual mastery is unusually high, the coincidence of these two response processes seems to occur more frequently among boys than among girls. It is suggested that the motives and conflicts behind intellectual achievement in boys may differ somewhat from those that mediate high levels of intellectual achievement in girls.

There is one element of communality between the high achieving boys and girls in our sample. These children did not adopt the traditional sex-role attitudes and behaviors. The boys were noncompetitive, nonathletic, and fearful; the girls were fearless, independent, and competitive. It may be that intense involvement in intellectual activity is facilitated by a weak identification with the traditional sex-role values of the majority peer group.

THE RELATION OF ACHIEVEMENT THEMES TO
ACHIEVEMENT BEHAVIOR

The availability of an independent index of achievement concern—
stories to TAT pictures—enabled us to assess the relation between
achievement imagery and the child and adult behavior ratings. These
results have been presented in an earlier report (Moss and Kagan, 1961)
and will be summarized briefly here.

TAT achievement themes

Early adolescent (median age of 14–6) TAT protocols were available
for 67 of the 71 adults, and all 71 subjects were administered 13 TAT
stimuli after the adult interview. The adolescent protocol was based
on 7 cards from the Murray (1943) series (cards 1, 5, 14, 17BM, 3BM,
6BM, and 3GF). The adult male protocol included cards 4, 8BM,
7BM, 6BM, 12M, 17BM, 13MF, 14, 3BM, 5, 1, 3GF, and 18GF. The
adult females were administered cards 4, 6GF, 12F, 2, 8GF, 17BM,
13MF, 14, 3BM, 5, 1, 3GF, and 18GF.

For both the adolescent and adult protocols achievement themes
were scored according to the scheme described by McClelland, Atkinson, Clark, and Lowell (1953). Since incidence of the subcategories of
the McClelland scoring system was infrequent, only stories in which
achievement behavior was the major aspect of the plot were considered.
These are scored *Ach Th* in the McClelland scheme. For the adolescent
protocol there was a lack of comparability among the examiners with
respect to the inquiry questions, and only the spontaneous verbalization
of the child was scored. Agreement between two independent coders
for *Ach Th* was 95 per cent. As noted earlier, both the longitudinal and
interview ratings of achievement and recognition behaviors were made
without knowledge of the subjects' adolescent or adult TAT stories.
Since occurrence of achievement themes was not normally distributed,
contingency coefficients were used to test the association between
achievement themes and child and adult achievement behavior.[1]

Stability of TAT achievement themes

Although different sets of TAT pictures were administered to the
adolescents and adults, the three stimuli that usually elicited achievement stories were presented at both administrations. Cards 1, 14, and

17BM, which elicited 77 per cent of all the achievement themes, were common to both protocols. The strong tendency for these particular cards to elicit achievement themes has been noted in an earlier study (Kagan and Moss, 1959a). A typical achievement theme to Card 1 concerned a boy who wanted to master the violin and/or become a famous violinist. A typical achievement story to Card 17BM involved a person who was in a rope-climbing contest and wanted to do his best to win. A common achievement story to Card 14 concerned an artist or student who had been working hard and was looking forward to fame and success as a result of his accomplishments.

The stability of occurrence of achievement stories between the adolescent and adult protocols was moderate. The contingency coefficients were $+.34$ for boys, $+.36$ for girls ($p < .10$), and $+.31$ for the total group ($p < .05$), indicating that achievement themes showed some degree of stability over this 10-year period. These data extend the findings of an earlier investigation (Kagan and Moss, 1959 [a]) in which the authors reported a three-year stability coefficient of .32 ($p < .05$) for achievement themes obtained at median ages of 8 and 11 years. The stability coefficients between the adolescent and adult protocols are of the same magnitude as those found for the earlier age period.

Validity of achievement themes: Relations with child and adult behavior

The relation between adolescent or adult achievement themes and the longitudinal and adult achievement behavior ratings is presented in Table 7.

The highest and most consistent relations were between the adult achievement themes and the adult interview ratings. Achievement and recognition behaviors in adulthood were associated with achievement themes for both males and females.[2] The only significant relation between adult themes and childhood behavior held for mechanical achievement, positive for boys and negative for girls.

Adolescent achievement themes were also more predictive of adult than of childhood mastery. Adolescent achievement themes predicted adult achievement behavior for women and concern with intellectual mastery for men. Adolescent achievement themes showed minimal association with the child's achievement behavior, although mechanical achievement among girls was negatively associated with achievement themes. This negative correlation may be due to the fact that this is the only variable for which markedly different behavioral referents

TABLE 7. RELATION BETWEEN TAT ACHIEVEMENT THEMES AND CHILD AND
ADULT ACHIEVEMENT BEHAVIOR

Contingency coefficients

Child variable	Age	Adolescent TAT (Median age 14–6)		Adult TAT (Median age 25)	
		Male	Female	Male	Female
Achievement	0–3	−.15	−.25	−.20	.16
	3–6	.42*	.19	.19	.36
	6–10	.24	.15	.13	.30
Achievement					
Intellectual	10–14	.30	−.25	.26	.16
Mechanical	10–14	.31	−.62**	.63***	−.50**
Athletic	10–14	−.20	.12	.12	.17
Adult variable					
Achievement		.19	.44**	.37*	.52***
Recognition		.17	.25	.40**	.52***
Intellectual					
concern		.44**	.25	.31	.59***

* $p < .10$; two tails
** $p < .05$; two tails
*** $p < .01$; two tails

were used in rating the two sexes. For boys, involvement in carpentry,
engines, motors, and model airplanes was emphasized in the rating.
These activities are sex typed, and girls showed no interest in them.
The rating manual designated involvement in craft work and sewing
(making jewelry, leather articles) as evidence of involvement in mechanical activities, and girls chose these behaviors.

In sum, the adult and adolescent TAT stories showed moderate
correlations with adult achievement behavior but minimal association
with childhood achievement.

RELATION BETWEEN INTELLIGENCE AND ACHIEVEMENT

It might be anticipated that the child's tested intelligence would be
related to the intensity of his involvement in mastery behavior, es-

pecially intellectual mastery. Moreover, Sontag et al. (1958) have reported that highly competitive and mastery-oriented children have larger increases in IQ during the early school years than less competitive or achievement-oriented children. The child and adult ratings were made without knowledge of the subjects' intelligence test scores, and an analysis of the relation between IQ and the achievement variables seemed worthwhile. It will be recalled from Chapter Two that the child was administered the Stanford-Binet (Form L or M) semiannually from ages 2½ to 5, and annually from ages 5 to 12.[3] The Wechsler-Bellevue Scale (Form I) was administed at 13 years of age, and the 71 adult subjects were given eight subtests from the Wechsler Adult Scale (Form I) as part of the adult assessment.

Each of the nine child and adult achievement behavior variables was correlated with the child's average IQ at five different ages, and his change in IQ during ages 6 to 10. The average IQ score for ages 3, 6, and 10 was based on the average of the three Stanford-Binet scores around that age. That is, the child's IQ at age 3 was the average of his scores at ages 2½, 3, and 3½; the score at age 6 was the average of his score at ages 5, 6, and 7; the score at age 10 was the average of his scores at ages 9, 10, and 11. There were some cases where only two scores were available at one of these ages. In these cases, the two scores were averaged. The score at age 13 was the Full Scale Wechsler IQ; the score at adulthood was the prorated Full Scale Wechsler IQ. The child's IQ change score was obtained by subtracting his average IQ at 6 years of age from his average IQ at age 10.

Table 8 presents the correlations between the child and adult achievement ratings and each of the five IQ scores. Table 9 presents the relations between child and adult behavior and amount of increase in IQ score from ages 6 to 10.

The child's intelligence from *age 6 on was highly correlated with achievement behavior and intellectual mastery during both childhood and adulthood for both males and females.* In most cases the child's IQ at age 6 or 10 was as good or better a predictor of adult concern with intellectual competence as the rating of the child's behavior during Periods III and IV. For this particular group of children, tested intelligence was a highly sensitive predictor of current and future achievement.

There are several reasons for this. First, the average IQ of the group was 120, and although there were a few subjects with scores below 100, the great majority had intelligence quotients between 100 and 135. It is suggested that, for children with this restricted range of scores, the

TABLE 8. RELATION BETWEEN INTELLIGENCE AND ACHIEVEMENT BEHAVIOR DURING CHILDHOOD AND ADULTHOOD

Child's Intelligence

Child Variable		Age 3		6		10		13		Adult	
		M	F	M	F	M	F	M	F	M	F
Achievement	0–3	−.26	−.27	.04	−.20	.11	−.09	.31	.01	.37	.03
	3–6	.66****	.39**	.58***	.65***	.39**	.62***	.35**	.56***	.34*	.72****
	6–10	.40*	.42**	.38***	.66***	.63*****	.71*****	.57****	.77*****	.51***	.68*****
Achievement											
Intellectual	10–14	–	.31	.60***	.76****	.78*****	.74*****	.71****	.73****	.65***	.60***
Mechanical	10–14	–	–	.21	.42*	.45**	.38***	.45**	.37*	.51**	.24
Athletic	10–14	–	.17	−.58***	.20	−.40**	.11	−.34*	.25	−.33	.05
Adult Variable											
Achievement		−.01	.24	.10	.63***	.55***	.56***	.50***	.52***	.50***	.54***
Recognition		.00	−.01	.17	.70****	.54***	.55***	.54***	.50***	.48***	.52***
Intellectual concern		−.01	.13	.41**	.62***	.73****	.62***	.70****	.67*****	.66*****	.61****

* $p < .10$; two tails   ** $p < .05$; two tails   *** $p < .01$; two tails   **** $p < .001$; two tails

TABLE 9. RELATION BETWEEN INCREASE IN IQ SCORE AND ACHIEVE-MENT BEHAVIOR DURING CHILDHOOD AND ADULTHOOD

Child variable	Age	Male	Female
Achievement	0–3	.13	.04
	3–6	−.02	.24
	6–10	.39**	.47**
Achievement			
Intellectual	10–14	.37*	.41**
Mechanical	10–14	.15	.14
Athletic	10–14	−.16	−.46**
Adult interview variable			
Recognition behavior		.48**	.25
Achievement behavior		.38**	.38**
Intellectual concern		.49**	.42**

* $p < .10$; two tails
** $p < .05$; two tails

child's motivation to master intellectual skills is a major determinant of individual differences in test score. For certain populations the IQ can serve as an index of achievement concern.

Amount of increase in IQ was also a moderately good predictor of concern with intellectual mastery during both childhood and adulthood for both sexes. However, absolute level of intelligence at age 10 was a better index of future intellectual mastery than amount of IQ increase between 6 and 10 years of age.

The positive relation between an increase in IQ and intellectual achievement support and extend earlier studies from the Institute (Sontag et al., 1958; Kagan et al., 1958). In these early studies increases in IQ were correlated with behavioral indexes of achievement strivings for ages 6 to 10 and with early adolescent (age 10 to 14) achievement stories. These relations were significant even when the influence of the child's IQ at age 6 was statistically controlled.[4]

The reader should note that the boys' IQ scores at age 10 were a better predictor of intellectual concern in adulthood than the scores obtained at 6 years of age. This difference reflects the fact that boys with strong desires to master intellectual skills gained in IQ score during the early years of school, while those with low mastery motivation remained stable or showed slight decreases in IQ score. This difference in the predictive power of the IQ at age 6 versus age 10 did not occur for girls. This is consistent with the fact that the girls' IQ scores remained more stable than the boys' during this period. For twice as many boys as girls had major increases in IQ score during the early school years (Sontag et al., 1958).

In sum, when one is working with children whose IQ scores are average or above, level of intelligence and increases in test score appear to be good indexes of the strength of overt achievement behavior during childhood, adolescence, and adulthood, and a reflection of intensity of motivation to master intellectual tasks.

EVALUATIVE DISCUSSION

Achievement behavior displayed evidence of adequate stability from childhood to adulthood. The sizes of the correlations were consistently high for both males and females, in contrast to the patterns obtained for passivity, dependency, and aggression. It was possible to make fairly accurate guesses about intensity of strivings for intellectual competence in high school and college from the child's behavior or tested intelligence in the third and fourth grades.

We have alluded to two factors that may contribute to the stability of this behavior. First, achievement is a socially approved behavior or at least a behavior that is not punished by the social environment. Second, mastery behavior often leads to status, acceptance by parents and parental surrogates, material rewards, as well as personal satisfaction and inner feelings of adequacy and competence. For men, mastery of a special skill is necessary for a satisfactory vocational adjustment. Finally, intellectual achievement, unlike dependency and aggressive behavior, is highly correlated with educational level of the family. Thus a middle-class child's concern with intellectual competence is supported by most of the significant others in the child's life space.

Table 10 presents the correlations between child and adult achievement behavior and the educational level of each of the parents.

Adult concern with intellectual competence as well as general achievement behavior were highly correlated with parental educational level. Intellectual mastery during adolescence was more highly associated with parental educational level for boys than for girls.

Mastery behavior during Period I showed no relation to parental educational level, supporting the previous statements that early persistence with simple materials is not related to the behaviors characterizing school age or adult achievement.

TABLE 10. RELATION BETWEEN EDUCATIONAL LEVEL OF EACH PARENT AND
ACHIEVEMENT BEHAVIOR IN CHILDHOOD AND ADULTHOOD

Child Variable	Age	Boys		Girls	
		Father	Mother	Father	Mother
Achievement	0–3	−.03	.17	.10	.11
	3–6	.36**	.15	.36**	.33
	6–10	.39**	.37**	.23	.19
Achievement					
Intellectual	10–14	.71****	.54***	.09	−.11
Mechanical	10–14	.53***	.41	.19	−.04
Athletic	10–14	−.22	−.34	.09	.34
Adult variable					
Achievement behavior		.39**	.34**	.53****	.49***
Recognition behavior		.62***	.45***	.47***	.43***
Intellectual concern		.64***	.55****	.68****	.63****

** $p < .05$; two tails
*** $p < .01$; two tails
**** $p < .001$; two tails

The substantial association between adult achievement in men and
educational level of the family did not occur for the dependent and
aggression clusters. In a later chapter (Chapter Seven), the relationship
between ratings of maternal acceleration and the child's achievement
behavior will be discussed. However, in this context, we wish to note
that those correlations with adult achievement are not as high as
those which used parental education as the predictor of adult achievement behavior. In an earlier report (Kagan and Moss, 1959b), it was
demonstrated that maternal education was a better predictor of the
child's IQ than the mother's own intelligence quotient. The predictive
power of parental educational level rests on its implications for the
total life experiences of the child, in addition to its implications for
specific behavior on the part of the father and mother. Parental education is an index to the type of peer group the child will enter, the
identification models he will encounter, the opportunity for extrafamilial intellectual stimulation, and, for our sample, the type of
school he will attend.

The importance of social-class membership in determining areas of
mastery is supported by the work of Thorndike and Hagen (1959),
who found that some college training, which is social-class correlated,

provided the best clue to future occupational choice. Hobbies, athletics, or types of work experience during early adulthood were all inferior to this social class variable (i.e., college training) as predictors of occupational choice 13 years later.

The entire social environment of the child acts as a continuing source of encouragement or discouragement for intellectual mastery. The negative correlations between athletic mastery for adolescent boys and parental educational level indicates that the area of mastery behavior chosen is specifically related to the values of the child's social class and the groups with which he interacts.

The significance of Period III behavior

As with dependency and aggression, achievement behavior during age 6 to 10 was a moderately reliable predictor of future behavioral predispositions. Prior to school entrance, the establishment of stable goal-related responses in these areas is still in flux, and some of the critical situations and experiences that crystallize adult motivational dispositions either have not occurred or have not had sufficient time to exert their effect on the child's behavior.

The first four to five years of school appear to be a critical period for the child. He is forced to resolve some of his dependent ties to his family, to learn academic skills, and to work out relations with peers. Moreover, he is exposed to the values and attitudes of new social agents (i.e., teachers and peers) who either support existing goals and values or create conflict in the child. As preadolescence approaches, many children have formulated stable behavioral strategies in the areas of passivity, aggression, and intellectual mastery. This is a time when one can obtain a moderately accurate preview of what the young adult might be like.

Footnotes

1. The contingency coefficients were based on χ^2s computed from Mood's likelihood ratio test for a 3×2 distribution (Mood, 1950, p. 257).

2. These data raise some question concerning the validity of the hero hypothesis. Cards 1, 14, and 17 BM all picture a male in a potential achievement situation, and one might expect that achievement themes for women would not be highly correlated with their achievement behavior. The present results indicate that the production of achievement themes may be more influenced by the subject's conception of what behaviors are appropriate for the hero than by the degree of identification of storyteller with hero. If this assumption is valid, it would appear

that high achievement-oriented girls tend to conceptualize the male role as more concerned with task mastery more than the low achievement-behavior girls do.

3. Dr. Virginia L. Nelson administered all the Stanford-Binet childhood tests and the adolescent Wechsler-Bellevue Scale.

4. In the present sample of 71 Ss, 50 per cent of the males and 20 per cent of the females overlapped with the group of 70 subjects used by Sontag, Baker, and Nelson (1958) in their study of the correlates of IQ change. However, their data only dealt with the period from 3 to 10 years of age. The present behavioral material covered adolescence and early adulthood.

CHAPTER SIX

Stability of Behavior: IV

Sexuality, Social Interaction,

and Selected Behaviors

Passivity, dependency, aggression, and achievement were variables for which the longitudinal and interview data were most extensive. Other variables, which are of pivotal importance in a description of human behavior, were also evaluated from the longitudinal records. However, the childhood observations for these behaviors were typically less detailed, and, usually, it was only possible to rate one or two general variables.

This chapter will consider the stability of heterosexual behavior, traditional sex-role interests, social-interaction anxiety, compulsivity, nurturance, fear of bodily harm, hyperkinesis, and introspectiveness. Some of the variables were only rated for one or two of the longitudinal periods; others for all four age periods.

HETEROSEXUAL BEHAVIOR AND SEX-ROLE INTERESTS

The development of a mature sexual orientation is of major significance for adult functioning. However, the behavioral signs that delineate this complicated process are often difficult to observe. Achievement and dependent responses are open to the community and are frequently manifested during the preschool years. The child's attempts to obtain sexual gratification, however, are concealed, and the initiation of heterosexual relations does not usually emerge until preadolescence or later. Thus the longitudinal observations for this area of behavior were not as complete as one would wish. The limited treatment of this variable is a function of the available material and not a reflection of its developmental relevance.

Two types of behaviors were evaluated. The first involved a rating of amount of interaction with members of the opposite sex during the years 6 to 14. Prior to school entrance, the differentiation of sex roles is diffuse, and reciprocal play with peers is not organized or well structured. It is not until age 11 or 12 that interaction between boys and girls acquires a sexual connotation.

Admittedly, amount of contact with opposite sex peers is not the most sensitive index of the tendency to seek sexual gratification. However, it was believed that the initiation of dating and the attempt to establish heterosexual bonds during early adolescence might have some relation to future sexual behavior and attitudes with love objects.

A second variable associated with sexual behavior was the adoption of traditional sex-typed interests and behaviors—a measure of the construct of *sex-role identification*. Success or failure at the task of winning the affection of a love object is one of the primary characteristics of an individual's sex-role identification. For adolescent males, in particular, sexual conquest, in addition to athletic prowess, independence, dominance, and courage, form the foundation for an adequate assumption of the traditional male role. A boy whose recreational and avocational interests were traditionally masculine might be expected to establish heterosexual relations earlier and with more zeal than a boy who had not adopted traditional male attitudes.

It is true that the adolescent girl's ability to attract a boy forms a major support for her sex-role identity. However, the girl is not allowed as much license as the boy in initiating sexual contacts, and the *opportunity* for dating is a more influential variable in the heterosexual behavior of girls than of boys. During the years 1929 to 1954 the middle-class sexual mores in southwestern Ohio differed somewhat from those gaining dominance today. It was clearly inappropriate for a 14-year-old girl to be sexually aggressive with boys, and the dominant sex-role prescription for the female called for modesty and propriety in heterosexual situations. Thus the adoption of traditionally feminine characteristics by a girl might be minimally related to her sexual behavior.

The longitudinal records were used to rate two variables involving heterosexual behavior and sex-role identification.

Variable 21: Heterosexual interaction

This variable, rated for Periods III and IV, evaluated the frequency and quality of interaction with members of the opposite sex. Particular emphasis was given to interactions in which the child related to opposite sex peers as love objects (e.g., dating behavior).

Variable 27: Opposite sex activities

This variable, rated for Periods II, III, and IV, assessed the child's interest in and practice of activities that are traditionally associated with the opposite sex (i.e., interest in athletics, mechanical objects, and highly competitive activities were regarded as masculine; involvement in gardening, music, cooking, and noncompetitive activities were viewed as feminine). The stability coefficients for these two variables are presented in Table 1.

TABLE 1. STABILITY OF HETEROSEXUAL INTERACTION AND SEX-ROLE ACTIVITIES FOR CHILDHOOD PERIODS II TO IV

Variable	II–III	II–IV	III–IV
21. Heterosexual interaction			
Boy			.40*
Girl			.21
Total			.29**
27. Opposite sex activities			
Boy	.79****	.38*	.82****
Girl	.71****	.38*	.56****
Total	.70****	.36**	.71****

* $p < .10$; two tails
** $p < .05$; two tails
*** $p < .01$; two tails
**** $p < .001$; two tails

Heterosexual interaction

The amount of contact with opposite sex peers was not highly stable over the years 6 to 14, although the pooled coefficient did reach statistical significance ($r = .29$; $p < .05$). This is not too surprising. There is a discontinuity between the child's heterosexual interactions during the latency period and early adolescence. During the years 6 to 10 most boys and girls coalesce into same sex groups and usually avoid contact with opposite sex peers. Those children who preferred to play with opposite sex peers during this time were often rejected by peers of the same sex. At age 12 to 13 these "gangs" break down, and a shift to a more heterosexual orientation emerges. It is not reasonable, therefore, to expect a high degree of stability for this variable over these years.

Opposite sex activity

The degree to which the child's sex-role interests remained masculine or feminine was quite stable over Periods II to IV. The boys who preferred music and reading to team athletics and mechanical interests—the girls who preferred climbing trees to baking cookies—retained this orientation from school entrance to adolescence. The child's sex-role identification, which has been one of the most important explanatory concepts for many of our findings, appears to be a relatively enduring aspect of the child's personality.

PREDICTION OF ADULT BEHAVIOR

The interview variables relevant to sexuality assessed erotic behavior and anxiety over sexuality as well as opposite sex activities.

Variable 21: Avoidance of premarital sexuality

This variable assessed S's reluctance to establish heterosexual relationships during late adolescence and early adulthood and the degree of inhibition placed on erotic behavior (necking, petting, coitus). Table 2 presents the correlations between the longitudinal variables and the avoidance of sexuality in adulthood.

TABLE 2. RELATION BETWEEN CHILDHOOD BEHAVIOR AND ADULT AVOIDANCE OF PREMARITAL SEXUALITY

Childhood Variable	Age	Males	Females	Pooled
Heterosexual interaction	6–10	.06	−.27	−.04
	10–14	−.47**	−.06	−.26*
Opposite sex activities	3–6	.49***	−.14	.25*
	6–10	.65****	.13	.47****
	10–14	.35*	.22	.31**

* $p < .10$; two tails
** $p < .05$; two tails
*** $p < .01$; two tails
**** $p < .001$; two tails

The relationship between preadolescent behavior and adult sexuality was more consistent for males than for females. *The boys who avoided dating during age 10 to 14 did not establish intimate heterosexual relationships or engage in erotic activity during late adolescence and adulthood.* Furthermore, failure to adopt traditional masculine interests among boys was also associated with avoidance of erotic behavior in adulthood. The boys who chose masculine interests and vocations and entered into competition activities during the early school years were the men who established frequent sexual relationships with women.

It was impossible to predict the character of adult sexuality in women from their preadolescent and early adolescent behavior. There are two reasons for this lack of continuity in the women.

First, frequency of dating is more dependent on opportunity in girls than in boys. Some of the girls in the present sample were the daughters of upper middle-class families. These girls were attending a small high school where very few upper middle-class boys were in attendance, and dating was infrequent for this group. Had the population of eligible male adolescents been larger, the dating behavior of this group might have been different.

Second, participation in erotic activity is more anxiety arousing for females than for males. The traditional ego ideal for women dictates inhibition of sexual impulses. The stronger sexual conflict in women would be expected to oppose expression of sexual behavior and attenuate the stability of this response system.

The tachistoscopic data gave some minimal support to the assumption that the women were more conflicted over sexuality than the men. The men accurately recognized the "beach scene" earlier than the women ($\chi^2 = 6.01; p < .05$). Furthermore, the women who avoided erotic activity as adults and heterosexual interaction during Period IV had the greatest difficulty recognizing the beach scene ($p < .01; < .05$ respectively).

For men, erotic behavior in adulthood was not associated with ease of recognition of either of the romantic scenes. However, failure to adopt the masculine traits of ambition, daring, and rebelliousness was associated with delayed recognition of the sexual scenes (i.e., the average recognition threshold for the two sex pictures). For example, recognition strivings in adulthood were correlated with early recognition of the romantic scenes ($r = .33; p < .05$). Conformity to adults for age 10 to 14 was predictive of late recognition ($r = .41; p < .05$), as was avoidance of potentially dangerous games (e.g., bodily contact sports, hunting) during Period IV ($r = .64; p < .01$). In sum, boys who adopted traditional masculine interests showed early recognition of the sexual scenes. Indeed, the adoption of these sex-role behaviors was a better predictor of recognition threshold than was the rating of sexual behavior. This finding is congruent with the fact that interest in masculine activities for age 6 to 10 was a better predictor of adult sexuality than was heterosexual behavior for Periods III or IV.

Occurrence of sexual behavior in the young male appears to be influenced by the degree to which the individual has adopted those characteristics advertised by the culture as masculine. To be athletic, competitive, and fearless are defining characteristics of the traditional male sex. Rejection of these attributes is associated with avoidance of premarital sexuality. Acceptance or rejection of traditional sex-role characteristics is less crucial in the occurrence of sexuality in adolescent and adult women.

Two contrasting cases illustrate the association between early masculine identification and an active seeking of heterosexual gratification during adolescence and adulthood.

Subject 2283 was the first-born son of a middle-class family and a boy who clearly showed a masculine orientation during the preschool years. As early as age 3 he was described as follows:

"In the nursery school S was extremely energetic. Even when he was pushing small cars around the floor he seemed to be putting the greatest possible force into it. He talked loudly and accompanied his car and train play with plenty of imitations of engine noises and whistles. Outside he ran around furiously some of the time and played fearlessly on the apparatus. He also played construction games in the sandpile. In the house, he built garages, roads, and usually used blocks in connection with cars or trains. He was interested in small locomotor toys and did the best building of any of the children. S was definitely the leader in the group. He was bright, original, and full of ideas."

Three years later a description of S was similar in flavor.

"S was strong, vigorous, agile, and quite capable on all the apparatus. He rode his bike, used the sand, the swings, and jungle gym in very dramatic play and competition. During routines S was independent and capable. With adults he usually tried to get his own way, and he required supervision when some desire was inconsistent with the requirements of adults. S was outstandingly curious, alert, and vocal. He could not stand to be out of anything and had to know, to run, to see, to examine, to question. He was impetuous and unrestrained in his vocalizations, interrupting others and arguing right through a peer's explanation. He indulged in a lot of competitive word-games in which he compared ability, possessions, hurled insults, challenges, experiences, and stories. Often he directed the best building and dramatic play that went on, and there was a strong interest and concern with construction of different sorts. To others in the group S appeared as aggressive, dominating, and rejecting. He had a tremendous drive to boss, to get things done his own way, and to tell everyone how to act."

When he was 7 years old he was observed at his elementary school. "S is a well-built, attractive looking youngster; a real little boy. When I saw him, he was building a barracks with blocks. There was a good deal of give and take between the children. S had built the barracks, and another boy built a torpedo boat. This quite naturally led to war-play. In a very short time all the children in the room were machine-gunning each other. S yelled to another boy, 'I'm the Japs and you're the Germans. No, what I mean is him and me are the Japs and you're the Americans. All guns turn this way.' "

At age 7½ his day-camp behavior combined the aggressiveness, dominance, and competitive gross-motor activity that characterize traditional male-role behavior.

"For S everything he does is excitable and highly competitive. He has a fund of physical energy. Bouncing, rushing around, wanting to do things, and a great deal of talk about his own abilities. For the races, he announced before hand that he was not going to do them and, yet, strained himself to the limit to try to win. He loves to play and exert himself physically but does not like to lose. His honesty in competitive situations is sketchy, not listening to the directions and seeing how much he can get away with. There is much compensatory clowning and bravado, and S might say, 'I let him beat me because I thought there would be more races and I could have beat him in there if I had wanted to.' While S is a terrific *alibi ike*, he would argue over every score he received. S would be a much better athlete if he did not try so very hard to win."

S started dating about age 12 and did an average amount of dating during high school. At 16 he began to go steady. He dated one girl frequently and consistently during his last two years of high school, and there were episodes of erotic activity. When S went to college, dating increased, and there were frequent occurrences of coital activity. Some of his comments during the interview follow.

E: "Can you tell me a little bit about your dating history?"
S: "I can give you almost a complete history, down to how many girls I have taken out."
E: "What about dating during college?"
S: "In my sophomore year I went on a rampage, I guess—I mean, I went out every weekend. For a while, different girls, then I would take out one girl

for 3 or 4 weeks and then another girl, usually for a semester, once a week or sometimes twice a week if I was dating two girls at the same time."

E: "Did you neck with them?"

S: "Of yes, a little bit, depending on the girl."

E: "Any intercourse?"

S: "Some. Do you mean on dates, premeditated dates? There weren't many girls I took out on a premeditated date that I didn't know I couldn't lay before I took them out. Some girls I know go; some girls I'm not sure about. Some girls I know don't. Those I wasn't sure about, I didn't—very few of them I ever laid."

E: "Did you try?"

S: "Well, most of the time I didn't try."

E: "This first group that you knew would lay, you took them out occasionally?"

S: "I would take them out to get laid."

E: "Only for that reason?"

S: "Yeh, but not very often, 'cause that's not my philosophy. I was, I can name about 60 girls that I have taken out on a premeditated basis."

E: "By premeditated you mean what?"

S: "I mean I've called them up in the middle of the week and said, 'Let's go out on Saturday night.' That's what I mean. I mean like when you walk into a bar and walk up to somebody and start dancing with them; now, that to me is not premeditated; that's what I mean."

E: "Have your intercourse experiences been with girls whom you always took out for this one purpose, or are there some girls whom you like and didn't take out specifically for sex?"

S: "Most of the girls that I have had intercourse with I have taken out purely for that purpose."

E: "Have there been exceptions?"

S: "Yes, there have been exceptions, a couple."

At the time of the interview S felt that he was in love with a girl he had known for several years. He was ambivalent about becoming engaged because his schooling was not completed.

Let us contrast this man with another first-born, middle-class boy who showed a much different pattern. This boy had difficulty assuming an aggressive, competitive, or power role during the preschool and early school years. During late adolescence and early adulthood he experienced strong anxiety over dating and the initiation of erotic activity.

Subject 2373

At 3 years of age S's nursery-school summary read:

"S is a pale, bleached-out looking child with blond hair, light blue eyes, and very little color in his face. He is tall, thin, and stoop-shouldered. He lacks compactness and sturdiness of muscle or body build. He gave the general impression of being gangling, and this was accentuated by the fact that he did not have good control over his body. During the entire nursery-school period S was uneasy. He was not relaxed and very dissatisfied. He showed tension in many ways. He has many mannerisms and nervous habits. In his use of materials, and in his approach to other children, S was almost constantly on edge. Whenever he was stimulated, he overreacted. His body tensed, his face showed some strain, and there were many excess movements. S sometimes would fall into a very deep lassitude and almost collapse. He would drop in a chair or swing inertly and become very difficult to arouse. He was not very purposeful or creative in his play, and he used materials socially.

At age 4 these traits were more firmly established.

"During this nursery-school period S was thin, tall, and stringy looking. He was rather wooden in his movements, resembling an unfinished marionette during his inactive periods. He seemed weary and empty of animation, like a child who lived perpetually indoors. He was an overly dressed boy, always very trim, and never approaching the usual group dishevelment at the end of the day. S was also able to sustain a thoroughly fatuous smile for long periods of time. S seemed to be on the sedentary side, and in most activities he showed no vigor."

At age 6 he was described as:

"Pasty-skinned, skinny, a loiterer, a slumper, and given either to frozen periods or taking queer gangly or stiff poses. He seemed less like a nursery-school child than a miniature caricature of an adolescent with self-consciousness and emotional difficulties getting in the way of whatever motor controls he might have. S was picked on a good deal, and much of his behavior invited teasing. When someone turned on him, he became helpless, cried, ran to an adult, or sat with a mute grin. He seemed to have no resistance against verbal attacks. S often commented that there was no reason for him to make anything because the other kids would break it. S did not seem to quite fit into the group. He was much like a 2-year-old in his reaction to pain and was helpless when someone else was hurt. In contrast to the interest of most boys in athletics or construction, S became interested in flowers. He was very careful as he picked them so that the stems wouldn't be hurt, sorting out a bunch of beautifully contrasting colors and making up names for the flowers. Hyacinths, for example, were, 'those sparkly, purply flowers.' He quickly caught on to the use of the magnifying glass and eagerly brought in specimens of flowers to examine. Occasionally he took delight in the dolls or tiny dishes when he thought no one was looking at him."

At 9 years of age he was interviewed, and the staff psychologist wrote the following summary:

"Throughout the interview S was in constant motion, sliding about in his chair, moving arms and legs, peering about the room. I asked him how he was doing in school and he said he had an 'A,' 'B,' 'C,' and two 'F's,' S shows a preoccupation with threats at night and still shows much fear. Ever since Christmas he has taken a pistol to bed with him, and for a long time he has taken several animals to bed: a bear, a chicken, and a panda. S said, 'Sometimes I get scared because everyone else is asleep. I get up and turn on the light and go to the bathroom. I get scared because everybody's asleep. Sometimes I think there's a man in the house and every night I close the venetian blinds.' "

The isolation from peers, the lack of interest in competitive sports, and the fear of peer aggression were apparent in the description of S at 11 years of age. The summary was written after a visit to S's school and talking with S's teacher.

"S has plenty of ability but does not use it. He has to be pressured all the time and does not volunteer very much. He is slow and seems to have no pep, steam, or temper. He fools around a great deal in class, fiddling with a little car, comic book, or daydreaming. S does not participate at all on the playground with the other boys. The teachers often find him in the schoolroom when he should be out on the playground with his peers. He does not seem to care about being active and would rather be by himself. He has become more interested in reading lately, and he likes books."

As an adult of 20 years S was tall, thin, and very tense. He was in college but was unsure about a career because of excessive doubts over his intellectual ability. He reported much tension and anxiety with girls and a strong reluctance to initiate erotic activity with them. He was afraid that a girl would reject him if he were to become sexually aggressive, and he usually waited for her to initiate any romance. He had never petted with a girl or experienced sexual intercourse. He disliked competitive situations and was thinking of teaching as a vocation.

These two cases illustrate the association between the failure to adopt traditional masculine behavior and apprehension over sexual activity.

The interpretations of the scene of the "couple on the beach" given by these two men reflect their differential conflict over sexuality.

On the first exposure at 0.01 seconds, the sexually aggressive subject replied:

"Male and female lying on the beach. They're necking. The female was in the front, the male was sort of laying behind her."

On the first exposure the second man replied:

"Looks like a couple of boys. They are on a trampoline, and they've been doing some stunts and they've fallen down. They are in the middle of the trampoline on top of each other."

On the third exposure he perceived the content correctly but placed the male in a passive posture in relationship to the woman. He reported:

"Well, it's a fella and his girl on the beach and they're laying there, and she's laying partly on top of him with her arm around him, and they could be talking or kissing. Well, it looks like they might be talking."

The easy availability of sexual associations for the sexually aggressive male is manifested in his blatantly sexual interpretations of two TAT stimuli that are not strongly suggestive of sexuality.

To picture 18GF (often seen as a person strangling a younger person), *S* replied:

"This is a scene from Peyton Place. The mother is scolding her daughter for being out in the woods with this fellow. In so many words, she is accusing her of having intercourse. Do I have an intriguing imagination or am I sexually inclined?"

To picture 4 (a man and woman looking forward), *S* reported:

"This is a picture of a guy in a whore house—the girl is trying to talk him into a higher price and he's holding out for a lower price. He wants to pay $3.00 and she wants $5.00."

The interpretations of these TAT scenes by the passive male were more conventional. To 18GF he said:

"I can't make out if it's a woman or man or either one. Looks like he's fainting. She's catching him. This one's falling, and the other one is catching her."

To card 4:

'Well, that pretty well applies to me right now. Say they have been going together for a long time and he's leaving and she wants him back—she doesn't want him to leave and they're breaking up."

Even to the modified ink blots, the preoccupation with sexuality was unambiguously expressed by the sexually aggressive subject. To ink blot stimulus 7 (bottom part of Plate VII) *S* replied:

"What we call a snatch, a vagina."

The sexually inhibited male offered a neutral response:
"Looks like a bell, the Liberty Bell."

It is not implied that the sexually aggressive subject necessarily had a stronger *desire* for sexual gratification than the sexually inhibited adult. Rather, it is suggested that one of the concomitants of maintaining a traditional masculine identification is a preoccupation with and an ostentatious display of sexual ideas. The individual gains support for his masculinity by announcing his concern with sexuality.

The men who, either out of choice or conflict, had not adopted the traditional masculine ego ideal were more conflicted over sexual urges, less likely to impose a sexual interpretation on ambiguous stimuli, and more reluctant to reveal to others their sexual associations. However, their desire for sexual gratification may have been as strong as that of the sexually aggressive adults.

The open advertisement of sexual behavior and ideation in a male is associated with a masculine sex-role identification. It should not necessarily be taken as an index of the intensity of motivation for sexual gratification.

Sex anxiety and repression of sexual ideas

These two variables are analogous to the variables, "aggression anxiety and repression of aggressive ideas" described in Chapter Four. The former assessed anxiety over anticipation or commission of sexual behavior. The latter evaluated denial of sexual thoughts and absence of any conscious concern with sexual gratification.

Table 3 presents the correlations between the child variables and sexual conflict in adulthood.

The pattern of correlations was similar to that found for the previous interview variable, with the results more striking for males than for females. *For males, failure to adopt masculine behavior during age 3 to 10 was predictive of high sex anxiety. For girls, sex-role interests were not highly related to adult sexual anxiety.* This supports the previous suggestion that practice of masculine activities by the adolescent girl (athletics, for example) is more independent of sex-role identification and sexual conflict in the female than are feminine interests in the male. The adolescent girl is allowed some masculine interests without violating her position as a female; the boy is not allowed to enter into traditionally feminine activities with as much psychic freedom.

TABLE 3. RELATION BETWEEN CHILDHOOD BEHAVIOR AND ADULT SEXUAL
CONFLICT

	Sex Anxiety			Repression of Sexuality		
Childhood Variable	Male	Female	Pooled	Male	Female	Pooled
Heterosexual interaction						
Age 6–10	.15	−.34*	−.02	−.01	−.18	−.08
Age 10–14	−.39*	.15	−.12	−.40*	−.04	−.13
Opposite sex activity						
Age 3–6	.41**	−.23	.12	.18	−.09	.00
Age 6–10	.61****	−.11	.34***	.30*	−.07	.12
Age 10–14	.18	−.01	.11	.02	.07	.04

    * p < .10; two tails
   ** p < .05; two tails
  *** p < .01; two tails
 **** p < .001; two tails

Interview Variable 24: Opposite sex interests

The interviewer also assessed the degree to which the adult's current activities were masculine in nature (athletics, hunting, fishing, gambling, concern with power roles) or feminine (music, reading, gardening, cooking, noncompetitive activities). Table 4 presents the correlations between childhood behavior and opposite sex interests in adulthood.

TABLE 4. RELATION BETWEEN CHILDHOOD BEHAVIOR AND OPPOSITE SEX
ACTIVITIES IN ADULTHOOD

Childhood Variable	Age	Male	Female	Pooled
Heterosexual interaction	6–10	.35*	−.04	.13
	10–14	−.05	−.32	−.11
Opposite sex activities	3–6	.54***	.10	.22*
	6–10	.63****	.44***	.52****
	10–14	.57***	.10	.37***

    * p < .10; two tails
   ** p < .05; two tails
  *** p < .01; two tails
 **** p < .001; two tails

The stability of these sex-typed activities was consistently high for the males, but not for females. Opposite sex interests during ages 6 to 10 correlated .63 ($p < .001$) for men and .44 ($p < .01$) for women with adult sex-typed activities. The sex-role content of the boys' play *as early as age 3 to 6* was predictive of adult sex-role interests ($r = .54$; $p < .01$). Competitiveness and involvement in mechanical, gross-motor, and aggressive games during the preschool years were prognostic of sex-role activities 20 years later. This association for men was the highest obtained between any behavior rated for age 3 to 6 and a related interview variable.

The degree to which an adolescent or adult male will adhere to traditional masculine values can be previewed during the preschool years, even before the boy comes into contact with the school environment. The extraordinary continuity of sex-typed traits is dramatic evidence of its importance in the individual's psychological development. These data, together with similar findings by others (Mussen, 1961), strengthen our conviction that the sex-role appropriateness of a behavior is a primary determinant of the probability of its assimilation into the individual's behavior repertoire.

One potentially important derivative of sex-role identification involves the adult's vocational choice. We compared the vocational choices of the 10 boys who were given the highest ratings on masculine activities during age 3 to 6, with the choices of the seven boys whose behavior was least masculine during the preschool period. The vocational choices of these two groups showed no overlap. Each of the 10 masculine boys had chosen traditional masculine careers (3 businessmen, 2 farmers, 2 athletic coaches, a carpenter, a machinist, and an engineer). Every one of the seven preschool boys who avoided gross-motor games and preferred sedentary, noncompetitive activities *chose an intellectual career* (3 secondary school teachers, a chemist, a biologist, a physicist, and a psychiatrist). The relationship between non-masculine behavior during age 3 to 6 and the selection of an intellectual career is related to the previously reported correlation (for males) between fear of physical harm for age 3 to 6 and adult concern with intellectual competence ($r = .50$; $p < .01$).

Moreover, the adult recreational pursuits of these two groups paralleled their career choices. The masculine men spent their time building amplifiers, working with machines, or on the athletic field. Art, music, and reading were the dominant pastime choices of the men who chose intellectual vocations.

The rating of opposite sex interests during age 3 to 6 was not significantly associated with the social class of the child's family. The correlations between education of the family and opposite sex interests ranged from .10 to .22. However, opposite sex activities during age 10 to 14 were more positively related to parental educational level. For boys, the correlations with parental education were .56 for father ($p < .01$) and .45 for mother ($p < .05$). The corresponding correlations for girls were .29 and .53 ($p < .01$) *Preadolescent boys and girls from lower middle-class backgrounds were more likely to adhere to traditional sex-role interests.* This finding is congruent with the fact that lower-class parents are more likely than middle-class ones to encourage traditional sex-typed traits (Kohn, 1959).

Although a preference for sex-typed activities during age 6 to 10 predicted similar adult interests for both sexes, the relationship over the childhood span 3 to 14 was better for men than for women. This is due, in part, to the fact that many girls with some masculine interests (sports, competitiveness) during the early school years dropped these behaviors and assumed the feminine roles of wife and mother after marriage. Other girls inhibited their masculine interests during adolescence in an attempt to increase their attractiveness to boys.

The unusual degree of persistence of masculine or feminine behavior in boys is related to the degree of passivity shown by the child during the first three years of life. Passivity (Variable 13) during age 0 to 3 was correlated with opposite sex activities in boys for ages 3 to 6 and 6 to 10 ($r = .68$; $p < .01$ and .36; $p < .10$, respectively). The passive girls, on the other hand, were feminine in their interests during ages 3 to 6 and 6 to 10 ($r = .18, .39$; $p < .05$). Thus adoption of traditional masculine traits may not simply be a function of the pattern of social reinforcements during the school years. It is possible that other variables—acting early in development—may give some direction to the sex-role identification the child eventually adopts. This point will be discussed in more detail in Chapter Nine.

Social class and sexual behavior

The relations between the longitudinal variables and the educational level of each parent were only significant for opposite sex activities during Periods III and IV. It has been noted that older boys with well-educated parents had less traditional masculine interests during age 10 to 14 than the boys from the less well-educated (lower-class) families. The girls with well-educated parents, on the other hand, had more masculine interests than the girls from less well-educated families. Table 5 presents the correlations between the educational level of each parent and the four adult variables.

TABLE 5. RELATION BETWEEN EDUCATIONAL LEVEL OF PARENT
AND SEXUAL BEHAVIOR IN ADULTHOOD

	Males		Females	
Adult Variable	Father	Mother	Father	Mother
Avoidance of sexuality	.36**	.39**	.06	.03
Sex anxiety	.25	.33**	.13	.17
Repression of sex	.21	.28*	—.15	—.19
Opposite sex activities	.33**	.39**	.46***	.49***

* $p < .10$; two tails
** $p < .05$; two tails
*** $p < .01$; two tails

The social class of the family is clearly related to the sex-typed interests of the adult. The higher the educational level of the family, the less likely was the individual to prefer the traditional attitudes appropriate to his or her sex-role. The upper middle-class men rejected orthodox masculine traits; the upper middle-class women rejected orthodox feminine traits.

Moreover, avoidance of premarital sexuality was much greater for men from well-educated families. This result agrees with Kinsey's (1948) finding that premarital intercourse was more frequent for lower-class than for middle-class men, and with a recent study of 200 psychiatric out-patients (McCulloch and Stewart, 1960). In both studies, occurrence of premarital coitus was inversely related to social-class status in men but independent of social class in women.

In the present sample, also, premarital sexual experience in women was relatively independent of their social-class standing. Since social class was correlated with sex-typed interests for men and women, the lack of association between social class and premarital sexual experience for women supports the previous suggestion that the child's sex-role identification is more directly related to overt sexual behavior in men than in women.

In sum, the frequency of heterosexual behavior in our men was positively associated with the adoption of a traditional masculine identification and lower middle-class standing. For women, sexual behavior was more independent of sex-typed interests and social-class background. It was more often a function of the desire and opportunity to establish a love relationship with a man.

SOCIAL INTERACTION ANXIETY

Most of the social interaction behaviors that have been considered up to now (e.g., dependency, aggression, dominance, competitiveness, and sexuality) are directed toward the attainment of a specific goal. This section deals with the stability of social interaction anxiety—the degree of spontaneity or inhibition that accompanies interaction with others. The occasional perception of threat in an interpersonal situation is a common experience. However, when an individual is continually apprehensive about meeting and talking with others, he is likely to withdraw from these activities. In the organization of western society, a prepotent tendency to withdraw from others carries some liability as far as heterosexual and vocational adjustment are concerned.

Young children often show signs of fear in the presence of strangers, and it would be of interest to determine if these childhood reactions are prodromal signs of later social anxiety. The longitudinal variables that were rated dealt with inhibition, anxiety, and withdrawal in social situations, in contrast to a spontaneous and uninhibited orientation to others. The definitions of the five child variables follow.

Variable 23: Anxiety with the Fels visitor

This was a highly specific variable, rated only for Periods I and II, that assessed anxiety in the presence of the Fels home visitor. The major sources of evidence included sudden crying when the visitor arrived, withdrawal or freezing, and seeking proximity to the mother or a familiar adult.

Variable 24: Anxiety in novel situations

This variable, also rated only for Periods I and II, assessed anxiety displayed when the child was in a novel situation (other than a home visit). The indexes of anxiety were the same as those described for the previous variable. Some typical novel situations included visits to Fels for examinations, initial visits to the nursery school, or entrance into elementary school.

Variable 31: Social spontaneity

This variable, rated for all four periods, evaluated the child's responsiveness and affective ease with peers and adults (i.e., laughing, smiling, eagerness to interact) in contrast to signs of inhibition and shyness in interpersonal situations.

Variable 89: Expectancy of peer rejection

This variable, rated for Periods III and IV, evaluated behavior which suggested that the child anticipated rejection from peers. Some evidence included statements that peers did not like the subject, absence of friends, and manifestation of reserve and constriction with peers. The final child variable was rated only for Period IV.

Variable 102: Withdrawal from social interaction

This variable assessed the child's tendency to withdraw from social situations with peers. Typical evidence included reluctance to attend peer functions and remaining on the sidelines in group situations.

Table 6 presents the stability of the child variables for Periods I to IV.

TABLE 6. STABILITY OF SOCIAL INTERACTION BEHAVIOR FOR CHILDHOOD PERIODS I TO IV

Variable	I–II	I–III	I–IV	II–III	II–IV	III–IV
23. Anxiety Fels visitor						
Boys	.44**					
Girls	.05					
Total	.22*					
24. Anxiety novel situations						
Boys	.60****					
Girls	.20					
Total	.41****					
31. Spontaneity						
Boys	.59***	.46**	−.45	.57****	.00	.57***
Girls	.47***	.16	.12	.37**	.00	.53***
Total	.54****	.30**	.03	.48****	.00	.55****
89. Expect peer rejection						
Boys						.54**
Girls						.47***
Total						.48****

* $p < .10$; two tails
** $p < .05$; two tails
*** $p < .01$; two tails
**** $p < .001$; two tails

Variables 23 and 24: Anxiety with the Fels visitor and in novel situations

Situational fear and inhibition during the first six years were moderately stable for boys but not for girls. This sex difference was not anticipated, and no simple explanation comes to mind. The boys who were protected by their mothers during age 0 to 3 showed more fear of the Fels visitor during Period I than the nonprotected boys ($r = .67$; $p < .001$). This relationship did not occur for girls.

Variable 31: Spontaneity

This variable showed moderate stability for boys over the first 10 years and for girls over the first six years. The stability coefficient for Periods III to IV was equally high for both sexes. However, social spontaneity during age 10 to 14 was unrelated to spontaneity during the first six years for both sexes. Apparently some children showed a marked change in degree of social inhibition between the preschool and adolescent years. Thus it was not until age 10 or 11 that social anxiety became stable for both sexes and, as we shall see in a moment, predictive of adult behavior.

Since expectancy of peer rejection was related to timidity and apprehension with others, it is not surprising that expectancy of rejection was also stable for both sexes over the years 6 to 14.

PREDICTION OF ADULT BEHAVIOR

One interview variable assessed adult inhibition in social situations.

Interview Variable 29: Social Anxiety

This variable assessed the degree of tension and discomfort the individual experienced in social situations: the degree to which he approached interaction with strangers with caution and apprehension due to an expectancy of rejection. Table 7 presents the correlations between the childhood variables and the adult rating.

Inhibition and apprehension with peers during the early school years were predictive of social anxiety in adulthood for both sexes. For boys, the beginnings of this source of anxiety were traceable to the first three

TABLE 7. RELATION BETWEEN CHILDHOOD BEHAVIOR AND ADULT
SOCIAL INTERACTION ANXIETY

Childhood Variable	Age	Male	Female	Total
Anxiety Fels visitor	0–3	.29	−.33	−.06
	3–6	.30*	.25	.25**
Anxiety novel situation	0–3	.07	−.08	.06
	3–6	.53***	.02	.34***
Spontaneity	0–3	−.45**	.35	.01
	3–6	−.27	.09	−.06
	6–10	−.41**	−.30*	−.38***
	10–14	−.50**	−.56***	−.53****
Expect rejection	6–10	.18	.09	.06
	10–14	.41*	.48**	.45***
Withdrawal from social interactions	10–14	.65***	.54**	.64****

   * $p < .10$; two tails
  ** $p < .05$; two tails
 *** $p < .01$; two tails
**** $p < .001$; two tails

years of life. An inhibited and nonspontaneous approach to strangers during Period I was associated with social anxiety in adult men
($r = .45$; $p < .05$). For girls, however, this relationship did not emerge
until Period III, for spontaneity during the first six years was unrelated
to adult social anxiety. In sum, lack of spontaneity and social withdrawal during pre- and early adolescence were predictive of adult social
anxiety.

The developmental observations on one of the men document the
continuity of social anxiety.

Subject 045

S was the second-born child of a lower middle-class family. He usually
showed distinct signs of fear when he came to Fels for a physical or
mental examination, or for the nursery-school sessions. When he came
for his examination at 2 years of age, the following summary was written.

"S gave the appearance of being frightened at first. When taken
downstairs for the physical examination following the mental test, S

would not allow the doctor to take his hand to guide him. He was shy and remained very timid throughout the procedure. He cried when the examination began and cried at new items in the procedure. He was suggestible and responded to distraction. He recovered quickly from his tears, was attentive to the toys given him, and was interested in their construction. Although the mother was present during the mental test that preceded the physical exam, S was shy and apprehensive."

At 4 years of age S attended the Fels nursery school for the first time. His initial reactions to this new setting were characterized by timidity and caution. The following notes were written after the three-week period.

"This was S's first visit to the nursery school and probably his first time away from home for any length of time. It took the entire period for S to make the adjustment. S was very apprehensive and insecure during his first days. He cried a lot and stood about looking sad in the interim between his howls. Initially he did not enter into any of the play but was entirely concerned with his unhappiness. He objected to coming and cried in the car. Once at the school he stood about weeping or sobbing and followed the teacher around for comfort. He was not in a tantrum of anger, but appeared to be showing fear and apprehension. For the first two weeks S made no attempts to get into any of the groups. He was shy with the other children and timid with the new equipment."

"During the period he was highly emotional and did not try to control his fears at all. He was somewhat sober and depressed most of the time, although he got friendly and happy toward the very end. He showed no anger, little jealousy, and no excitement. With adults he was very conforming and obedient. Even though unhappy, he was not especially rebellious."

One year later, at 5 years of age, S again attended the nursery school for a three-week period. His behavior continued to reflect caution and apprehension.

"S was one of the gentlest creatures in the group. He seemed to be like a delicate plant in the vivid world of the nursery school, meekly and solemnly acquiescing to whatever other children or adults suggested. He would often stand on the edge of the group with wide eyes watching the others. Only as the group dispersed would he get to the front and examine the object the group might have been playing with. At times S would stand helplessly crying and shielding his face while he was pelted with snowballs. S spoke in an exceedingly low voice, barely above a whisper, and never really laughed outright or came near a shout. The words he spoke were spaced with long pauses, and the last words of the sentence were even softer than the first, sometimes drifting into silence. His crying was soft too, with heavy sobs in his chest. S's behavior was much more characteristic of a 2- or 3-year-old, showing immense ranges over the month. He went from tears and hiding in the corner in the beginning of the nursery-school period to a gradual staring and sideline participation. Shyness is a word that really seems to fit him; he has vulnerability to any contact with new people. He would hang his head and edge off when any strange adult was present or give apprehensive glances toward the children in the other groups. He was slow to warm up to the materials and would look at them from a distance, gradually finger them, and when the sanction for their use was established, he would then use them with some gusto. S was the only one in his group to react, as the younger children frequently do, to a change of cars or to a change of drivers. He would cry and resist going in the car until an older girl led him. His hard crying occurred only the first day, but tears came sporadically during the whole first week of nursery-school attendance. His reliance on a familiar person to carry through an unfamiliar situation showed in the car episodes and in any experimental situations. During one experimental session, when he was taken from the room, he came back and saw the nursery-school room deserted. He began to cry, but once I got him playing contentedly with me, he came up willingly again to the experimental room. He was not frightened as long as I was with him. S was quietly and consistently conforming, never laying down the law for others or being shocked at the transgressions of other peers. He did what was expected of him immediately and without supervision. Sometimes with adults there was a quality of extra politeness in his obedience."

When he entered school at 6 years of age, there was occasional crying during the first half-year. His older sister was attending the same school, and he followed her about during the initial month of school. The following notes were written after a visit to the home soon after S had started school.

"The mother says that S would rather be at home than with people, and his shyness is very slow to wear off. Last spring at a big family picnic at the school, where all the children and families had attended, the mother suddenly recognized that S was gone and couldn't find him. They finally discovered that he had gone home, changed his clothes, and was quietly playing in his own yard."

When S visited Fels for an examination at 7 years of age, he was still socially apprehensive.

"S was still on the subdued side, although a less shadowy person than he had been at nursery school the year before. His voice is more audible than it was and his movements less limp. In the morning he cried a little, with the subdued swallowing of tears that he often shows in a new situation. The mental tester reported that he was quite pleasant and cheerful. When he was tested in psychophysiology, he was a little stiff. He lay flat on his bed, quite silent, rolling his big brown eyes. When he was downstairs playing, he just stood around for the first 10 minutes, looking over the familiar rooms but touching nothing. When he went to lunch with another child and a staff member, he didn't know what he wanted to eat but ate what was put in front of him."

During subsequent observations in the following year at home, in the nursery school, and in his public school setting, S seemed afraid of interaction with other boys. During a recess period at school, S typically stayed inside and played with the girls while the rest of the boys were outside running around. When called on to recite, the observer noted, "his wee, small voice could scarcely be heard; he missed so many words, he was asked to reread the last half of the page."

At 8 years of age S attended the Fels day camp.

"S is still a shrinking violet, avoiding any situations where he might be hurt, by physical contact with others, hard objects, high places, etc. He seems to show a social diffidence and an unsureness, and these two things reinforce each other. The first morning S disappeared from the group and was discovered all alone in the front yard quietly sobbing to himself. He explained his presence there in terms of a sore foot, and while he had, in fact, hurt his foot, his generalized discomfort at the newness of the day-camp situation probably reinforced the pain and reduced him to tears. He was continually ignored or shoved around by the more energetic and outspoken children. In any close contact situation, such as a crowded car, S completely withdrew and became self-effacing."

When S was 10 years old, he was interviewed by a staff psychologist, who wrote the following summary.

"S was very quiet and very cooperative during the physical examination and hardly said a word. He warmed up a little afterwards and talked in a friendly way but still without much spontaneity. He talked about school and had a bright smile when he mentioned his teacher, whom he likes very much. He prefers English the best and has a desire to become a school teacher. His general behavior during the interview was placid and rather feminine."

At 16 years of age S was again interviewed.

E: "What are some ways in which you would like to be different from the way you are now, some of the things you would change about yourself?"

S: "I'd like to be more forward, I mean, to be able to meet people and talk."

E: "Any other ways that you would like to change?"

S: "I'd like to feel like I could take on responsibilities which I don't. I don't feel like—I don't feel self-confident. *That's it in a nutshell,* self-confidence."

S was 20 years old when he was seen for the adult interview. He was thin and slight of build, with a bony, pale face. He looked more like an adolescent than a young adult. He spoke in a very low, high-pitched voice, and he was uneasy and tense during the three interviews. He was restless and very eager to please and to cooperate with the interviewer. At the time of the interview he had completed several years of college. As he indicated during preadolescence, he was still interested in becoming a teacher. He had made few friends at college, and he habitually expected rejection and aloofness from authority figures as well as peers. He was tense in his interactions with others, and he had intense feelings of personal inadequacy. Excerpts from the adult interview reveal his extreme social anxiety.

E: "Did you tend to be afraid of your boss on the job when he came around?"

S: "Yeah, I was kinda afraid of him."

E: "What about this fellow you are working with now? Do you feel relaxed with him, or tense?"

S: "No, I don't feel relaxed with him. I just as leave he's not around."

E: "You feel tense when he's around?"

S: "I'm not afraid of him, see; I just don't like to have him around. That other guy down there; at first I couldn't talk to him, ah—not at all, but it's getting a little bit better now."

E: "What about Dr. _____; the man that you worked for in college? Did you feel tense when you were with him?"

S: "It's a funny thing; I wasn't exactly at ease with him, but he was nice and I really liked him and I still do. I think I am in awe with him. You know, he was a big professor, something that I'd like to be, and I was really never friendly with professors. Well, I was really never friendly with any school teachers."

E: "Did you talk much in classes?"

S: "Well, that all depends on the professor. In Dr. _____ class I always had my mouth open, but in other classes—I never said a word."

E: "Why was that? Because you had no questions or because you just didn't want to say anything?"

S: "I don't know, I just didn't want to talk. In history I never said a word unless he asked me."

E: "If you ever had any questions, did you go up after class or during office hours to ask professors about your work."

S: "I didn't do that. I don't know if I could do it yet or not."

E: "Have you ever thought about doing it and decided not too?"

S: "Yeah."

E: "Why did you not go?"

S: "I don't think I would. I never knew professors, any professors that you would say personally, except Dr. _____. Well, of course, I asked him things 'cause I worked with him, but, ah—not any of the others, like Dr. _____. I wanted to talk to him, and I think if I had talked to him, my problems would have been solved."

E: "Why didn't you talk to him?"

S: "I don't know; I couldn't. He had such a way about him that I couldn't get my point across. He would persuade his opinion on me. He would, and I don't want his opinion. I mean he would try to tell me that he was right and I'm wrong and believe me he's right. He had a way about him that my opinion had no value. It was like going in and talking to a blank wall. He would have such a better argument than I would that I would lose, that's what I thought anyway."

E: "Who do you feel more comfortable with, more relaxed with, men or women?"

S: "Older women I don't like, older men, ah—too. Because, you know, they don't talk about the same things I do. Older women don't either—I—I couldn't go in a room with an older woman and talk to her."

E: "How about people your own age? With whom do you feel more comfortable, boys or girls?"

S: "Boys. I don't talk to girls much. I mean, I couldn't go up to a strange girl and talk to her as well as I could a strange boy. But if I know the girl, then I can talk to her."

E: "Can you tell me about your friends, the kind of friendships you have?"

S: "Well, you know, I don't think I have any close friends. When I came home from college, any friends I had in high school were gone, and—ah— I didn't have any people that were more than acquaintances, they weren't close friends. A couple of people that I work with are classified as friends more than acquaintances, but not what I would call a close friend. When I was in school I had, oh, three real close friends and a lot of acquaintances, _____ was a very close friend."

E: "What made you and _____ such close friends?"

S: "Like I said before, he's like me. Neither one of us was very good in sports and it seemed like everyone else was, and I envied them."

E: "You say you envied these other people and he didn't?"

S: "He did. Oh, I don't know if he did or not; I don't know if he cared. But I did. I mean, I'd like to have been good sportswise, but, ah, he wasn't either. You see, we had to go someplace else. I couldn't go with the gang of boys and talk about sports and, ah, there didn't seem to be so many places to go, and I like to talk about books that I've read that other people have read and, ah, argue about 'em. But I couldn't do that with very many people. That's the way I like to talk."

E: "Could you do that with _____?"

S: "No, he didn't read books, but there were a few more people on campus that I could argue with. But, yet he would listen to me and give me his ideas if he had read the book. But we could talk about serious things."

E: "Was there something else about him personally, another reason that might account for the fact that you and he were close friends?"

S: "Well, in the first place, when I first got to know him, we both didn't know any people. It was hard for us to get to know any people, and I sat beside him in class, see, and that's how I got to know him. We didn't know anyone, and it was hard for both of us to get to know people. I think it was even harder—more hard for him to get to know people than it was even for me. Because he lived off campus and it's extra hard then. He didn't know many people and I didn't know anyone and—so we just sorta went together."

E: "In college were you the kind of person who actively sought to make a lot of friends?"

S: "No, I didn't make a lot of friends."

E: "Was that out of choice or because of no time?"

S: "It's probably cause I didn't know how; I couldn't. In the dorm we were in sections and I was in section 5. I lived with these guys, and I know all of them real well, but I was hardly on speaking terms with some of them in the other sections. I have to be with people a long time before I get to know them. I just couldn't go up to a person and enter into a conversation with him, even if I knew him."

E: "Why not?"

S: "I don't know."

E: "Would you say that you feel uncomfortable in this sort of situation?"

S: "I wouldn't have been if I had known all of them. If I had known all of them, I could have gone up to them. If there were several that I didn't know and they wanted to talk, then I did."

E: "What would you be thinking or feeling that would prevent you from doing this?"

S: "Um (pause) I think mostly it was—(long pause) you know, I think it was mostly that maybe I kept thinking that they didn't want me in their group."

E: "You anticipated that they didn't want you?"

S: "Uh-huh."

E: "To join them?"

S: "I think that was it. You know, I always thought that someone should ask me to do something instead of me offering to do it. You know, like, if they had asked me to come in the group, I'd have gone willingly. But I wouldn't have just gone up by myself."

E: "Are you still like that today?"

S: "Same way. I try to change, but I can't. I mean, I'd like to go up and be able to talk to people that I don't even know, but I can't."

E: "You feel uncomfortable when you're with strange people?"

S: "I think it's because I try too hard to think of what to say. They say that you don't, but you've got to say something—you can't stand there like an ox. People talk about me and say how much I talk. But I talk only when I know the people real well. Then I can—you know, but not with strangers, with strangers I don't talk at all. Same way with eating in the cafeteria. If I would have to sit at a table with no one I knew well, I wouldn't say a word. Last year I worked in the cafeteria and—uh—so I got down there on Thursday night on the third shift, and I saved the whole table for my friends. They all came there to sit and they'd wait for me. Maybe I should've got out and met other people, but I liked it that way."

E: "Did you ever look forward to meeting new people or are you rather indifferent?"

S: "Now, you know, I have such mixed emotions about that. Now, I want to meet them, but it's difficult to meet them. And sometimes I'd rather avoid it."

These excerpts capture the chronic social anxiety this man feels in interpersonal interactions. The enduring social inhibition exhibited by this particular man provides some flesh to the correlation of .53 between anxiety in novel situations during age 3 to 6 and social anxiety in adulthood.

There is no relation, however, between preschool and adult social anxiety among women. One *post hoc* explanation for this sex difference rests on the following assumptions. The basis for social acceptance (or rejection) for boys remains rather constant from the preschool years through adulthood. In order to gain peer acceptance the boy must be competent in gross-motor activities, capable of retaliation when attacked, and generally autonomous and counterphobic in the face of frustrations. Absence of these masculine characteristics predisposes the boy to rejection by both males and females during adolescence and adulthood. Since passivity and nonmasculine interests are highly stable for boys from school entrance through adolescence, we would expect that the anticipation of social rejection (which is a likely consequent of passivity and nonmasculine interests) would also be an enduring disposition.

The bases for social acceptance among girls, on the other hand, are more varied and do not emerge until late childhood. Attractiveness or intelligence facilitates popularity and leads to confidence in interpersonal relations. These characteristics do not emerge as clear assets until the school years. Thus it should be more difficult to predict adolescent and adult social anxiety from preschool interaction patterns for women. A study of those girls who showed marked shifts in level of social anxiety from Period II to adulthood confirms this hypothesis. There were six girls who showed a major shift from high anxiety during age 3 to 6 to low anxiety during adulthood. All of them were quite attractive as adults, and five of the six had better than average academic records in high school and college.

Three girls shifted from minimal anxiety during preschool years to unusually high social inhibition as adults. All three were unattractive as adolescents and adults. One of them had recently left college in an acute anxiety attack; the remaining two did poorly in high school and felt intellectually inadequate.

Social class and social interaction anxiety

The degree of timidity in social situations during the first 10 years was generally unrelated to the educational level of the child's family, although the boys with high anxiety in novel situations for age 3 to 6 came from families with lower levels of education. The correlations with parental and maternal education were $-.47$ ($p < .05$) and $-.39$ ($p < .05$), respectively. The corresponding correlations for girls were $+.07$ and $+.01$.

There was a moderately high correlation between educational level of each parent and the girls' social spontaneity during age 10 to 14 ($r = .40$; $p < .05$). Spontaneity at adolescence was independent of social-class standing for the boys. Adult social anxiety was unrelated to the educational level of the family; the correlations ranging from $-.15$ to $+.12$.

Summary

People comprise the most relevant set of stimulus objects to which we react. When social objects elicit anxiety, the individual's freedom for productive and satisfying behavior is considerably restricted. A perception of others as threatening has its historical roots in the early school years and, in selected cases, even earlier in the developmental sequence. The distorting lenses through which adults view their social environment apparently acquire their astigmatic character long before the individual has sampled a wide variety of social objects. The child's labeling of people as cruel or kind, rejecting or accepting, resists change to a remarkable degree.

COMPULSIVITY

Ever since Freud introduced the phrase obsessive-compulsive neurosis into the channels of psychological communication, students of child development have attended to evidence of compulsive habits in young children. Since these habits are strong in some adults and notoriously resistant to alteration, it might be expected that they are established early in development.

Ritualistic attempts at order and cleanliness are not uncommon during childhood. Repeated washing of hands after minimal soiling, the careful piling of blocks in a corner, and the reluctance to smear with fingerpaints seem to reflect anxiety over dirt and disarray. The longitudinal material was used to rate one variable related to compulsivity. This variable was rated for all four age periods.

Variable 26: Compulsivity

This variable evaluated the child's concern with neatness, cleanliness, order in his environment, and preciseness in working with materials. Table 8 presents the stability of this behavior over the four longitudinal periods.

TABLE 8. STABILITY OF COMPULSIVITY OVER LONGITUDINAL PERIODS I TO IV

Variable	I–II	I–III	I–IV	II–III	II–IV	III–IV
Compulsivity						
Boy	.62**	.47**	.72**	.61****	.39*	.73****
Girl	−.12	.34	.32	.52****	.27	.61****
Total	.27*	.38**	.51***	.55****	.40***	.69****

* $p < .10$; two tails
** $p < .05$; two tails
*** $p < .01$; two tails
**** $p < .001$; two tails

Compulsive habits were moderately stable for boys over all four longitudinal periods, and the stability coefficient for the pooled sample increased linearly with age. For the Period III to IV comparison, the pooled coefficient was +.69 ($p < .001$). Over the first six years, however, compulsivity was less stable for girls than for boys. For the Period I to II comparison, the difference between the boys' and girls' correlations was statistically significant ($p < .05$).

One plausible explanation for this sex difference rests on the assumption that habits of neatness and cleanliness are encouraged for almost all preschool girls but only for a proportion of preschool boys. That is, mothers will be less tolerant of dirt and disarray in the behavior of their daughters than in their sons. The boy is permitted greater license to continue practicing the habits he has adopted by age 3. If he happens to be concerned with order and cleanliness, this disposition will be accepted; but so will the converse. Girls will be pressured, however, to become clean, orderly, and neat. This pressure will necessarily reduce the stability of this variable during the first five or six years. One half of the girls rated for both Periods I and II were classified as more compulsive for age 3 to 6 than for age 0 to 3. Moreover, four of the five girls who showed the greatest increase in compulsivity from Period I to II came from traditional middle-class homes where cleanliness was considered "next to Godliness."

PREDICTION OF ADULT BEHAVIOR

The interviewer rated two relevant variables.

Interview Variable 30: Compulsivity

This variable assessed the subject's need for order in his possessions; his tendency to be unusually neat in the organization of his clothes, tools, records, financial receipts, etc.

Interview Variable 31: Impulsivity

This variable assessed the degree of impulsivity, in contrast to caution and vacillation, in decision-making situations (e.g., choice of college and career, major purchases). Table 9 presents the correlations between childhood compulsivity and these two adult traits.

TABLE 9. RELATIONSHIP BETWEEN CHILDHOOD BEHAVIOR AND ADULT COMPULSIVITY AND IMPULSIVITY

Variable	Age	Compulsivity			Impulsivity		
		Males	Females	Pooled	Males	Females	Pooled
Compulsivity	0–3	.08	.02	.06	.07	.02	.02
	3–6	.25	−.03	.11	−.36*	.17	−.06
	6–10	.18	.00	.07	−.23	.00	−.06
	10–14	−.13	.18	.05	.05	.16	.11

* $p < .10$; two tails

Compulsive habits in childhood were not highly related to compulsivity or caution in adulthood for either sex. The only relation that even approached borderline significance involved impulsivity in adult men. The adult men who vacillated with decisions were rated as more compulsive during age 3 to 6 ($r = .36$; $p < .10$).

Compulsivity is one of the few variables we have considered that has not shown moderately high stability from Period III or IV to adulthood. This lack of continuity could be due, in part, to the fact that the nursery-school and day-camp settings were not the best places to observe the private rituals that the child may practice in the solitude and familiarity of his own home. The childhood ratings may not be sensitive indexes of this trait. Moreover, the interviewer experienced more difficulty in making this rating than he did for most of the other adult variables.

Finally, the definition used in rating adult compulsivity was restrictive in scope, for it only assessed compulsive handling of personal possessions (clothes, tools, papers). This restriction may have attenuated the stability coefficients, especially for the men. Of the boys who were rated as highly compulsive in childhood, only about one-half remained compulsive in their personal habits. The remaining half were minimally concerned with order in their personal possessions. However, these men chose vocations that required order and precision (e.g., physicist, engineer, geneticist, mechanic, newspaper editor). These vocational choices may have served as an adequate outlet for compulsive needs. The men who were compulsive neither as children nor as adults chose vocations requiring less concern with order (e.g., business, elementary school teaching, and athletics—job situations not necessarily requiring a compulsive orientation). Perhaps if we had evaluated the degree to which the adults' work situation required a compulsive attitude, the stability coefficients might have been higher.

The suggestive relation, for males, between childhood compulsivity during age 3 to 6 and adult vacillation and reflection in problem situations is consonant with the hypothesis that a need for order reflects fear of an unpredictable environment, and leads to an attempt to control potential environmental dangers. If the environment is viewed as threatening, the individual may be reluctant to make impulsive decisions. For a commitment to action may lead to dangerous consequences.[1] Thus vacillation, like ritualistic hand washing, can reflect a need for control over a potentially dangerous environment.

For the women, compulsivity showed no evidence of stability, perhaps because the roles of wife and mother ordinarily call for order and neatness. One group of females who were not compulsive as children became highly compulsive when they married. A second group of wives and mothers seemed to be rebelling against the extreme compulsivity they showed during childhood and early adolescence.

Social class and compulsivity

Compulsivity during childhood or adulthood was unrelated to the girls' social class. The correlations between educational level of each parent and compulsivity or impulsivity during adulthood were close to zero and ranged from −.12 to +.11.

Compulsivity among the adult men was also independent of social-class background (correlations ranged from −.07 to +.04), but there was a slight positive relationship between educational level of the father and compulsivity among boys for age 3 to 6 ($r = .44$; $p < .05$).

Summary

Compulsivity was the first variable to show high stability during Periods III to IV and minimal relationships with analogous adult behaviors. There are several possible interpretations of this discontinuity, aside from the obvious one that this trait is, in fact, not highly stable. We favor the possibility that the restrictive definition of the adult compulsive variable plus the greater difficulty in reliably assessing this behavior during the interview were responsible for the low and equivocal stability coefficients.

NURTURANCE

The attempt to help, encourage, and display concern for the welfare of younger siblings and peers is a potential index of the degree to which the child has identified with a nurturant adult role. Since the child views the maternal role as primarily nurturant in character, it might be anticipated that acts of assistance and solace toward other children might reflect the adoption of a variety of socialized behaviors that characterize the adult female role.

Variable 86: Nurturance

One variable was rated for Periods III and IV. It assessed the degree to which the child spontaneously gave assistance, sympathy, or showed concern for siblings or peers when the latter had difficulty in a task, or requested help or comfort.

This variable showed no stability over the period 6 to 14 years of age. The correlations for the Period III to IV comparison were .25 and −.05 for males and females, respectively.

About one third of the girls shifted from high nurturance for Period III to low nurturance for Period IV. The girls who showed this change became concerned with their attractiveness to boys during early adolescence, and this increased narcissism was associated with a decreased nurturant attitude. A smaller group of more aggressive girls shifted from low nurturance during 6 to 10 to high nurturance during 10 to 14 years of age. The degree of shift for the boys was less marked.

PREDICTION OF ADULT BEHAVIOR

There was no adult interview variable that was directly analogous to childhood nurturance. In order to assess the relationship between childhood nurturance and adult behavior, we selected the major variables from the four socialization areas described in the previous chapters: dependency, aggression, sexuality, and achievement. Appendix 4 presents the correlations between nurturance for Period III or IV and the interview variables related to these four areas.

Nurturance during age 6 to 10 was associated with high aggression anxiety in both sexes (i.e., low retaliatory aggression, a high threshold for anger arousal, high aggression anxiety). *Nurturance during age 10 to 14,* on the other hand, was associated with *low* aggression anxiety in adult women and low sexual anxiety in both sexes.

Thus, nurturance during age 6 to 10 appears to have a different significance for later development than nurturance during 10 to 14 years of age, especially for the females. It is possible that Period III and Period IV nurturance are the products of different sets of forces and, like Period I and Period II mastery, have different meanings during development.

PHYSICAL HARM ANXIETY

The development of anxiety over potentially dangerous objects and situations and the avoidance of activities that may lead to bodily injury are characteristic of the behavior of many young children. Fear of darkness, lightning, thunder, and large animals, as well as apprehension over climbing jungle gyms or entering into bodily contact play, are some of the more common evidences of this source of anxiety.

During the first year of life, sudden and unexpected changes in the external environment lead to a reaction that resembles fear. By the time the child enters school, however, many of his fears are closely related to objects and events that can cause bodily harm (Dunlop, 1951; England, 1946; Jersild, Markey and Jersild, 1933). When he is directly questioned about sources of fear, the child names most frequently dangerous animals, accidental injury, being struck by a peer, ghosts, and witches. When school-age children were asked to draw the most important event in their lives, one third of the drawings illustrated fearful experiences (England, 1946).

The conditions that nourish the acquisition of school-age fears are, of course, multiple. Specific parental warnings about dangerous objects provide one route by which fears are established. An oversolicitous mother, constantly exaggerating the potential dangers of the outside world, will impress her child with the probability of bodily damage. However, the frequency and intensity of irrational fears of ghosts, witches, and the dark suggest the possible symbolic meaning of these fears.

The traditional interpretation of children's irrational fears has been that feared objects represent parental punishment; they symbolize expected adult retaliation for the contemplation or commission of prohibited acts. For example, guilt over hostility toward the parents is presumed to lead to an expectation of punitive retaliation. These expectations may find expression in the exaggerated fear of injury at the hands of the external environment. The cross-cultural research of Whiting and Child (1953) supports this point of view.

Childhood fears might be regarded, therefore, as an index of guilt over aggressive or sexual motives or the product of a close tie to an oversolicitous mother who exaggerated environmental dangers.

During the first two age periods, one variable was used to assess signs of general fearfulness over potential bodily harm. During Periods III and IV, two variables were rated. The first dealt with avoidance of dangerous activities; the second with irrational fears and phobias. The definitions of these three variables follow:

Variable 7: Anxiety over bodily harm

This variable, rated for Periods I and II, evaluated the degree of apprehension over possible injury, sickness, or bodily harm. The specific behaviors used in making this rating included (a) fear of and avoidance of cars, animals, the dark, and activities that were potentially dangerous and (b) excessive disturbance over injury or illness.

Variable 70: Irrational fears

This variable, rated for Periods III and IV, assessed the intensity and frequency of irrational fears and phobias (e.g., the dark, strange animals, large objects), the occurrence of nightmares, and excessive concern with the health and illness of the self or others.

Variable 90: Avoidance of dangerous activity

This variable was also rated for Periods III and IV. It assessed the child's avoidance of games and activities that involved the risk of physical injury (e.g., contact sports, climbing, swimming).

Table 10 presents the stability coefficients for the three variables over the first four longitudinal periods.

Fear of bodily harm was relatively stable over the first 10 years for both sexes, and the coefficients for Periods II to III and III to IV were moderately high. Fear of harm during the preschool years was predictive of avoidance of potentially dangerous activities during age 10 to 14.

It is interesting to note that the presence of irrational fears was more stable for girls (Variable 70), whereas the avoidance of dangerous activities (Variable 90) was more stable for boys.

PREDICTION OF ADULT BEHAVIOR

There was no specific interview variable that assessed physical harm anxiety. However, a self-rating inventory was administered to each adult after the interview (see Appendixes 14 and 31). One of the scales of the inventory assessed fear of bodily harm, and the subject indicated the degree to which he was afraid of speeding autos, airplanes, atomic fallout, etc. These data will be discussed after we consider some relevant interview variables.

Since theory suggests that childhood fear of bodily harm should be associated with a variety of personality dimensions, the stability correlations between this longitudinal variable and the interview variables related to aggression, dependency, achievement, and sexuality will be presented. Appendix 5 contains these correlations.

TABLE 10. STABILITY OF PHYSICAL HARM ANXIETY OVER THE LONGITUDINAL PERIODS I TO IV

Variable	I–II	I–III	I–IV	II–III	II–IV	III–IV
7. Anxiety over bodily harm						
Boys	.52***					
Girls	.54***					
Total	.51****					
70. Irrational fears						
Boys						.37
Girls						.61***
Total						.49****
90. Avoidance of dangerous activities						
Boys						.56**
Girls						.39
Total						.48****
7–70.						
Boys		.13		.66****	.24	
Girls		.02		.34**	.29	
Total		.07		.50****	.31*	
70–90.						
Boys		.34*		.68****	.49**	
Girls		.25		.36**	.24	
Total		.29**		.56****	.39**	
70–90.						
Boys						.54***
Girls						.42**
Total						.44***
90–70.						
Boys						.36
Girls						.43
Total						.41*

* $p < .10$; two tails
** $p < .05$; two tails
*** $p < .01$; two tails
**** $p < .001$; two tails

The boys who showed evidence of intense physical harm anxiety during the preschool years were, as adults, anxious about sexuality, uninvolved in traditional masculine activities, and highly concerned with intellectual competence and status goals. This cluster has an intuitive consistency. Anxiety over bodily harm in the 5-year-old boy is prognostic both of future withdrawal from competitive activities with other males and with inhibition of heterosexual behavior; it is associated with failure to adopt the traditional masculine ego ideal in adolescence and adulthood.

Fear of harm during the girls' first 10 years was not highly associated with any of these adult behaviors. However, the girls who avoided dangerous activities during age 10 to 14 were, as adults, dependent on love object and family, aggressive in the face of attack, and unconcerned with intellectual goals or social recognition.

Childhood fearfulness was associated with different adult behavior patterns for males and females. The fearful boys tended to be concerned with intellectual competence as adults; the fearful girls were not. The fearful boys were reluctant, as adults, to retaliate in the face of aggressive attack; the women were likely to retaliate. The fearful boys were reluctant to remain dependent on their family as adults; the women were highly dependent.

The social class correlates of the fear variables supplied some clues to the reasons for the sex differences in the pattern of correlations. Table 11 contains the correlations between childhood fear and educational level of each parent.

The boys who showed fear of bodily harm during age 0 to 6 came from well-educated families. This relation did not occur for girls. Fear of harm during the school years was independent of social class for boys. However, the girls who avoided dangerous activities during age

TABLE 11. RELATION BETWEEN EDUCATIONAL LEVEL OF PARENT AND CHILD'S FEAR OF BODILY HARM

Childhood Variable	Age	Boys		Girls	
		Father	Mother	Father	Mother
Fear of harm	0–3	.50**	.40	−.26	−.13
	3–6	.38**	.31	.13	.15
Irrational fears	6–10	.09	.17	−.28	−.21
	10–14	.00	.01	−.39	−.06
Avoidance of danger-ous activity	6–10	.14	.05	−.12	−.28
	10–14	.12	.26	−.53**	−.48**

* $p < .10$; two tails
** $p < .05$; two tails
*** $p < .01$; two tails
**** $p < .001$; two tails

10 to 14 came from poorly educated families. *It will be recalled that the girls' avoidance of danger during age 10 to 14 was the variable most predictive of adult behavior.* This was the period when the correlation with social class was high. The fearful girls, who came from lower middle-class families, displayed adult dependency on love object and family, and minimal strivings for achievement or intellectual competence. Adoption of these behaviors could have been determined, in large measure, by the values, reinforcements, and role models associated with the child's social milieu.

The self-rating scale

After the interview each subject was asked to fill out a self-rating scale devised by the authors and dealing with a variety of behaviors (see Appendix 31). The scale consisted of 110 items, each to be rated on a four-point scale, and the subject indicated the degree to which he agreed or disagreed with the item. A group of six items, randomly dispersed throughout the scale, dealt with fear of bodily harm. These items appear in Appendix 31.

Each subject's mean score for the six items was computed; the mean for the males was 1.8; for the females, 2.3 ($t = 3.63$; $p < .001$).

The higher anxiety score for women parallels the result found with school-age children (Sarason et al., 1960; Castaneda, McCandless, and Palermo, 1956), for school-age girls admit to more test and general anxiety than school-age boys.

The average self-rating score for physical harm anxiety was correlated with the longitudinal variables. *There was no significant relation between childhood fear of harm for any of the four age periods and the self-rating score.*

HYPERKINESIS

The term *hyperkinetic impulsive* originated in clinical child psychiatry and describes those children who are unable to inhibit impulses to action, especially uncontrolled aggressive outbursts. These children react to minimal tension with immediate motor discharge, and they frequently have difficulty adjusting to the required sedentary character of the school situation.

Even in a group of children who are not extreme or pathological on this dimension, there are some who are perennially restless. When brought into a nursery school, these children are likely to dash around aimlessly for 5 minutes; they are constantly moving some part of their body, and they fidget when forced to rest.

At the other pole of this dimension is the pokey, lethargic child, who rarely displays restless, impulsive, or aimless motor discharge.

It is difficult to rate this variable for the first three years because the typical child does not begin to walk and run until the middle of the second year. Furthermore, it was difficult to rate this variable for all the children because of lack of relevant information. Thus the average sample sizes for the longitudinal ratings for Periods II, III, and IV included about 25 boys and 25 girls, less than the sample size for the other longitudinal variables. Table 12 presents the stability of hyperkinesis (Variable 69) for Periods II to IV.

Hyperkinetic behavior showed a high degree of stability over the years 3 to 14 for both sexes.

As with nurturance and fear of harm, there was no specific interview variable that evaluated hyperkinesis in adulthood. Thus we will present the correlations between hyperkinesis and the 17 interview variables from the four major clusters of dependency, aggression, sexuality, and achievement. Appendix 6 contains these correlations.

The boys who were hyperkinetic during ages 6 to 14 were, as adults, competitive, sexually active, and not highly involved in intellectual pursuits. Their behavior was in sharp contrast to the adult behavior of the boys who showed fear of physical harm during the preschool years. *The predictive value of childhood hyperkinesis in females was less impressive. A hyperkinetic tendency in girls, during age 10 to 14, predicted adult dependency on the family.* Hyperkinesis during ages

TABLE 12. STABILITY OF HYPERKINETIC BEHAVIOR OVER CHILDHOOD PERIODS II TO IV

Variable	II–III	II–IV	III–IV
69. Hyperkinesis			
Boy	.58****	.58**	.72****
Girl	.50***	.50**	.45**
Total	.57****	.57***	.62****

* $p < .10$; two tails
** $p < .05$; two tails
*** $p < .01$; two tails
**** $p < .001$; two tails

3 to 10, however, was unrelated to adult dependency, but associated with minimal involvement with intellectual mastery in adulthood. Thus hyperkinesis during the preschool or early school years was associated, in both sexes, with a rejection of intellectual mastery in adulthood.

The negative correlation of $-.61$ ($p < .001$), for males, between hyperkinesis for age 3 to 6 and adult dependency on love object parallels the positive correlation of $+.69$ ($p < .001$) between fear of harm for 0 to 3 and adult dependency on love object, and the positive correlation of $+.47$ ($p < .05$) between Period I passivity and adult dependency on love object. These are remarkably high correlations considering the fact that they link a response manifested during the first six years of life with a complex multidetermined adult behavior. The men who were dependent on their sweetheart or wife were passive, fearful, and motorically placid during the preschool years. The men who were least likely to adopt a dependent posture with love objects were fearless, retaliatory, and hyperkinetic during this early period.

Social class and hyperkinesis

There was no marked relation between the parents' educational level and the child's hyperkinetic tendencies. For boys, the correlations ranged from $-.34$ to $+.08$; for girls, from $-.11$ to $+.30$. None of the coefficients was statistically significant.

INTROSPECTIVENESS

The last variable to be considered describes the individual's ability and willingness to discuss motives, goals, conflicts, and sources of anxiety during the interview sessions. This variable is becoming popular in psychology. There is a growing recognition that an individual's self-understanding and freedom to discuss conflictual and anxiety-arousing topics influence the content of his responses during an interview and to most personality tests.

Most of the children were interviewed several times during age 10 to 14, and the summaries of these interviews provided information on the child's ability and willingness to discuss his personal feelings and motives. We have called this tendency "introspectiveness" (Variable 108).

The comparable adult rating (Interview Variable 32) was based on the subject's skill and willingness to discuss his goals, affect states, and sources of anxiety. The correlation between these two ratings indicated the stability of an introspective tendency over a 10-year period.

The correlations between the ratings of an introspective attitude for age 10 to 14 and adulthood were .35 ($p < .10$) for males; .27 for females, and .32 ($p < .05$) for the pooled sample.

Introspectiveness, therefore, remained moderately stable from adolescence through adulthood. Recent research (King, 1958; Kagan and Moss, 1960b; Singer, Wilensky, and McCraven, 1956) indicates that the human-movement response in ink-blot interpretations is associated with an introspective attitude and the ability to discuss the self and others in terms of motives, feelings, and conflicts. The stability of the introspectiveness ratings is parallelled by the stability of the human-movement response for this sample over a similar time period. A group of 63 adolescents were administered the standard Rorschach stimuli at ages 13½ and 16½. The stability of the human movement response over these two administrations was .40 and .38 ($p < .05$, for males and females respectively, ϕ coefficients).

Moreover, the human movement score from the adolescent Rorschach (administered at 16½ years) was predictive of human movement interpretations on the modified Rorschach that was administered in adulthood. For a total of 53 subjects, the ϕ coefficient was .42 ($p < .01$). Thus human-movement scores showed moderate stability during adolescence and from adolescence to adulthood. Finally, the human-movement scores obtained during both adulthood and adolescence were each predictive of the rating of introspectiveness in the adult interview. The correlations (ϕ coefficients) between the adult human movement score and adult introspectiveness were .60 for men ($p < .01$), .42 for women ($p < .05$), and .54 ($p < .01$) for the total group. Moreover, the human-movement score obtained at age 16½ also predicted the adult introspectiveness rating ($\phi = .30$; $p < .05$ for the total group).

This cluster of correlations strengthens the conclusion that an introspective attitude is relatively stable from adolescence through adulthood. In a later discussion of styles of conceptualization (Chapter Eight), this issue will be considered in another context.

As might be expected, introspectiveness was highly correlated with the educational level of the subject's family (correlations in the fifties for both sexes ($p < .01$)). The relation between introspectiveness and social class agrees with other research indicating that the human-movement response is moderately correlated with intelligence and that well-educated patients adapt more easily than poorly educated ones to the introspective requirement of psychotherapy.

EVALUATIVE DISCUSSION

As with dependency, aggression, or achievement, sex-role interests and social anxiety during age 6 to 10 were moderately good predictors of similar adult characteristics.

Second, the pattern of adult derivatives of childhood behavior revealed important sex differences. Childhood hyperkinesis was associated with adult competitiveness in males but not in females. Childhood fear of bodily harm was predictive of low aggression in men and high aggression in adult women. Boys who were nurturant during Period III rejected the traditional masculine role as adults; nurturance in girls was independent of sex-typed behaviors. Thus responses that were similar on the manifest level had different psychological correlates for males and females.

Finally, this chapter provided some instances of what we shall call the "sleeper effect." This phrase refers to a pattern of correlations suggesting that behavior appearing during the early years (Periods I or II) is a better predictor of an adolescent or adult characteristic than similar behavior during the school years. This phenomenon was noted for the relation between Period I passivity in boys and adult dependency on love object (see Chapter Three). In this chapter we noted that fear of bodily harm during Period I and hyperkinesis during Period II showed high relationships with adult dependency on love object for men, whereas ratings of these variables for the subsequent periods were not related to love-object dependency.

There are two possible interpretations of this finding. It is possible that the data for these variables were more adequate during Periods I and II than during the subsequent two periods. The failure to find correlations between the Period III behavior and adulthood might be due to methodological deficiencies. This interpretation is not persuasive, since the majority of the correlations between child and adult behaviors involved the ratings made for Period III and IV. It seems more reasonable to assume that selected behaviors (such as passivity, hyperkinesis, fear of harm) are subject to restrictive ego controls when the child enters school. These behavior tendencies are not easily detected in the everyday behavior of the school-age child, and we do not yet know what derivative responses to code in order to assess this disposition. Prior to school entrance, these responses are less disguised in form and can be assessed with more accuracy. Of course, this phenomenon only holds for a select group of behaviors, for most of the variables rated for Period I did not display this effect. It may be significant that the three behaviors that have shown this effect involved the active-passive dimension in boys. This finding supports the suggestion made in Chapter Three that early passivity may prove to be a critical developmental disposition.

ADULT DERIVATIVES OF EARLY BEHAVIOR

The primary question directed at the longitudinal data involved an assessment of the stability of passivity, dependency, aggression, achievement, sexuality, sex-role identification, and social anxiety. These relationships were examined first. However, it is reasonable to argue that a specific response might not be predictive of a phenotypically similar analogue in adulthood and yet may be associated with a behavior that was theoretically consistent with the early response. These related reactions, which are not manifestly similar to the childhood responses, might be regarded as derivatives of the early behavior.

Childhood passivity, for example, was not highly related to adult passivity or dependency in men. However, early passivity might be predictive of adult reaction patterns in the area of aggression, sexuality, or achievement. Since a search for derivative behaviors had the flavor of a fishing expedition, it was decided to preselect a core set of child and adult behaviors for study.

We selected as predictors those childhood variables that had both satisfactory inter-rater reliabilities and the most adequate longitudinal information for Periods I, II, and III. The variables chosen were passivity, dependence, aggression to mother, indirect aggression to peers, behavioral disorganization, and mastery behavior. The adult derivatives of physical harm anxiety and hyperkinesis have already been discussed, and these data appear in Appendixes 5 and 6. Mastery during age 0 to 3 was not considered because it was difficult to rate for Period I and was unrelated to mastery during later childhood.

The adult derivative behaviors included dependency, withdrawal, aggression, achievement, sexuality, sex-role interests, and social interaction anxiety.

In order to be on the side of caution we will only present and discuss the correlations that were significant at the .05 level or better for two tails. Appendixes 7, 8, and 9 present the significant correlations between the child ratings for passivity, dependence, aggression, and achievement for Periods I through III and the adult behaviors. Dependency for Periods I and II (Variable 14) is not listed because none of the correlations with adult behavior was significant at the .05 level. Of the 600 odd correlations computed, over 13 per cent were statistically significant (some at the .001 level), suggesting that these coefficients were not the result of chance alone.

DERIVATIVES OF PASSIVITY AND DEPENDENCY

The boys who were passive during the first 10 years adopted non-masculine interests as adults. This association was significant even when passivity during the first three years was the predictor ($r = .44$; $p < .05$). Moreover, passivity among boys during age 6 to 10 predicted, noncompetitiveness ($r = .58$; $p < .001$), avoidance of sexual behavior ($r = .57$; $p < .001$), and apprehension in social situations ($r = 46$; $p < .01$). This cluster is internally consistent and suggests that these men typically withdrew from the anxiety associated with (a) competitive situations with other men, (b) initiation of heterosexual behavior, and (c) interactions with strangers.

The child's dependent behavior during this period was much less predictive of this cluster of adult traits. Dependency during the first six years showed no significant relationship with adult behavior. Although Period III dependency was associated with nonmasculine interests, it was not associated with sexual anxiety, social anxiety, or competitiveness.

A passive orientation to frustration, social stress, and attack may be a more significant characteristic of childhood (as far as prediction of these adult traits is concerned) than the seeking of affection or instrumental assistance.

Passivity among girls during the first six years was unrelated to any of these adult behaviors. Passivity during Period III, however, predicted low dependency conflict, noncompetitiveness, feminine interest patterns, and repression of sexual motives in adult women. Thus passivity, which is an acceptable orientation for females, was associated with traditional feminine characteristics in adult women.

DERIVATIVES OF CHILDHOOD AGGRESSION

The boys who were aggressive toward their mothers during ages 3 to 10 were aggressive as adults and had adopted traditional masculine attributes. The girls who expressed aggression toward their mothers during the preschool years had, as adults, high fear of failure, feminine sex-role interests, and low social recognition strivings. Thus aggression to mother during the preschool years was predictive of traditional sex-role identification in adulthood for men and women.

Verbal aggression to peers, among boys, had correlates in adulthood similar to those found for mother-directed aggression (i.e., masculine interests, frequent sexual episodes, low sexual anxiety, and competitiveness). Peer-directed aggression among girls during the first 10 years was not clearly related to a consistent cluster of adult variables, although it did correlate with ease-of-anger arousal and low sex anxiety.

Behavioral disorganization during the *first six years* was not clearly associated with any of the adult behavior clusters. Disorganization during age 6 to 10 had markedly different associations with the adult behavior of men and women. *For the men, disorganization predicted overt aggressivity. For women, on the other hand, disorganization was unrelated to direct aggression but predictive of intellectual mastery, dependency conflict, and masculine interests—characteristics of the intellectually competitive women.*

Thus passivity, which is unacceptable to the male, did not predict adult passivity or dependence but did predict theoretically reasonable derivatives (noncompetitiveness, nonmasculine interests, social anxiety, and avoidance of sexuality). Passivity among women, which is congruent with female sex-role standards, had positive associations with the phenotypically similar adult responses of withdrawal and dependency.

Behavioral disorganization showed the reverse pattern. Rage reactions and low frustration tolerance, which are congruent with traditional masculine sex-role standards, were primarily associated with aggressive behavior in adult men—a phenotypically similar class of behaviors. Behavioral disorganization more clearly conflicts with acceptable behavior for women and was associated with the theoretically reasonable derivatives of intellectual mastery, status striving, and conflict over dependency.

The differential sequelae of passivity and disorganization for men and women suggest an hypothesis related to one formulated previously. *When a behavior is congruent with the traditional definition of sex-appropriate behavior, it is likely to be predictive of phenotypically similar behavior in adulthood. When it conflicts with traditional sex-role standards, the relevant motive is more likely to find behavioral expression in derivative or substitute responses that are socially more acceptable.*

The high correlation, for men, between indirect aggression to peers during age 3 to 6 and masculine interests in adulthood ($r = .66$; $p < .001$) supports the previous suggestion (see Chapter Four) that peer-directed verbal aggression in young boys may be less an index of hostile motivation and more a reflection of the boys' choice of a traditional masculine identification. It is suggested that when a response, which is often regarded as an index of motive intensity, is also one of the defining attributes of a child's sex-role identification, occurrence of the behavior may not be a sensitive index of motivational strength. Thus verbal aggression in boys and girls may have different significance with respect to intensity of hostile motivation.

This argument can be extended to include other areas of behavior. Specifically, sexual behavior among male adolescents and adults is often used as a means of strengthening the individual's sex-role identification. When used in this way, it cannot be regarded as a valid measure of intensity of sexual motivation (i.e., the desire for genital stimulation). The work of Kinsey and his colleagues (1948) indicates that premarital coitus is more frequent among lower-class men than among middle-class men. It seems reasonable to interpret this finding as indicating that lower-class men regard sexual conquest as an instrumental response whose aim is to support their conception of themselves as masculine. It would be foolish to conclude that lower-class men have stronger biological needs for sexual gratification. This argument is not restricted to overt behavior but is also applicable to the content of projective and questionnaire protocols.

In sum, phenotypically similar responses in males and females may often be the result of different antecedent processes. Many psychologists are concerned over the frequent discovery of puzzling sex differences in the patterns of correlations among identical test scores or behavioral ratings. It is possible that attention to the differential sex-role appropriateness of the response may help to explain away some of these enigmatic results.

This argument also has implications for the assessment of motive constructs from behavior. Psychologists acknowledge that anxiety and conflict over a goal can lead to inhibition of goal-oriented behavior and repression of goal-related imagery. They are wary, therefore, of equating frequency of goal-related behavior with strength of motivation in areas where conflict is presumed to be high. Absence of a response does not necessarily mean low motivation. We are suggesting further that *occurrence of a goal-related response* may be misleading, for aggressive and sexual behavior in a male may be executed in the service of bolstering a sex-role identification, instead of being a reflection of the desire to injure another or obtain orgastic discharge.

DERIVATIVES OF ACHIEVEMENT BEHAVIOR

As noted in Chapter Five, mastery behavior during age 6 to 10 predicted adult achievement for both sexes. However, for women, childhood achievement was associated with a cluster of adult characteristics outside the achievement area. Achievement-oriented girls were, as adults, counterphobic in problem situations, competitive, masculine in their interests, and self-confident. None of these adult variables was associated with childhood achievement in boys. It appears that a high level of intellectual achievement in females has implications for many sectors of psychological functioning. To know that a woman is heavily invested in intellectual achievement allows one to make predictions about many other aspects of her personality. In males, intellectual mastery is not as clearly linked to other response systems, suggesting greater heterogeneity in personality among high achievement men than among high achievement women.

The pattern of associations between child and adult behaviors is consistent with the importance we have attributed to the sex-role appropriateness of a response. When the behavior was congruent with sex-role standards, derivatives were less likely to occur and the child's behavior was generally predictive of a manifestly similar response in adulthood. When the behavior conflicted with social prescription, it was often linked with adult characteristics that were theoretically consistent with the original reaction but socially more acceptable.

The data on derivatives lend more importance to the child's preschool behavior than did the stability correlations reported in Chapters Three through Five. The latter set of stability coefficients indicated that age 6 to 10 was the period when the correlations with similar classes of adult behavior became moderately high. However, preschool passivity, achievement, fear of harm (see Appendix 5), and aggression each had theoretically reasonable associations with aspects of adult behavior. For example, aggression to mother during age 3 to 6 was associated with ease-of-anger arousal and masculine interests in adult men. Masculine behavior in girls during age 3 to 6 was predictive of competitiveness, counterphobic defenses to anxiety, and masculine interests in adulthood.

Preschool behavior, therefore, is not without significance for later functioning. Perhaps the most important implication of this entire study is the reinforcement it gives to the assumption that adult character formation begins to take form during the the first 10 years of life. Habits and attitudes learned during this period give a direction to the child's development—guiding him toward specific goals and making him selectively receptive to specific environmental experiences.

Footnotes

1. The relationship between childhood compulsivity and adult vacillation among men is supported by some supplementary test information. The men who showed high levels of cardiac arrhythmia at rest (i.e., above median on spontaneous heart rate variability) were rated as more compulsive and less impulsive as adults ($p < .01$) than the men below the median on cardiac arrhythmia. *Moreover, compulsivity during Periods II and III was also predictive of heart rate arrhythmia in adulthood* ($p < .05$). The four most compulsive children during ages 3 to 10 were all above the median on cardiac arrhythmia as adults, and all chose vocations requiring a concern with order and precision (architect, engineer, musician, and newspaper editor). Of the four boys who were least compulsive during ages 3 to 10, three of them had the lowest heart rate variability scores. The vocations of these three noncompulsive, low arrhythmia men included an athletic coach, an unskilled laborer, and a white-collar worker. One boy who was not compulsive as a child, yet who was high on heart rate variability as an adult, was in conflict over a career. He was vacillating between farming and engineering. The fact that adult cardiac arrhythmia was associated with compulsivity during both childhood and adulthood lends support to the continuity of this trait.

The possible link between heart rate arrhythmia and conceptual vacillation gains some minimal support from the relation between reaction time to the modified Rorschach ink-blot stimuli and the subject's arrhythmia score. Since the ink blots were both novel and fairly challenging, the subject's latencies to these stimuli might be associated with vacillation tendencies and, therefore, with cardiac arrhythmia. When the subject's median reaction time to the 32 modified ink blots was compared with his cardiac arrhythmia score, a curvilinear relationship emerged.

The subjects with high arrhythmia scores were either fast (median of 0 to 10 seconds) or slow (16 to 28 seconds) in responding to the ink blots ($\chi^2 = 12.99$; $p < .05$). The men with low or moderate arrhythmia scores showed moderate reaction times. The high arrhythmia men were at the extremes of the reaction time distribution; they either reflected a long time or responded quickly.

CHAPTER SEVEN

Maternal Practices and
the Child's Behavior

The acquisition and continued practice of a given response are determined by a variety of familial and extrafamilial experiences. The attempt to master intellectual skills, for example, is no doubt influenced by a number of factors, including success experiences in school, peer and teacher recognition for intellectual competence, character of the role models available to the child, and parental encouragement and reward. The nature of the longitudinal data and the existing theoretical climate directed our attention to the influence of one class of antecedent events on the child's developing personality: maternal treatment of the child.

Theory and research have acknowledged the profound importance of the mother as a determinant of the child's behavior. She inculcates goals and values and, by so doing, acts as a mediator of her culture. She influences the child's development through the relationship she establishes with him. She may, for example, be cold and detached or so lavish with affection that the child is infantilized; she may allow him autonomy or control his every activity. Finally, she acts as a model, and the ways in which she is perceived by the child determine many of the behavioral choices he will make.

The mother has been the family member most scrutinized in studies of child development. This choice has been jointly determined by the theoretical importance ascribed to her role and her availability and cooperative attitude toward research. This is not to deny the relevance of the father, and, more recently, investigators have included assessments of him in studies of developmental processes. However, our data were gathered at a time when the mother was the focus of inquiry.

As part of the Fels program, observations and interviews with the mothers of our children occurred during the first 12 to 14 years. The sources of these data were described in Chapter Two and consisted primarily of home visits and interviews. From these protocols, four types of maternal practices were evaluated: (a) maternal protection, (b) maternal restrictiveness, (c) maternal hostility and criticism, and (d) maternal acceleration of the child's developmental progress.

These variables were defined and rated on a seven-point scale. The maternal ratings, made simultaneously with the child's ratings, were repeated separately for the first three developmental periods, 0 to 3, 3 to 6, and 6 to 10 years of age. The maternal ratings for age 10 to 14 were omitted because of inadequate information. The ratings of the mother's behavior pertained specifically to the child under study. For example, a mother might be rated as hostile toward her first child but more accepting toward her second. The definitions of the maternal variables follow:

Maternal protection

This variable assessed the degree to which the mother rewarded dependent overtures and prevented independent development. Major sources of data included (a) unsolicited and unnecessary nurturance of the child, (b) consistent reward of the child's requests for help and assistance, (c) encouraging the child to become dependent on her, (d) overconcern when the child was ill or in danger.

Maternal restrictiveness

This variable assessed the mother's attempts to force the child, through punishment or threat, to adhere to her standards; the degree to which she punished deviations (which were not necessarily asocial) from her standards. In essence, this variable measured the mother's rigidity with respect to the child's development of idiosyncratic interests. Major sources of data included punishment for any deviation from maternal standards and channelling the child into activities the mother valued, without regard for his abilities or interests.

Maternal hostility

This variable assessed maternal criticism of the child and hostile statements expressed directly to the child or to other adults. It reflected both expression of dissatisfaction with the child as well as active rejection. Major sources of data included (a) criticism of the child's behavior and derogation of his skills and personality, (b) statements of preference for another sib, and (c) active rejection or

BIRTH TO MATURITY: A STUDY IN PSYCHOLOGICAL DEVELOPMENT

neglect. The latter behavior was infrequent, and this variable was measuring primarily an openly critical attitude toward the child.

Maternal acceleration

This variable assessed the degree to which the mother showed excessive concern for her child's cognitive and motor development and her tendency to place excessive expectations on his level of achievement. It reflected the degree to which the mother pushed the child's developmental level beyond his abilities and her concern with his achievement level. Major sources of data included (a) concern over the age when the child talked, walked, rolled over, (b) showing off of the child's skills and abilities, (c) maternal dissatisfaction with the child's cognitive development, and (d) maternal encouragement of the child to master various skills.

The inter-rater reliabilities for the four maternal variables were assessed with product moment correlations as well as essential percentage of agreement. The reliabilities appear in Appendix 1. The product moment correlations ranged from .41 to .88, with a median correlation of .75. Essential percentage of agreement ranged from .71 to .91, with a median of 83 per cent. There were no significant sex differences in means or variability for any of the maternal variables.

Several factors directed the choice of these particular maternal behaviors. First, frequent discussions of these practices appeared in the longitudinal reports. Second, these variables were essentially behavioral and did not require extensive inference on the part of the rater. Finally, maternal protectiveness, restrictiveness, hostility, and acceleration were theoretically tied to the classes of behaviors that were rated for the children. The development of dependent tendencies is generally assumed to be a function of parental rewards for this behavior as well as of severe restrictions on the child's independent, problem-solving activity. Similarly, achievement strivings in the 10-year-old are assumed to be facilitated by parental acceleration and encouragement of mastery behavior.

Further support for the relevance of these variables comes from a recent statistical analysis of ratings of maternal behavior. Schaefer (1959), using Guttman's circumplex model, analyzed ratings of maternal behaviors made by a variety of investigators. Schaefer concluded that the same two orthogonal continua emerged from his many analyses. He labeled them as love versus hostility and autonomy versus control. Maternal protection, restriction, and hostility are intimately related to the variables defining Schaefer's two dimensions.

Baldwin, Kalhorn, and Breese (1945, 1949), as well as Crandall and Preston (1955), identified similar clusters of maternal variables from an analysis of the Fels Parent Behavior Rating Scales. Moreover, variables of this flavor were critical in the study of patterns of child-rearing by Sears, Maccoby, and Levin (1957).

Finally, Levy (1943) evaluated the role of maternal protectiveness and hostility in the development of severe emotional disturbances in childhood. Unlike Levy's sample of mothers, who were extreme in these behaviors, the Fels mothers were typically within normal limits on the dimensions of protection or hostility. A high rating on protectiveness should not be equated with the pathological overprotection characteristic of Levy's population. Similarly, maternal hostility usually reflected a critical attitude toward the child rather than severe rejection or neglect.

The intercorrelations among these four variables suggests the relative independence of these dimensions. Table 1 presents the intercorrelations among the maternal variables for boys and girls, respectively, for each of the first three developmental periods, the only ones for which reliable ratings could be made.

TABLE 1. INTERCORRELATIONS AMONG MATERNAL VARIABLES

	Protection	Restriction	Hostility	Acceleration
Period I				
Protection	–	.29	–.21	.28
Restriction	.14	–	.08	.11
Hostility	–.50**	.29	–	–.11
Acceleration	–.22	.22	.47*	–
Period II				
Protection	–	.16	–.22	.46*
Restriction	.13	–	.36	.20
Hostility	–.22	.56**	–	–.09
Acceleration	.05	–.26	–.34	–
Period III				
Protection	–	.24	–.52**	.56**
Restriction	.12	–	.54**	.14
Hostility	–.45**	.45**	–	–.44*
Acceleration	.13	.40*	.14	–

* $p < .05$; two tails
** $p < .01$; two tails
Male data to right and above diagonal; female data to left and below diagonal.

The maternal variables were relatively independent of each other for boys during Period I. For Period II, the only significant correlation was between protectiveness and acceleration ($r = .46$; $p < .05$), and this positive association became more pronounced by Period III ($r = .56$; $p < .01$). *Thus, during ages 3 to 10, the mothers who were protective of their sons were also acceleratory.* The maternal behaviors showed more clustering during Period III; hostility was negatively correlated with both protectiveness ($r = -.52$; $p < .01$) and acceleration ($r = -.44$; $p < .05$).

For the girls, hostility and protection during Period I were negatively correlated ($r = -.50$; $p < .01$), while hostility and acceleration were positively correlated ($r = .47$; $p < .05$). These relationships were not significant for Period II. For Period III, hostility was again negatively correlated with protectiveness ($r = -.45$; $p < .01$) and positively associated with restrictiveness ($r = .45$; $p < .01$).

In summary, the four maternal variables were relatively independent of each other for the first six years, and different patterns of maternal behavior emerged for boys and girls. Specifically, protectiveness and acceleration were positively correlated for boys for Periods II and III. Hostility and acceleration during Period I were positively associated for girls but were independent for boys. The relative independence of these four variables during the first two age periods supports our decision to use each of them as independent predictors of child behavior.

STABILITY OF MATERNAL VARIABLES

The stability of maternal behaviors was determined for Periods I to II, I to III, and II to III. The stability correlations for the four variables appear in Table 2.

Protectiveness was moderately stable for boys but not for girls. Restriction, on the other hand, was highly stable for girls over the first 10 years, while only the Period II to III comparison was significant for boys.[1] The stability of maternal hostility toward girls parallels that found for restriction. All of the girls' correlations were significant, whereas only the Period II to III comparison was significant for boys. Maternal acceleration was not stable for girls but moderately stable for boys.

These correlations also provoke speculation over differences in maternal behavior toward boys and girls. Acceleration and protection

TABLE 2. STABILITY OF MATERNAL VARIABLES

Variable	Age Period		
	I–II	I–III	II–III
Protection			
Boy	.35*	.53**	.54***
Girl	.29	.12	.26
Restriction			
Boy	—.11	.24	.64****
Girl	.57***	.77****	.84****
Hostility			
Boy	.36	.11	.64****
Girl	.45**	.36*	.66****
Acceleration			
Boy	.49**	.27	.49**
Girl	.07	.08	.25

* $p < .10$; two tails
** $p < .05$; two tails
*** $p < .01$; two tails
**** $p < .001$; two tails

were stable for boys, whereas maternal restriction and hostility were more stable for girls. This sex difference in stability parallels the intercorrelations among these variables; for acceleration and protectiveness were more clearly associated for boys than for girls. It is possible that girls and boys receive different patterns of maternal treatment during the childhood years, and a more rigorous, microscopic examination of the mother-child interaction might reveal the details of these differences.

SOCIAL CLASS AND MATERNAL BEHAVIOR

The mother's social class showed some relation to her behavior. The mother's educational level was correlated with the maternal ratings for each age period, and these correlations appear in Table 3.

The mother's behavior toward her son for the first three years was independent of her social class. But the better educated mothers were slightly more critical and more acceleratory toward their daughters

TABLE 3. CORRELATION BETWEEN MOTHER'S EDUCATIONAL LEVEL AND
MATERNAL BEHAVIOR

Variable	Period I		Period II		Period III	
	Males	Females	Males	Females	Males	Females
Protectiveness	.05	−.22	.13	.01	.05	−.16
Restrictiveness	−.03	−.11	−.56****	−.09	−.16	−.38**
Hostility	−.10	.32*	−.05	.28	−.02	.25
Acceleration	.04	.33*	.54***	.17	.05	.13

  * $p < .10$; two tails
 ** $p < .05$; two tails
 *** $p < .01$; two tails
 **** $p < .001$; two tails

than the less well-educated mothers ($r = .32, .33$, respectively; $p < .10$).

For Period II, the better educated mothers were less restrictive and more acceleratory toward their sons than the poorer educated ones. For Period III, restriction of daughters was negatively related to maternal educational level, an association that may be due to the fact that the better educated mothers were more familiar with the popular child-rearing practices that encouraged freedom and permissiveness in school-age girls.[2]

In general, the mother's educational level was not highly correlated with her treatment of the child. It was anticipated that maternal education might be consistently related to acceleratory behavior, but this relation was minimal for Period III and not consistent for Periods I and II. Mothers pressured their children to master tasks for different reasons, and these reasons varied during different developmental periods. Some mothers emphasized mastery because they wanted the child to develop the ability to deal effectively with the world. Some viewed their child's achievement as a method of vicariously obtaining status in the community. Still others began to show an intense, but transient, involvement in their child's competence because of pressures brought on by the child's sudden failure in the school situation. Several mothers showed a pattern of indifference to the child's achievement during the infancy and preschool period. When the child began to do poorly in the second or third grade, however, the mother suddenly became concerned and exerted acceleratory pressures on the child. Acceleration at this time in the child's development has a different impact than similar pressures exerted when the child is 3 years of age. Early acceleration seems to be more characteristic of the well-educated mother. Once the child has entered school, attempts to encourage achievement behavior are less clearly related to social-class standing for the present group of predominantly middle-class parents.

MATERNAL TREATMENT AND THE CHILD'S BEHAVIOR

The remainder of the chapter will focus on the relationship between maternal and child behaviors. Each of the maternal variables for the three age periods was correlated with the child's behavior during that and subsequent periods as well as with the adult interview ratings. The data are organized according to the behavioral clusters of dependency, achievement, aggression, sex, social interaction, compulsivity, and anxiety over physical harm.

Each of the maternal variables (for Periods I, II, and III), was correlated with a large number of child and adult behaviors. In order to keep the presentation pointed and manageable, only those correlations that are consistent with current theory and research, and statistically significant, will be discussed. The complete sets of coefficients appear in Appendixes 10 to 13, and the interested reader can consult them.

There is, of course, a serious danger in attributing causality to associations between maternal treatment and child behavior. Although most of the significant correlations were congruent with theory, some relationships were clearly inconsistent with contemporary notions regarding the consequences of particular maternal practices. In some cases we attempted to rationalize them.

However, even when a result matches expectation, caution is necessary. For example, a positive correlation between maternal acceleration and the child's mastery might be a result of the action of other factors that were highly related to maternal acceleration but not measured by us (e.g., degree to which the mother and father were active in mastery behavior).

Since psychologists are not free to manipulate experimentally parental behavior, we are forced to rely on theory, albeit weak theory, to justify the occasional use of cause-effect statements.

MATERNAL TREATMENT AND PASSIVE AND
DEPENDENT BEHAVIOR

Each of the maternal variables for each of the age periods was correlated with the child passivity and dependency variables (for all four periods) and with the relevant interview variables. These correlations appear in Appendix 10.

Protection

Maternal protection of sons during the first three years predicted passive and dependent behavior in the boy for the first 10 years of life. It is of interest to note that protection of sons during Period I was as good a predictor of school-age passivity or dependency as the mother's behavior during Periods II or III.

Maternal protection of daughters was not as sensitive a predictor of childhood passivity or dependency for girls as it was for boys, although there was a positive relation between protection during Period II and passivity in girls during Period III. Protection of girls during Period I, on the other hand, was highly associated with adult withdrawal behavior in women ($r = .52$; $p < .01$), whereas protection for Periods II and III showed negligible relationships with adult withdrawal.

Restriction

The boys whose mothers were restrictive during Period I were *minimally* dependent on love object or friends as adults; whereas restrictiveness during Period II had a slight *positive* association with dependence on love object in adulthood. The absence of a relationship ($r = -.11$) between restrictiveness of sons for Periods I and II suggests that some mothers made major shifts in degree of restrictiveness toward sons over the first six years of life. Apparently restrictiveness during the first three years has different consequences than restrictiveness during the preschool and school years.

Restriction of girls during all three periods was associated with childhood passivity and dependence. It will be recalled that, in contrast to boys, maternal restriction of girls had the highest stability coefficients over the first 10 years. If the mother initially placed severe restrictions on her daughter, she was likely to continue this regimen and lay the foundation for a dependent orientation to others. To our surprise, however, the relation between early restrictiveness of daughters and adult dependent behavior was minimal.

Hostility

Maternal hostility toward sons showed minimal associations with childhood passivity or dependency in boys. *Hostility toward girls during the first three years, however, predicted independence with love objects and a reluctance to withdraw from stress during the adult years.* Hostility toward girls during Periods II and III showed no relationship with these adult behaviors. The mothers who were excessively critical of their daughters during the early years tended to be the better educated women who valued self-reliance and counterphobic posture with problem situations. The relationship between early dissatisfaction with the girl and the adult woman's reluctance to withdraw from stressful situations may reflect the mother's early pressure for independence and autonomy in problem situations.

Acceleration

Maternal acceleration showed no striking relationship with dependency for boys. Maternal acceleration of daughters during Period III predicted an independent approach to problems in childhood and high dependency conflict during early adulthood.

Summary

Despite some suggestive trends, the four maternal behaviors were not highly predictive of adult dependency, especially for men, and were poorer predictors of adult passive or dependent behavior than the child's own behavior during age 6 to 10 or 10 to 14. Dependent behavior in adulthood is not simply a function of the degree of maternal protection or restriction imposed on the child.

Protectiveness was a slightly better predictor of passivity for boys, whereas restriction was a better predictor of passivity for girls. It will be recalled that maternal protection was more stable for males than for females, whereas maternal restriction was considerably more stable for females over the first 10 years. These sex differences are perplexing, and we do not have an easy explanation for them.

The relationship between protectiveness and the boys' dependent behavior during the school years is consonant with hypotheses regarding the effect of this class of maternal treatments. The regular reward of dependent overtures strengthens the child's tendency to make this response in time of crisis. Moreover, a protective mother prevents the child from learning how to deal with environmental crises on his own and facilitates the development of a feeling of helplessness in the child.

It should be noted, however, that the frequency of the mother's protective reactions *is not independent of the child's requests for nurturance.* A mother is more likely to exhibit this behavior when the child signals for help or affection. Thus an unusually passive or dependent child may elicit more protective behaviors than a self-reliant one.

One of the more provocative although tentative findings was that maternal behavior during the first three years was, in some cases, more highly associated with child and adult behavior than evaluations of similar maternal treatment during Periods II or III. The most dramatic example of this phenomenon involved the tendency to withdraw from anxiety-arousing situations in adult women. Protection and hostility toward girls during Period I were the best correlates of adult withdrawal (positive for protection and negative for hostility). Similarly, maternal protection of sons during Period I was a slightly better predictor of passivity in boys age 6 to 10 than protection for Periods II or III.

We have called this phenomenon the "sleeper effect," implying that the mother's early interactions with the child may be more prognostic of his future behavior than contemporaneous assessments of the mother's behavior. The "sleeper effect" argues for the unique value of a longitudinal design. In cross-sectional investigations, a maternal treatment is correlated with the child's contemporaneous behavior. However, the mother's current treatment of her 10-year-old may be less clearly related to what the child is like at age 10 than her treatment of him during earlier years. Behavior, unlike most physical phenomena, has a long-time course, and the critical antecedents of a response may have occurred many years prior to its occurrence.

There are at least two possible interpretations of this phenomenon. It is possible that our early assessments of maternal behavior were based on more adequate data and were more valid than the ratings for Periods II or III.

A second possibility is that the mother's initial attitude to her infant, before his distinctive personality has emerged, was a more accurate index of her basic child-rearing values and attitudes than her reactions toward her school-age child. Many of the mother's reactions toward a school-age child are determined by how dependent, independent, aggressive, conforming, or mastery oriented he is at that age. That is, her treatment of the 7-year-old, in contrast to her treatment of the 1-year-old, is more likely to be influenced by the child's personality. If he is too aggressive, she may try to curb this disposition by becoming more restrictive. If he is not sufficiently independent, she may increase her demand for independence and decrease her reward of the child's passivity and dependency. In comparison with the early years, the mother's behavior during the school years is more directly governed by the degree to which the child's behavior deviates from her idealized conception of how he should behave.

Moreover, the early reward of dependent responses, before incompatible habits have been learned, is likely to have a greater effect on the strength of dependent behavior than similar reward during the preschool or early school years.

The first three years, therefore, may be a critical time to observe the mother-child interaction, for it is likely that some basic maternal attitudes can be observed most clearly during this developmental period.

CASE HISTORY IN MATERNAL RESTRICTIVENESS

A series of excerpts is presented below in order to illustrate the stability of maternal restrictiveness and its association with the acquisition of a passive and dependent predisposition in one girl. The mother and father had high school educations; the father was a skilled laborer; and the girl had an older and younger sister.

Home visit: Age 20 months

"As soon as the mother brought S into the front door downstairs, she started to cry; a subdued, whining note. The mother carried her up the stairs and held her in her arms for a few minutes."

"S wanted to take a doll downstairs with her; she gathered it up in her arms. In so doing, she caught up her dress in front. The mother said, 'Put your dress down.' S showed no response other than looking at her mother. 'I see your stomach. Shame, shame,' said the mother. This had no effect, and the mother pulled the dress down herself."

Home visit: 3 years, 1 month

"The mother told S not to pick the ears off a toy rabbit. S said, 'I did pick it off,' with some evidence of impudence. Mother said, 'What are you doing, defying me or something?' and she struck S two or three light blows with a knitting needle, which brought on a few tears."

Home visit: 3 years, 4 months

"The mother states that S has not had so many temper tantrums lately. The home visitor asked what treatment is used, and mother says in a prompt, matter-of-fact tone, 'I give her a good spanking—a good slap usually brings her out of it.' Meanwhile S is up, whimpering, and pushing the porch glider back and forth idly. Mother says cajolingly, 'Come in here a minute.' S comes in and climbs into mother's lap, still whining. The mother says that S usually comes when she is called; if not, she gets slapped."

Home visit: 4 years, 7 months

"In general, S seemed to me to be somewhat more subdued than on previous visits. I could not tell how much of this was due to the presence of the grandmother. Thinking back, it seems that S is becoming a little more listless and withdrawn, with brief interludes of noisy play, which may have been initiated by her mother."

Home visit: 5 years, 1 month

"The mother does not think the nursery school is good for S. After she has been attending, it takes several weeks to cure her of being 'fresh.' This is definite evidence of a parental attitude that is different from that of the average mother in the sample; she expects her children to obey implicitly; there is no treating them as equals."

Home visit: 5 years, 6 months

"S's younger sister had skinned her face when S had pushed her off the front steps that morning. The older sister and S 'fight like cats and dogs,' S usually starting it. Her mother slaps her, always producing tears. Occasionally S is required to sit on a chair. Most punishment is ineffective, for S thinks it is funny and giggles. She is always a follower, either with her older sister or the other children in the neighborhood. The mother blames Fels Nursery School for S's 'sassiness,' and she is not going to send her this year for that reason. According to the mother, S seeks attention and affection and is sulky when she doesn't get it. However, she plays well alone."

Nursery-school summary: 5 years, 8 months

"S was not a talkative child. She seemed to be silent most of the time. She played with other children as a follower. She usually cooperated with them and with adults. After her initial shyness, she seemed to enjoy nursery school thoroughly."

"S gave the impression of being constantly on the alert for adult interference. She seemed to play most freely when she felt most free from adult scrutiny. She seemed distrustful of any new situation and paused to size it up carefully before entering into it. Her constant companion was Joan, with whom she was previously acquainted. S seemed very dependent on Joan. On one occasion Joan was absent and S was somewhat at a loss. In spite of her dependence on another child, she was at ease in the nursery-school situation and seemed to enjoy it quietly."

Home visit: 7 years, 9 months

"The mother said that she would not 'think of' letting the children go to the store alone or even on the street after twilight. She herself is very timid and insists that the girls take no chances. She has a particular horror of Negro men. She admitted that she was overcautious but said, 'It is better to be safe than sorry. My husband tells me that I am babying the girls.' "

Interview notes with the mother at 8 years

"The mother seems to believe in discipline for children; she thinks the school and the Sisters are too lenient with the children. She contrasted this school with another Catholic school, where strict discipline is maintained. She likened the teachers at S's school to herself, threatening but never carrying out the threats. The mother also seems to take a sheltering or protective attitude toward the children, not allowing or encouraging them to do things for themselves, such as take their baths, comb their hair, or care for themselves at the table.

She doesn't allow the children far from home, for she is afraid something will happen to them."

Interview with S at 10 years of age

"S seems to be very much afraid of adults. She was extremely shy with me and talked so low that I could hardly understand her even when she was trying to be understood. She was exceedingly inept at verbalization. At the slightest question that had to do with judgment of her position, relevant to someone else, she just would say that she didn't know. She didn't know who she liked or disliked and couldn't describe any aspect of her personality."

Interview with mother at 10 years of age

"After school S skates until evening. She is supposed to come home and tell them where she is but twice failed to do this. Once her allowance was stopped; once she was whipped (quite a spanking—a hard one), but it didn't do much good. The mother is apparently quite strict with the girls. She fears racial trouble in this city and will not allow the oldest girl to go to the movies anymore."

Day-camp summary: 10 years, 3 months

"S seems to be playing a passive role in relation to her environment. She is nonassertive, nonaggressive, not verbal. She is often dumbly patient and appealing, making silent requests and responses. Her outgoing moments seem to be mainly responses to objects and materials. She drinks in the activity of others and stays parallel, keeping a safe distance."

Home visit: 10 years, 5 months

"S was her usual shy, quiet, withdrawn self this afternoon, and she had little interaction with her mother, me, or the other children. She was finally sent upstairs by her mother to take her bath with specific and angrily delivered directions to clean up the bathroom when she was done and to put her clothes away. The mother always gives the impression of expecting the worst behavior from S, and she meets it aggressively ahead of time."

Interview with mother at 11 years, 1 month

"The mother said, 'I have always tried to suppress them (meaning S and her older sister), but I have let the younger one go.' The youngest girl, apparently, has a more spirited personality and gets away with so much that it 'simply drives the others mad; they would like to kill her.' This was said with much humor, as if she finds the rivalry between the girls an amusing spectacle. I had the feeling that she enjoys the youngest girl's spunk, and she is now contemptuous of the mild manner of the suppressed older girls. The oldest one is beginning to come out of it a little bit, but S is rather hopeless."

Home visit: 11 years, 10 months

"S had a friend visiting, and they sat coyly across the room from me and giggled at whatever was said. S was uncomfortably shy, very uncommunicative and took a long time to warm up. She and her older sister were eating peanuts, and once the mother suggested that she give me some. S came darting across the room at 5-minute intervals, thrusting the dish at me, usually before I had finished my previous handful."

"The mother is a tough customer. She continually insulted the girls, managed to toss off a continual string of withering remarks. Her commands to them are of the 'get here' and 'get there' variety. Their every move is noted and criticized. For example, S and her friend started upstairs, and the mother demanded, 'Now what are you going to do?' S mumbled, 'going to the bathroom.' The mother replied ominously, 'Well, mind what you do up there.' "

Interview with S at 12 years, 2 months

"Everything that S said about her family confirmed the mother's repression of any spontaneous activity and the child's resentment of this treatment. Hearing one of the older kids playing the piano, S tentatively expressed a wish to take piano lessons, but she added immediately that her mother wouldn't let her. When asked about fighting at home, S said, 'Mother's the one that does the hitting.' Her father sometimes takes part in the discipline, too, but he's on the night shift and sleeps all day. She seemed genuinely shocked at the idea of sassing back. S's home tasks are closely supervised. She is punished for getting the dishes only half dry or for staying out a little late. Her social life is also restricted by family verdict."

Home visit: 13 years, 1 month

"S seems to grow increasingly dull and solemn; she has lost most of her former winsome attractiveness with developing obesity. The mother now calls her fatty when addressing her. She is more slow moving and heavy-footed than ever, galloping and making funny noises whenever she moves around the house. She rarely does anything at home, seems very lethargic, giving the impression that, in face of the mother's restricting and interfering policies, it is easier to simply sit than to initiate any activity and have it squelched. S conforms to the mother's orders (e.g., 'Get that telephone,' or 'Go out on the porch and see where your younger sister went to') promptly and methodically. The mother's suggestions are staged in threatening tones, 'If you don't do it, you know what you'll get.' "

Home visit: 13 years, 8 months

"S has shown no interest in dating, and the mother feels as though there is plenty of time for that when the time comes. She seems to think that most young girls are led astray once they start going out with boys. She then went into a lengthy discussion about young girls being out on the street after dark. 'There are always a lot of girls grabbed around here.' She won't let them go anywhere at night in pairs, and she even thought of moving because she would like to be closer to the bus line so that her girls would be in less danger of being grabbed."

Interview notes with S at 14 years of age

"At the start of the interview S was extremely inhibited. As it progressed, she opened up a little bit, although, for the most part, she answered only in monosyllables and volunteered nothing. She said school was not going too well, although she is passing everything. Throughout the interview S bit nervously on her nails and seemed to finger her mouth considerably. She was dressed well for a girl with such a disadvantageous figure, and her hair was nicely combed. It was apparent that considerable care had gone into her grooming for this occasion. S is socially inhibited and one of the shyest children that I have seen in an interview."

Home visit: 14 years, 2 months

"The mother ignores S's presence in the room except to tell her to go get something, to stop doing something, or to make some derogatory statement about her appearance. In response to this biting sarcasm, S grins sheepishly. S was readily submissive to the few commands that her mother made this afternoon. For example, her mother told her in stentorian tones to close the garage doors and bring her the keys. S said meekly that she had already done so. The mother then felt called upon to say imperiously, 'Well, bring me the keys' and S jumped to do her bidding."

These excerpts capture the consistency, albeit in one mother, in the parental suppression of a child's autonomy. The content of the mother's restrictive demands necessarily varied with the age of the child, and different referents for restrictiveness were used at various developmental periods. Nevertheless, the mother's suppression was evident throughout the 15-year period. The timidity and dependence that characterized this girl's personality give concrete meaning to the correlation between maternal restriction and passivity in school-age girls.

MATERNAL TREATMENT AND ACHIEVEMENT BEHAVIOR

Appendix 11 contains the correlations between each of the four maternal variables and child and adult achievement.

Protection of boys during Period I was one of the best predictors of child and adult intellectual achievement. The correlation with intellectual achievement for Period IV was .76 ($p < .001$); the correlation with concern over intellectual mastery in adulthood was .42 ($p < .10$). The comparable correlations, when maternal protection for Periods II or III was the predictor, were low and ranged from .11 to .30. Thus protection of sons during Period I has special significance for the development of achievement strivings. Acceleration of boys for Periods II and III was associated with high levels of childhood achievement, low fear of failure, and concern with intellectual mastery in adulthood.

It will be recalled that acceleration and protectiveness were positively associated for boys. *It appears that the pattern most likely to lead to involvement in intellectual achievement in the boy is early maternal protection, followed by encouragement and acceleration of mastery behaviors.*

For girls, however, the pattern was quite the reverse. Maternal hostility toward the daughter during the first three years, together with acceleration during age 6 to 10, were associated with adult intellectual mastery in the woman. As with the boys, acceleration during Periods II and III was associated with childhood achievement.[3]

Why were different maternal behaviors associated with intellectual achievement in boys and girls? In order to explain these differences it is important to recognize that the rating of maternal hostility did not typically refer to the more severe forms of rejection that typify pathognomonic homes. Rather, a high rating on hostility usually indicated a critical attitude toward the child, a dissatisfaction with his or her performance and personality. Low ratings characterized those mothers who accepted their children as they were, without constantly harping on their faults and failures.

Acceleratory mothers tended to be aggressive and competitive women who were critical of their daughters and presented themselves to their daughters as intellectually competitive and aggressive role models. It is reasonable to assume that the girls identified with these intellectually aggressive women who valued mastery behavior. *It is suggested that these same kinds of women* (i.e., *women with similar personalities*) *reacted differently toward their sons.* They protected them during the first three years, and the boys' adoption of mastery motives was based, in part, on a desire to please an acceleratory mother.

The significance of maternal treatment during the first three years was clear for both sexes. The best predictors of adult achievement behavior for women were Period I hostility and Period I acceleration. For boys, the best correlates of adult intellectual mastery were low hostility and high protectiveness during Period I. Thus the sleeper effect applied to achievement as well as to dependent behavior.

The danger of attributing causality to correlations between maternal treatment and child behavior is illustrated in the positive association between maternal hostility and the girls' achievement behavior. On the basis of existing theory and empirical data, it would be fallacious to conclude that maternal hostility is essential for or leads to intellectual mastery. In the present sample, those mothers who were critical of their daughters during Period I and exerted acceleratory pressures on them were intellectually competitive role models. It is suggested that this combination of maternal traits and practices, and their timing in the girls' development, are both critical in the development of intellectual mastery in the girl.

One of the implications of these findings is that study of the mother-child relationship should assess the patterning, over time, of a variety of maternal dimensions, including affection, restriction, protection, and acceleration, as well as the mother's salient personality characteristics. The pattern of maternal behaviors and their timing, rather than one specific treatment at one particular time, may well be the critical processes to understand in explicating the effect of maternal behavior upon the child's developing personality.

MATERNAL TREATMENT AND AGGRESSIVE BEHAVIOR

The correlations between aggression during childhood and adulthood and the four maternal variables appear in Appendix 12. In general, the findings for aggression were less impressive than they were for dependency or achievement. *There were no consistent associations between maternal treatment of sons during the first six years and the child's aggression toward his mother. Acceleration of girls, however, was consistently associated with aggressive behavior toward the mother during preadolescence.* Acceleration of daughters during all three periods was associated with aggression to mother for age 10 to 14 ($r = .34, .44, p < .05$; and $.49, p < .01$ for Periods I, II, and III, respectively). Acceleratory mothers did not suppress rebellion and verbal aggression in their daughters, and this may be one reason for this association.

Maternal treatment during the first six years was not consistently related to peer-directed aggression in the child. Maternal hostility toward sons during Period III, however, was associated with peer-directed aggression for boys, and the highest correlations occurred when mother and child behaviors were assessed *at the same time* (Period III). Since these ratings were made contemporaneously, it is possible that the child's aggressive behavior provoked maternal criticism and hostility. This possibility is supported by the fact that the highest correlation between maternal hostility and nonconformity in the child occurred for the Period III ratings. Degree of maternal hostility could have been influenced, in part, by the frequency of the child's aggressive behavior; the more aggressive the child, the more critical the mother became.

Behavioral disorganization, which was one of the best predictors of adult aggression (see Chapter Four), was positively associated with maternal hostility. Maternal hostility toward girls during Period II was associated with disorganization in the girl for ages 3 to 6 and 6 to 10; hostility during Period III was correlated with disorganization for ages 6 to 10 and 10 to 14 in both boys and girls.

Conformity to adult authority (i.e., nonrebellion to parents and teachers) was the only variable that showed a clear relation to early maternal treatment. *Protectiveness during Period I predicted conformity during ages 6 to 10 and 10 to 14 for both sexes.* This finding suggests that the mother who rewarded the child's early dependency may have provided the conditions for effective socialization of rebellious tendencies. The earlier this maternal treatment occurred, the more effective this socialization.

As with dependency and achievement, the maternal variables were not highly correlated with adult behavior. The most significant associations linked Period III restriction of boys with both ease-of-anger arousal and aggressive retaliation in adult men ($r = .36, .35; p < .05$). Restriction during Period II was associated with aggressive retaliation in adult men and with ease-of-anger arousal in adult women. Thus restrictiveness during the preschool and early school years was a better predictor of adult aggressive tendencies than restriction during Period I.

The men and women who criticized their mothers most intensively during the adult interview had mothers who were not highly restrictive during Periods II and III. The men with restrictive mothers may have been openly aggressive with peers, but they were reluctant to find any fault with their mother's personality when talking with the interviewer.

In summary, maternal restrictiveness during ages 3 to 10 was the most consistent correlate of aggressive behavior in adult men and women. Maternal hostility was the best correlate of aggression to peers during childhood.

It has been suggested that the mother's hostility to the child may have been a *reaction* to the child's aggressive behavior rather than a cause. This assumption is relevant to the popular criticism of cross-sectional studies that find a relation between maternal rejection and aggressive behavior in the child. The possibility that the child's aggression elicited the mother's hostile attitude prevents any satisfying conclusion.

Restriction, which is a direct frustration of the child's autonomy, is generally assumed to lead to hostile feelings in the child, and the positive association between restriction and adult aggression in men might be interpreted as supporting this hypothesis. However, restriction of sons was moderately correlated with the mother's social class.

The poorly educated mothers were more restrictive than the better educated ones. It is possible that a variety of experiences associated with lower middle-class standing, but not measured by us, were influential in the development of aggressive tendencies.

MATERNAL BEHAVIORS AND OTHER
BEHAVIORAL DIMENSIONS

The remaining child behaviors include sexual behavior, sex-role interests, social interaction anxiety, compulsivity, and physical-harm anxiety. The correlations between these behaviors and the four maternal variables appear in Appendix 13. Since the hypotheses for these behaviors were less clearly formulated, only the salient findings will be summarized. The interested reader can study the complete list of coefficients.

Sexual behavior and sex-role interests

Although none of the maternal variables was associated with heterosexual behavior among early adolescent girls, maternal protection of daughters during Period III was positively related to sex anxiety in adult women ($r = .43$; $p < .05$).

Adoption of sex-role interests was more clearly associated with maternal practices. *Protection of sons was the major predictor of nonmasculine sex-role interests in boys.* Protection during Period I was correlated with nonmasculine interests in boys age 6 to 10 ($r = .40$; $p < .05$); protection during Periods II and III was also associated with nonmasculine activities during Period III and adulthood.

Protection of girls was associated with the adoption of feminine interests during childhood and adulthood. *Maternal protection apparently "feminized" both the boys and the girls.* Once again evidence of the sleeper effect emerged. Only Period I protection was significantly associated with sex-typed interests in adult women; the corresponding correlations for Periods II and III were negligible.

Adoption of masculine activities in adult women was highly associated with maternal hostility during Period I ($r = .61$; $p < .01$). Since the critical mothers accelerated their daughters and pushed them toward independence, it might be expected that these girls would not adopt traditional feminine interests.

Social interaction anxiety and maternal behavior

Anxiety over social interaction in adult women was associated with maternal protection during the first three years ($r = .41$; $p < .05$). Protection of daughters during the later periods was unrelated to adult social anxiety. Hostility toward girls for Period I, on the other hand, predicted low social anxiety in adult women. These findings agree with the earlier statement that mothers who were critical during Period I had daughters who were mastery oriented, independent, and competitive with peers.

Protection of sons during Period III was associated with an expectancy of rejection for age 10 to 14 and adult social anxiety. Restrictiveness for sons during Period III was also associated with social anxiety for Period IV. *Thus maternal protection and suppression of autonomy were related to uneasiness in social situations for both males and females.*

Compulsivity

Compulsive tendencies in adulthood were not highly related to any of the maternal treatment variables. Acceleration of sons during Period III was associated with low compulsivity in adulthood ($r = .48$; $p < .01$). Compulsivity in childhood, on the other hand, was positively related to maternal protectiveness of both boys and girls during the first three years of life.

Fear of physical harm

Maternal protection during Period I was associated with fear of harm in boys during ages 3 to 10. For girls, maternal restriction rather than protection, predicted fear of harm for this age span. This pattern was repeated for Period II, with protectiveness predicting fear of harm in boys and restrictiveness predicting this response for girls. This result compares with the data reported for passive and dependent behavior, where protectiveness was accociated with dependence in boys and restrictiveness with dependence in girls.

EVALUATIVE DISCUSSION

Many of the correlations reported in Appendixes 10 to 13 are either too low to discuss or, if significant, not easily explained. However, there are three tentative conclusions suggested by these data.

The most striking finding was that maternal protection of boys during the first three years was associated with a theoretically consistent set of behaviors during the years 6 to 14. This cluster included a passive reaction to frustration, emotional dependence on adults, conformity to adult demands, striving for excellence in intellectual tasks, fear of physical harm, and minimal adoption of traditional masculine interests.

The mother who initially established an overly nurturant relation with her son may have created the conditions that facilitated the adoption of dependent tendencies and the incorporation of the mother's values. If the mother valued intellectual achievement, as many of our mothers did, the child probably may have adopted this motive in order to retain the mother's nurturance. The tendency to be passive and fearful during the early school years could have resulted, in part, from the feeling of helplessness that was a consequent of the mother's protective attitude. Since protection of sons was not highly related to social-class position, this set of relationships implies that protection *per se* may be a significant maternal behavior.

A second implication of these data involves the differential patterning of maternal treatment for the sexes. We have suggested that mothers who valued intellectual competence for themselves and their children protected their sons but were more critical and nonprotective of their daughters. These data suggest the relevance of making detailed observations of mother-child interactions during the first three years, looking for subtle differences in the pattern of behavior toward sons and daughters.

A third provocative finding involved the "sleeper effect." In several instances, the mother's behavior during the first three years was the best predictor of school age or adult behavior. Evaluation of similar maternal practices during Period II and III was often unrelated to the adult's behavior.

It is possible, of course, that the observations for Periods II and III were not as adequate as those for Period I, and that the ratings for the later periods were not sensitive indexes of the mother's treatment.

This possibility is contraindicated, in part, by the fact that many child behaviors were related to the maternal ratings made for Periods II and III.

A second interpretation rests on the assumption that these maternal variables involved different behaviors at different age periods and were provoked by different situations. In effect, these maternal variables may have been measuring qualitatively different responses and, therefore, were not of comparable meaning during different developmental eras.

Protectiveness toward a 2-year-old child usually requires much more physical contact between mother and child than protectiveness at age 10. During the first three years, a typical protective act involves picking the child up after he falls or cuddling him when he runs for help. During Period II, protectiveness is more typically displayed in preventing actions that might be dangerous to the child or offering instrumental help with specific problems. Moreover, the mother's rewards and punishments during Period III are more dependent on the child's personality than they are during the first three years. It may be semantically misleading to apply the same label to a maternal variable over a 10-year period. The fact that selected adolescent and adult behaviors were highly related to Period I maternal treatment suggests that observation of mother and child during the first three years may provide some insights into this reciprocal system.

Footnotes

1. In a recent study, Schaefer and Bayley (1960) reported that maternal restrictiveness during the child's first three years was unrelated to restrictiveness toward the preadolescent. These correlations, however, were based on a pooled sample of boys and girls. It is possible that if separate correlations had been computed for the sexes, the results would have resembled the ones reported here (i.e., high stability for girls and low stability for boys).

2. The reader is referred to a study by Bayley and Schaefer (1960), which found a substantial relation between social class and maternal variables, similar to those described here. Moreover, Maccoby and Gibbs (1954) reported that middle-class mothers used reasoning and praise more often than lower-class mothers and were more affectionate than lower-class mothers.

3. It will be recalled from Chapter Five that TAT stories during both adolescence and adulthood were available for most of these subjects. Maternal acceleration during the first 10 years of life showed suggestive relationships with the adolescent achievement themes. For example, maternal acceleration during Period I predicted occurrence of achievement themes at adolescence for girls ($p < .05$), but not for boys. Maternal acceleration during Period III predicted achievement themes for adolescent boys ($p < .05$), and adult women ($p < .10$).

CHAPTER EIGHT

Sources of Conflict and Anxiety

Aggression, dependency, and sexuality comprise the classic trio of conflictful motives in western culture. Although the term conflict falls easily and frequently from tongue or pencil, it is difficult to define and even more difficult to measure. Conflict is traditionally defined as the simultaneous arousal of incompatible or mutually exclusive goal strivings. Dollard and Miller (1950) have described the psychological characteristics of different kinds of conflicts (approach-approach, avoidance-avoidance, approach-avoidance, and double approach-avoidance) and have suggested that in approach-avoidance conflicts, the closer the individual is to the conflicted goal, the more evident will signs of avoidant behavior become. This assumption forms the foundation for the measurement techniques that psychologists have devised to measure conflict in human and infrahuman subjects.

In an approach-avoidance conflict, the avoidance response is elicited by aversive goal-related stimuli or their symbolic surrogates. Typically *anxiety* is the hypothetical construct that is called on to explain why stimuli symbolic of a conflicted goal are aversive and lead to avoidant behavior. The strategies used to assess the presence and intensity of a conflict usually involve measurement of responses that are assumed to result from the experience of anxiety. Typically the psychologist presents a stimulus that contains a direct reference to (i.e., is associated with) a potentially conflictful goal and assumes that the processing of this information elicits differing degrees of anxiety among a sample of subjects. He then codes each individual's reaction to this information, using verbal behavior, motor reactions, response latencies, perceptual distortions, or autonomic reactivity as indexes of anxiety. We chose to measure the individual's reactions in two modes of functioning: perceptual recognition of tachistoscopically presented scenes and autonomic reactivity. We assumed initially that these reactions might provide a more objective and sensitive index of anxiety and conflict than the interview ratings.

The evaluation of overt behavior through interviewing has its difficulties. But with sufficient time and rapport, and for selected response classes, the interview is capable of yielding relatively valid data. When the interviewer asks the subject to recount his actions in specific situations (e.g., What did you do when you had to decide about college?), the individual's report usually has more truth than error. However, the assessment of conflict and anxiety constructs encounters special problems. Assessment of anxiety over specific behaviors requires an evaluation of feelings, not actions. These feelings are not always available to conscious verbal report, and direct questioning often yields ambiguous information. Moreover, the vocabulary of our language is not sufficiently differentiated to allow for a sensitive delineation and description of the presence and intensity of anxious, conflictful, and emotional states.

Finally, the inexperienced interviewer can be misled by individual differences *in the ability to verbalize areas of conflict*. The interviewer can overevaluate the intensity of a conflict area, merely because the subject described the problem in a language that was congruent with the interviewer's conception of the conflictful process.

We turned, therefore, to two popular, but more objective, methods of assessing anxiety and conflict. In the tachistoscopic situation, distortion or delayed recognition of conflictful scenes was presumed to be a consequent of anxiety in the area illustrated. It was assumed that if a specific content were anxiety arousing, ideational representations of this content would be more likely to be repressed and, therefore, less readily available for a correct perceptual hypothesis. That is, the strength of the perceptual hypothesis, "That is a man choking a man," should be weaker for adults highly conflicted over aggression than for those with low conflict. The order of recall of these scenes (90 minutes later) was used as a supplementary index of conflict (i.e., decreased availability of the anxiety-arousing ideas).

A second potential index of conflict-produced anxiety was a change in either heart rate or palmar conductance in response to an anxiety-arousing communication. The assumptions behind this use of autonomic reactions have a long history in psychology. Changes in the level of activity in the autonomic nervous system have been viewed traditionally as a reflection of emotional arousal (Duffy, 1957; Malmo, 1957; Malmo, 1958). Since *anxiety* is a state of affective arousal, it seems reasonable to conclude that the intensity of anxiety elicited by a stimulus should be reflected in a proportional amount of discharge in autonomic target organs.

Five sources of anxiety were studied: conflict over dependency, aggression, and sexual behavior, as well as anxiety over bodily harm and intellectual competence. The tachistoscopic task sampled the areas of dependency, aggression, sexuality, and bodily harm; the autonomic battery sampled anxiety over aggression, sexuality, bodily harm, and intellectual competence.

The assumption that delayed recognition of conflictful scenes or autonomic discharge to conflictful communications reflects anxiety is of questionable validity. Many investigators are attempting to prove or disprove these hypotheses. The data to be reported, therefore, bear directly on this important methodological problem: the validity of tachistoscopic perception or autonomic discharge as indexes of anxiety associated with behavior and goal states that are regarded as conflictful in this society.

In the introductory chapter we stated our hope that this rich source of information on a longitudinal sample might lead to conclusions about the meaning of some of the popular measuring instruments in psychological research. This wish was realized to some degree.

THE TACHISTOSCOPIC SITUATION

In the middle of the third test session, the S was brought into a light-proof room and dark-adapted for 10 minutes. The S was then shown a series of 14 line-drawings of people in various situations. The pictures were presented at seven different exposure speeds ranging from 0.01 to 1.0 seconds. The 14 stimuli contained 4 aggression scenes, 3 dependency scenes, 2 romantic scenes, 2 physical harm pictures, and 3 neutral situations. Separate sets of stimuli were drawn for the sexes so that the central figures in the conflict pictures were the same sex as the subject. A brief description of the pictures was presented in Chapter Two, and the scenes are illustrated in Figure 3.

ADMINISTRATION

The S sat 22 inches from a flash-opal glass screen, and the image was projected from the back of the screen. The visual field was constantly illuminated (30 foot-candles at the screen), the only source of light in the room. The subject was given the following instructions:

"We are now going to show you some pictures at a rapid speed, and we want you to tell us what is happening in the pictures. Who are the people, are they male or female? What are their approximate ages; that is, are they old, middle-aged, young adult, or children? Finally, what is each person in the picture doing?"

The instructions were intended to orient the subject to report objective facts about the pictures rather than a theme or inferences about the motives or feelings of the figures.

The subject was then shown three practice pictures to adapt him to the situation and to familiarize him with the responses required of him. The 14 test stimuli were first shown at the fastest exposure (0.01 seconds). After each stimulus the subject reported what he saw, and when all 14 scenes had been presented for the first time, he was told that he would now see all the pictures again at a slightly slower speed but in a different order. This procedure was repeated a total of seven times at exposures of 0.01, 0.02, 0.04, 0.10, 0.20, 0.50, and 1.0 seconds. The pictures were shown in six different orders; the orders for exposures 1 and 7 were the same. All exposures were *above threshold*, and the subjects typically reported seeing something at each exposure. The entire procedure usually took 45 minutes, and the protocol was electrically recorded and transcribed verbatim.

At the end of the third test session, which was approximately 90 minutes after the completion of the tachistoscopic task, each subject was asked to recall as many of the 14 scenes as possible.

RECOGNITION THRESHOLD

The verbatim protocols were scored for the trial at which the subject first described accurately the sex, approximate ages, and content of the scene, and after which he continued to produce correct reports for succeeding trials. This trial was designated as the subjects' recognition threshold. In a few cases the subject described the scene correctly at trial 3, distorted the stimulus on trial 4, and then described the scene accurately for trials 5, 6, and 7. In these cases the recognition threshold was five. If a subject failed to recognize the scene on the seventh exposure, a threshold value of eight was assigned to him. The percentage of agreement between two independent scorers assessing recognition thresholds was 94 per cent. The average recognition thresholds for the 14 pictures varied markedly, and Table 1 presents the average threshold values for each of the 14 scenes.

The control pictures generally had low thresholds (recognized early) for both sexes. The scenes illustrating aggression to mother (A-13) and dependency (D4, 5) had the highest thresholds for the men. For the women, aggression to peer (A-1), aggression to an older man (A-14), and the romantic beach scene (S-6) had the highest recognition thresholds.

Ease of recognition of aggression and dependency scenes was related to the sex of the subject. For three of the four aggression pictures, the women had significantly higher recognition thresholds than the men. On all three dependency pictures, however, the men had significantly higher thresholds. These results suggest that the women were more conflicted over aggression, the men more conflicted over dependency.

The threshold data for the two romantic pictures were equivocal. The "beach scene" did not produce a significant sex difference when the means were compared. However, a χ^2 analysis (median test) revealed a higher threshold for the women ($p < .05$; two tails). The picture of the couple embracing was recognized earlier by the women. This is not in accord with the assumption that conflict over sexual activity is greater for women. It should be noted, however, that the erotic content of this picture was much tamer than that of the beach

TABLE 1. AVERAGE RECOGNITION THRESHOLD FOR THE TACHISTOSCOPIC SCENES

Picture		Males	Females	p (two tailed)
Aggression	1	4.3	6.4	.001
	2	2.3	4.0	.01
	13	6.8	5.2	.05
	14	4.5	6.7	.001
Dependency	3	3.8	2.5	.01
	4	5.6	3.8	.01
	5	6.4	4.7	.01
Sex	6	5.3	5.6	–
	7	5.3	3.9	.05
Harm	8	3.1	2.7	–
	9	3.7	3.1	–
Control	10	1.9	2.9	–
	11	4.4	3.6	–
	12	2.2	2.0	–

scene. The reason for the higher threshold for the men was that the scoring manual required the subject to report that the *figures were kissing* in order for the perception to be scored as accurate. The men characteristically reported seeing a couple embracing but failed to add that they were kissing. The scenes depicting physical harm did not yield significant sex differences in recognition threshold, although the men had slightly higher thresholds.

DELAYED RECALL

Although recognition threshold was the primary score used in the analyses to follow, delayed recall of these scenes corroborates the sex differences found for the threshold data. Most of the subjects recalled the majority of the pictures; both the median and mean number of pictures recalled for men and women was 13. One third of the subjects recalled all 14 scenes, and all of the women and 32 men recalled at least 12 of the 14 pictures.

Each picture was assigned a rank of 1 to 14, depending on its order of recall, and the average rank for each picture is presented in Table 2. The higher the average rank, the later the picture was recalled.

TABLE 2. AVERAGE RANKED RECALL OF THE
TACHISTOSCOPIC SCENES

Picture		Males	Females	p (two tailed)
Aggression	1	5.8	7.9	.05
	2	8.0	12.2	.001
	13	9.7	10.2	–
	14	9.0	11.3	.01
Dependency	3	8.8	7.9	–
	4	8.8	8.5	–
	5	9.1	8.5	–
Sex	6	4.0	4.1	–
	7	8.6	6.2	.01
Harm	8	4.9	4.5	–
	9	5.7	3.3	.01
Control	10	5.4	5.9	–
	11	9.8	7.8	.05
	12	7.5	6.7	–

The men had markedly lower recall scores for all four aggressive pictures but only slightly higher recall scores for all three dependency pictures. For three of the four aggression scenes, the sex differences were statistically significant. Thus the sex differences in ease of recall of aggression and dependency were congruent with the recognition threshold information and supportive of the assumption of greater aggressive conflict for women and greater dependency conflict for men.

The men recalled the romantic scene of the couple kissing (S-7), the dog attacking the person (H-9), and the man lighting a cigarette (C-11) later than the women. The sex difference for control picture (C-11) was unexpected and not easily explained. An analysis of the early interpretations of this scene revealed that the men were more likely than the women to perceive the two male figures in an aggressive posture. By the seventh exposure, however, almost all subjects had recognized the scene accurately.

There was no systematic relationship between the recognition threshold for a scene and its order of recall. The only significant correlation occurred for women for the scene illustrating the two women with a coffee cup (C-12). The women who recognized this picture late tended to recall it early ($p < .05$).

SELF-RATINGS

The striking sex difference in recognition threshold and delayed recall for the aggressive scenes was supported by the subjects' self-ratings. Although this instrument was not used as a measure of conflict, these data on the self-ratings will be summarized, for correlations were computed between these scores and the tachistoscopic and autonomic measures. Appendix 31 contains a detailed presentation of the relation between the self-ratings and the interview and child ratings.

After the interview each *S* was administered a 110-item, self-rating inventory; the instructions for this instrument were described in Chapter Six. A series of eight scales was scored from the inventory: aggression, hostility, dependency, sex anxiety, affiliation, compulsivity, status needs, and physical-harm anxiety. The items comprising these scales appear in Appendix 31.

The subject's average score for each of these scales was computed, and Table 3 presents the mean scores for males and females on each of the scales.

Significant sex differences were present for aggression, status needs,

TABLE 3. AVERAGE SCORE ON THE SELF-RATING SCALE

Scale	Males	Females	p (two tailed)
Aggression	2.3	2.0	.05
Hostility	2.3	2.3	–
Dependency	2.7	2.8	–
Sex anxiety	2.1	2.0	–
Affiliation	2.5	2.7	–
Compulsivity	2.5	2.5	–
Status strivings	2.8	2.1	.001
Physical harm anxiety	1.9	2.4	.001

and physical-harm anxiety in a direction that might be anticipated. In comparison to women, men admitted to more aggression and more status-seeking behavior but denied anxiety over physical harm. The females had higher scores than the men on the affiliation and dependency scales, but these differences were not statistically significant. Thus the threshold, recall, and self-rating data all indicate greater conflict over aggression for women and greater conflict over dependency for men.[1]

INTERCORRELATIONS OF THRESHOLD DATA

In order to determine if the pictures illustrating similar content areas had similar threshold and recall scores, intercorrelations among the pictures were determined with ϕ coefficients (with Yates' correction). In general, the pictures illustrating the same conflict areas had similar recognition thresholds. Among the four aggressive pictures, the correlations (males and females pooled) between pictures 1 and 13, 2 and 14, and 13 and 14 were .31 ($p < .02$); .34 ($p < .01$), and .34 ($p < .01$), respectively. The relation between the thresholds for aggressive pictures 1 and 2 was low. For dependency, pictures 4 and 5 were positively related ($\phi = .28$; $p < .05$), but neither of these pictures showed any relationship to the threshold for picture D-3 (adult on stool, leaning on adult of opposite sex). The two sex pictures had similar thresholds ($\phi = .36$; $p < .01$), and the thresholds for the two physical-harm pictures were positively correlated but only significant for males ($\phi = .43$; $p < .01$). The thresholds for the control pictures had low, positive correlations among each other (ϕ coefficients in the .20's; $p < .05$).

On the basis of the above relationships, average recognition thresholds were computed for seven groups of pictures; A1–13, A2–14, A13–14, D4–5, S6–7, H8–9, C10–11–12. Appendix 14 contains the intercorrelations among the seven average threshold scores. The correlations between the mean thresholds for each of the pairs of conflictful scenes and the control pictures were generally low and nonsignificant. There were only two significant relationships involving mean threshold for the control scenes; the women who recognized the control pictures early also recognized aggressive scenes A1–13 and A13–14 early.

Recognition thresholds among the four conflict areas tended to be independent. The threshold for dependency scenes was unrelated to the thresholds for the aggressive, sexual, and physical harm scenes for the men (r ranged from $-.06$ to $+.31$). Similarly, threshold for the sex pictures was not highly related to the thresholds for the other three areas (r ranged from $-.04$ to $+.34$). The males who had difficulty recognizing the sex scenes, however, also had difficulty with one pair of aggressive scenes (A1–13).

Appendix 15 contains the correlations between each of the seven threshold scores and the educational level of the subject. In general, educational level was unrelated to recognition of the scenes, although the better educated men had greater difficulty recognizing the physical-harm scenes.[2]

INTERCORRELATIONS OF RECALL DATA

The distributions of ranked recall scores were split at the median and the intercorrelations computed (ϕ coefficients). Very few significant relationships emerged from this analysis. There was no clear tendency for scenes tapping the same conflict area to be recalled together. Moreover, there was no relationship between the order of presentation of the scenes on the last exposure trial (which was the same order as that used on the first trial) and the order of recall (rho $= -.01$). That is, the order of recall was independent of the order of stimulus presentation on the first and last series. The pictures presented first and last in the final exposure series had median recall values of nine and six, respectively.

Since the recall data did not yield consistent correlations within the same conflict area and since these data showed no relationship to the perceptual threshold scores, they will not be discussed in the sections that follow.

AUTONOMIC TEST SITUATION

A group of 30 males returned the morning after the tachistoscopic session for the final assessment session. During this two-hour session, psychophysiological measurements were made under various arousal situations. The test situation was divided into two parts, autonomic reactions to conflictful tape-recorded monologues and to physical and problem-solving stressors.

Procedure

After the subject had been prepared for autonomic recording of heart rate, palmar conductance (conductance rather than resistance will be the term used in the discussion), and respiration, tape-recorded instructions were given him. The subject was told that his physiological reactions to "a variety of physical stimuli and of mental and emotional tests" would be measured. The instructions were as follows:

"After a relaxation period we will administer a series of stimuli and tests. In the first series of tests we are going to play some tape recordings involving different emotional problem areas. We are going to measure your physiological reactions as a series of these emotional areas are depicted in brief dramatic recitations. Your job is to put yourself in the place of the man who is speaking, to feel what he is going through. You must listen very attentively and you must let yourself go—you must feel yourself into the situation so to speak. Put yourself in the man's place, feel what he is feeling. The point of this is that all people have problems and conflicts in at least some of these emotional areas and by measuring your physiological reactions we can see the impact of these problems on you."

"There is a fixed procedure we are going to follow in administering these tests. We use this procedure so that you will never be startled by a sudden stimulus, you will always know what is going to happen. At the appropriate time in the experiment, I will warn you that the tape recording will be turned on in exactly one minute, and I will briefly describe what the dramatic recording is going to be about. After exactly 60 seconds we will play the recording. With your eyes closed, listen attentively, and feel yourself into the situation. When the recording is over, I will tell you to relax again. When you are once more showing physiological stability, I'll announce the next tape recording, briefly describe its nature, and again allow exactly 60 seconds for you to get prepared. After this series of tests is over I will give you a few instructions concerning the rest of the stimuli and tests we are going to use."

The subject was then told that a masking noise would be present, and he was instructed to relax. During this 10-minute relaxation period, heart rate and palmar conductance were continuously recorded.

After the 10-minute relaxation, each subject listened to five 1-minute tape-recorded monologues by a male actor, with a 3-minute rest period between each monologue. The procedure and timing for each monologue were as follows:

1. A rest period of 3-minutes, the last minute of which was called the base period.
2. The tape-recorded announcement of the content of the monologue, the alerting communication.
3. A 1-minute alert period during which the subject waited for the monologue.
4. Playing of the 1-minute tape-recorded monologue.
5. A rest period of 3-minutes, etc.

The order of the monologues was as follows. A motivationally neutral monologue, the desperate cries of a man pinned under a beam, an angry outburst to a friend, a romantic appeal to a woman, and an angry outburst to a mother. Appendix 16 contains the verbatim monologues.

The alerting announcements for these monologues were as follows:

1. *Control.* "All right, that's the end of relaxation. In one minute we will play the first recording. This is a practice recording to give you an idea of what they are like. Keep your eyes closed throughout. Sixty seconds to go."
2. *Physical harm.* "The next recording deals with the fear of physical pain and loss of life. The man speaking is pinned down by a fallen log or beam. Put yourself in his place. Eyes closed throughout. Sixty seconds to go."
3. *Anger to a friend.* "The next recording deals with the emotion of anger. The man speaking is very mad at a friend. Put yourself in his place. Eyes closed throughout. Sixty seconds to go."
4. *Sex.* The next recording deals with sex—a man is making love to a woman. Put yourself in his place. Eyes closed throughout. Sixty seconds to go."
5. *Anger to Mother.* "The next recording deals with the feeling of anger at a parent. A man is expressing his irritation at his mother. Put yourself in his place. Eyes closed throughout. Sixty seconds to go."

A short break occurred after the playing of the last monologue, and the subject was then told about the remaining tests in the series. The tests in the order of administration were as follows.

1. *Cold pressor.* The subject placed his foot in an ice water bath for 60 seconds.

2. *Make-up sentences.* The subject was given a letter and requested to form as many sentences in one minute with at least five words as he could, each word beginning with the letter given to him. For example, if the examiner said the letter "A," a correct sentence might be "Albert and Alice ate apples." The subject was given a letter and instructed to

make up the sentences mentally without announcing anything until he was asked for the answer.

3. *White noise.* The subject was told to close his eyes and to listen to a high-intensity white noise for 60 seconds.

4. *Mental arithmetic.* The subject was asked to solve mentally a series of multiplication and addition problems, for example, 6×33 and add 58; 8×29 and add 69. The problems were administered for 2 minutes.

5. *Memory for rules.* The subject listened to and attempted to memorize a set of rules for a fictitious card game. The rules were administered during a one-minute period.

6. *Flickering light.* The subject closed his eyes while periodic photic stimulation was administered for 60 seconds. He was told that he would see colors and shapes, which he would be asked to report at the end of the experiment.

7. *Reversed spelling.* The subject was given a six-letter word spelled in reverse order and asked to announce the correct word. Illustrative examples would be, for example, egnaro, esraps. The reversed words were administered for a 2-minute period.

The measures: Resting lability

The measure of resting heart rate variability (i.e., arrhythmia) was obtained in the following manner. The amplitude of each trough to peak change in the cardiac cycle during the 10-minute relaxation period was cast into a frequency distribution. The 75th percentile was selected as the index of heart rate arrhythmia. Thus, if spontaneous changes in heart rate were small, this value would be small.

The measure of spontaneous sudomotor activity was defined as the number of half-minute periods during which a PGR of 600 ohms or more occurred.

Reaction to taped monologues and stressor episodes

For each of the five alerting announcements and tape recordings, two measures were used—alerting and total reactions.

Alerting reaction (changes from base period to alert period)

The base to alert score was the change in heart rate or palmar conductance comparing the one minute preceding the announcement of the tape with the one minute of rest immediately following the announcement before the tape was played. The heart rate measure was the difference between the average of the 12 fastest heart beats during the one minute of base compared with the average of the 12 fastest heart beats during the one minute following the announcement. For palmar conductance, the comparable measure was the highest conductance reading during the one minute of base compared with the highest conductance reading during the one minute following the alerting announcement. In each case the heart rate and conductance levels during the alert period were corrected for the subject's initial or base level reactivity by a regression analysis described by Lacey (1956). The change scores (i.e., base to alert) were transformed into McCall T-Scores.

Total reaction (base to stress)

Comparable measures were obtained for heart rate and conductance changes when the values obtained during the one minute of base were compared with the values obtained during the minute while the subject was listening to the tape-recorded monologue.

As with the taped monologues, changes in heart rate and conductance to the physical and intellectual stressors were obtained by comparing the one minute of base period activity prior to the stressor with the heart rate and conductance values obtained during each of the seven stressors (total reaction). These change scores were also based on a regression of level during stress on level during base period, and transformed into McCall T-scores.[3]

There was a high positive correlation between the alerting reaction (base to alert) and total reaction (base to stressor changes) for either heart rate or palmar conductance. However, the correlations between heart rate and conductance changes taken at the same time (either base to alert or base to stressor), were much lower. Appendix 17 contains the correlations between heart rate and conductance changes for the alerting reaction and total reaction.

Only 3 of the 12 stimulus conditions yielded significant positive correlations between heart rate and conductance increases for the base to stress comparison (aggression to peer, mental arithmetic, rules of game).

Several of the situations yielded essentially zero correlations between these two autonomic response channels (aggression mother, noise, sexuality). There appears to be, therefore, some degree of independence between these two physiological reactions.

Appendixes 18 and 19 contain the intercorrelations among increases in conductance and heart rate for the total reaction for the twelve stimulus conditions. Appendix 20 contains the intercorrelations within each of these channels for the alerting reaction for the five tapes. These data will be discussed in some detail later in the chapter.

The most salient conclusion suggested by the data in Appendixes 17, 18, and 19 is that large changes in heart rate tend to be more selective than changes in conductance with respect to the psychological nature of the stressor. Of the 66 intercorrelations over the 12 conditions, 75 per cent were significant for conductance increases, whereas only 26 per cent were significant for heart rate. *Moreover, a third of the significant cardiac correlations involved tasks requiring similar psychological processes.* Changes in conductance appeared to be general reactions to any change in the environment—be it light, noise, solving problems, or listening to tape recordings. As we shall see later, the subject's style of conceptualization was highly related to a general tendency to display large changes in conductance to most stressors.

THE SIGNIFICANCE OF THE CONFLICT MEASURES

The purpose of this chapter is to provide information on the meaning of tachistoscopic perception and autonomic change through study of the correlations between these variables and the interview ratings, prose report ratings, and selected test scores. We will consider these relationships for the areas of aggression, dependency, sexuality, physical harm, and intellectual competence.

AGGRESSION

In order to determine the relation between each of the aggressive conflict measures and aggression in childhood and adulthood, correlations were computed with the relevant (a) adult interview ratings, (b) self-ratings, and (c) the longitudinal ratings for Periods III and IV. The child's ratings for Periods III and IV were chosen because the stability of these behaviors was greatest from age 6 through adulthood. Appendixes 21 and 22 contain the correlations between perception of aggressive scenes or autonomic changes to aggressive tapes and independent indexes of aggressivity.

Recognition thresholds for the aggressive scenes

Ease of recognition of the aggressive pictures by the men showed no significant relationship to interview ratings of aggressive retaliation, ease-of-anger arousal, aggression anxiety, or repression of aggression.

For the women, aggression anxiety showed a slight association with late recognition of pictures 2–14 ($r = .31$; $p < .10$). Reluctance to criticize the mother in the interview was also associated with late recognition of all three pairs of aggressive pictures for the females.

Self-rated aggression was clearly associated with early recognition for the women, but less so for men. The women who admitted to verbally aggressive outbursts recognized the aggressive scenes earlier than those who denied overt aggression.

Recognition of the aggressive scenes had a complicated relationship to childhood aggression. For the men, aggression to mother during age 10 to 14 predicted early recognition of pictures 2–14 ($r = .48$; $p < .05$). However, indirect aggression to peers and behavioral disorganization for Period IV were associated with late recognition of pictures 1–13 ($r = .44$; $p < .05$; $r = .52$; $p < .01$).

For the women, adolescent aggressivity showed no relationship to perceptual thresholds, but high degrees of physical aggression and competitiveness with peers during age 6 to 10 each predicted early recognition of the aggression scenes in adulthood ($r = .61$; $p < .01$; $r = .43$; $p < .05$).

The female data were more consistent than those for males. Women who denied aggressive behavior in adulthood and inhibited overt aggression toward peers in early childhood showed delayed recognition of the aggressive scenes.

Since women appear to have more aggressive conflict than the men (as exemplified in lower self-rated aggression, higher recognition thresholds, and greater delay in recalling the aggressive scenes), a tentative hypothesis is suggested. *Delayed recognition of conflictful stimuli is most clearly related to independent signs of conflict (e.g., tendency to deny practice of the behavior, inhibition) for groups for whom the behavior contradicts sex-role standards, and conflict is presumed to be high. Delayed recognition is minimally related to external signs of conflict for groups for whom the behavior is congruent with sex-role standards and, therefore, of lower conflict potential.*

Autonomic changes to the aggressive monologue

The relationships between base to alert and base to tape autonomic changes to the aggressive tapes with the interview, longitudinal, self-rating, and recognition threshold data appear in Appendix 22.

The men who showed the greatest increases in heart rate or palmar conductance while listening to the peer-aggression tape rated themselves as aggressive and were openly competitive with peers during adolescence and adulthood. Thus the instructions, "Feel yourself into the place of the person speaking," produced the largest autonomic changes in those men who were aggressive and competitive rather than in the men who characteristically inhibited overt aggressive behavior with peers. The high correlation between heart rate and conductance change for this tape ($r = .72$) is one reason for the similar patterns of correlations obtained for these two variables.

The reaction to the mother-aggression tape, on the other hand, yielded different results. Increases in conductance while listening to this tape were unrelated to self-rated aggression or competitiveness during adulthood or adolescence. Heart rate increases, however, were positively related to peer-directed aggression during adolescence. Changes in heart rate to both aggressive tapes, therefore, were more similar in their association with overt aggressive behavior than were the changes in conductance. This conclusion is supported by the correlations between autonomic change for the two tapes (see Appendix 19). The correlation between cardiac increase to the peer-aggression and mother-aggression tapes was .46 ($p < .01$). For conductance, the correlation between the two tapes was only .06. Thus cardiac and conductance increases (which were relatively independent of each other in response to the aggressive-mother tape) had different patterns of correlates with overt aggressive behavior.

Finally, there was no consistent relation between tachistoscopic recognition of aggressive scenes and autonomic change to the aggressive monologues. However, the direction of the relationships for the total reactions suggested that men who displayed the greatest increases in conductance to the aggression-mother tape recognized the pictures *earlier* than those who showed minimal increases in palmar conductance while listening to this monologue.

DEPENDENCY

The correlations between recognition threshold for the dependency scenes and overt dependent behavior were generally low (see Appendix 23). In contrast to aggression, however, the significant relationships held for men rather than for women. Early recognition of the dependency scenes was unrelated to dependent behavior in childhood or adulthood for the women; the correlations ranged from $-.10$ to $+.26$. For men, however, interview ratings of dependency on love object, dependency on friends, and fear of failure were associated with early recognition of the dependency scenes $(r = .34; p < .05; 29; p < .10; 29; p < .10)$. Moreover, the men who were instrumentally dependent during Period IV recognized the dependent pictures earlier as adults $(r = .42; p < .10)$.

These findings lend some support to the previous hypothesis that delayed recognition of conflictful scenes is most predictive of behavioral signs of conflict for groups for whom the behavior in question is socially inappropriate (i.e., conflict is expected to be relatively high). Dependency on others violates the masculine ego ideal and delayed recognition of the dependent scenes was more closely associated with inhibition of dependent behavior for males than for females. In addition to the generally higher recognition thresholds for men, the correlations between self-rated dependency and the interview ratings of dependency were higher for women than for men. The men may have been less accurate in their self-report because they were more conflicted over rating themselves as dependent. The relationship between self-rated dependency and the interview rating of dependency on family was .46 $(p < .01)$ for men and .61 $(p < .001)$ for women.

SEXUALITY

Tachistoscopic perception

The relationship between recognition of the sex scenes and heterosexual behavior was somewhat similar to that found for aggression (see Appendix 24). Delayed recognition of the sexual scenes among women was associated with anxiety over erotic behavior in adulthood

$(r = .28; p < .10)$ and avoidance of heterosexual contacts for ages 6 to 10 and 10 to 14 $(r = .35; p < .10; r = .45; p < .05)$. There was no relationship for men between recognition of the sex scenes and heterosexual behavior in either childhood or adulthood. Once again, the data suggest that delayed recognition is related to behavioral inhibition for groups with generally high conflict. The assumption of greater sexual conflict for women is supported by the higher female recognition threshold for the beach scene and the lower correlations, for women, between self-rated and interview-rated sex anxiety. The correlation for men was .64 $(p < .001)$; for women it was .36 $(p < .05)$. The difference between these two correlations is of borderline significance $(z = 1.52; p = .12)$.

Autonomic reactions to the sex tape

The autonomic reactions to the sex tape were not highly related to the other sources of data (see Appendix 25). The men who admitted to frequent erotic activity (i.e., low sex anxiety on the self-rating scale) had the largest increases in palmar conductance $(r = .36; p < .05)$ to the alerting announcement for the sex monologue. Base to tape changes were in the same direction but were not significant.

Moreover, men who had masculine interests during Period IV had large increases in heart rate while listening to the sex tape $(r = .41; p < .10)$. It was noted earlier (Chapter Six) that the boys who adopted traditional masculine interests were most likely to engage in erotic behavior during adolescence and adulthood. Thus the relation between cardiac increase to the sex tape and adoption of masculine traits is reasonable.

PHYSICAL HARM ANXIETY

Fear of bodily harm is present in most individuals but denied to different degrees. Men are less consciously preoccupied with physical harm than women, and the sex differences in self-rated physical-harm anxiety and recall of the physical-harm scenes support this assumption. This decreased conscious recognition of anxiety over bodily harm could be the result of minimal anxiety in this area or repression of these thoughts because it is inappropriate for men to acknowledge fear of injury. If the latter assumption were true (i.e., men repress thoughts involving the possibility of physical harm), we might expect recognition threshold for the harm scenes to be more closely associated with independent signs of repression for males than for females.

Appendix 26 contains the correlation between delayed recognition of the harm scenes and adult and child behavior. *The men who were easily angered both as adults and adolescents showed delayed recognition of physical-harm scenes. Delayed recognition among men was also associated with aggressive, dominant, and competitive behavior with peers for Periods III and IV.* For example, the correlation between indirect aggression to peers for age 6 to 10 and delayed recognition was .53 ($p < .01$).

For women, adult aggressivity was unrelated to recognition threshold, but aggression and competitiveness toward peers for age 10 to 14 showed a slight association with *delayed* recognition of the harm pictures ($r = .39, .36; p < .10$). Furthermore, the women who showed *early* recognition of the harm pictures showed some avoidance of dangerous activity during Period III ($r = .35; p < .10$). This relationship did not occur for men.

The men who had the greatest difficulty recognizing pictures of an individual being attacked by an animal or falling from a cliff were, as children, aggressive with their peers and prone to disorganized aggressive outbursts when frustrated. Thus delayed recognition of scenes in which a man is helpless in the face of danger or physical attack was characteristic of subjects who, as children, were aggressive. Their overt behavior, therefore, did not suggest the presence of intense physical-harm anxiety.

Anxiety over bodily injury, unlike dependency, aggression, or sex, is an *ideational* response rather than an *overt* act. If we extend the hypothesis relating sex-role appropriateness and perceptual recognition to thought products, we might expect that delayed recognition of the harm scenes would be more closely related to independent signs of conflict for men than for women. For this class of ideas is less appropriate for and less acceptable to men than to women. The present data agree with this expectation. The men whose behavior seemed to reflect denial of possible bodily injury had difficulty recognizing the harm scenes.

Autonomic reaction to the physical-harm tape

The relations between autonomic changes to the harm tape and behavior are summarized in Appendix 27. The men with the greatest increase in conductance for the alerting or total reactions rated themselves as aggressive and were rated as competitive and dominant with peers during childhood.

However, large changes in heart rate or conductance to the harm tape were highly correlated with the changes that occurred to the aggression peer tape. Moreover, the aggressive men showed high reactivity to both tapes. It is difficult, therefore, to interpret the psychological significance of these correlations. On the one hand, it is possible that similar psychological mechanisms underly the similar autonomic reactions to both tapes. Men who are overtly aggressive like to perceive themselves as bold and are apt to relish dangerous situations. Therefore they should have become highly involved in the situation described by the physical-harm monologue.

On the other hand, the aggressive peer and physical-harm tapes were both highly charged communications, and it is possible that aggressive men tend to react with large autonomic discharges to any affectively charged communication. The tendency to react autonomically may be related, in part, to a fundamental characteristic of the individual. That is, some people may be more labile than others and likely to show large autonomic discharges in a variety of situations. This possibility will be discussed later.

INTELLECTUAL ACHIEVEMENT

The final behavioral area tapped by the autonomic situation dealt with intellectual achievement. Four of the tests administered in the second part of the autonomic session involved intellectual problems (make-up sentences, mental arithmetic, rules of the game, and reversed spelling). The subject was given a clear picture of the nature of these tasks prior to their administration and was told that they were tests of intelligence. Changes in autonomic discharge between the base period and the time during which the tests were administered (base to stress changes) were correlated with intelligence, concern with intellectual mastery, and confidence over intellectual ability in childhood and adulthood. Appendixes 28 and 29 contain these correlations.

As a control for the psychological relevance of the intellectual stressors, the correlations between autonomic discharge to noise, cold pressor, and flickering light, and the personality and intelligence variables are also presented. The results are less ambiguous than those found for the conflict tapes.

The pattern of correlations suggests two conclusions. First, *the men who were of above average intelligence,* who *actively sought status goals as adults and who were interested in and confident about their intellectual competence as adolescents had the greatest increases in heart rate during the administration of most of the intellectual tasks.* The men who were of less adequate intelligence and who were less involved in intellectual mastery as adolescents, had minimal increases in heart rate. Men with high fear of failure in the intellectual area during Period IV (i.e., anxious about their intellectual competence) showed minimal increases in heart rate.

It is suggested that the largest heart rate increases to the intellectual problems occurred in those men who actively tried to solve them—the men who were interested and who became highly involved in the challenge of the problem-solving process. Minimal increases in heart rate characterized the men who apparently withdrew affective involvement from the problems because they doubted their intellectual ability.

These data are concordant with the results obtained for the peer-aggression tape. The men who showed minimal increases in heart rate to that tape were nonaggressive; the men who showed minimal increases in heart rate to the intellectual tasks avoided involvement in intellectual challenges. Heart rate increase under these laboratory conditions seems to be not an index of anxiety but an index of affective involvement in the situation. The absence of any relationship between intelligence or intellectual involvement ratings and cardiac increase to the physical stressors (i.e., loud noise, cold pressor) indicates that these heart rate changes were specific to the intellectual content.

Conductance changes while solving the intellectual problems produced a slightly different pattern of correlations. First, the brighter men displayed the larger increases in conductance to both the intellective and nonintellective stressors. Thus autonomic reactivity in this channel was not *specific* to the intellectual stressors. Second, the correlations with ratings of intellectual mastery, or fear of failure in adolescence, were not as consistently high as those obtained for heart rate changes.

The pattern of intercorrelations among conductance or heart rate change for all seven stressors casts some light on the reason for the difference in these correlation patterns (see Appendixes 18 and 19). For palmar conductance, 19 of the 21 intercorrelations among the seven stressors were significant at the .05 level or better. For heart rate change, only 6 of the 21 correlations were significant, and 5 of these involved the intellectual tasks. Thus heart rate change displayed a consistency across the four mental tasks and appears to be a reaction that is *relatively specific* to tasks requiring concentration. There was no consistency in heart rate response across the three nonintellectual stressors (cold pressor, noise, flickering light).

Increases in heart rate were more discriminating with respect to the content of the stressor and were elicited by tasks requiring mental concentration and elaboration. Increases in conductance were more frequently a generalized reaction to any new stimulus event and, in this study, were more characteristic of men with above average intelligence.

In sum, increases in palmar conductance and heart rate appear to be mediated by somewhat different intrapsychic mechanisms. Cardiac acceleration seems to be more closely related to specific kinds of psychological requirements than increases in conductance. It has been suggested that affective involvement in a task requiring mental elaboration is one condition that leads to cardiac acceleration. Thus individuals who showed the largest increases in heart rate to symbolic tasks were those who became most involved in the verbal communication or problem. This is not equivalent to saying that the most *anxious* individuals showed the greatest cardiac acceleration. As a matter of fact, since anxiety might lead to avoidance and withdrawal from the aversive situation, highly anxious individuals might be expected to show minimal heart rate increases to conflictful communications. It would appear that the presence of high anxiety over a class of responses may lead to detachment from communications that are symbolic of the conflictful area and, concomitantly, minimal autonomic reactivity.

Increases in palmar conductance are a more general reaction and less clearly tied to specific psychological inputs. Moreover, there appear to be individual differences in degree of GSR reactivity. One of the correlates of this tendency to react with large increases in palmar conductance to diverse situations will be discussed in the next section.

COGNITIVE CORRELATES OF AUTONOMIC REACTIVITY

The data presented thus far suggest that individuals differ in their tendency to display changes in level of autonomic activity, especially increases in palmar conductance. The consistently high intercorrelations among conductance increases across all twelve stressors support this hypothesis. Moreover, tasks that require or induce mental concentration appear to produce cardiac increases. It is possible that individual differences in the *tendency to become ideationally involved* in a communication may determine, in part, the amount of cardiac increase to various situations.

Relation between preferred mode of conceptualization and autonomic reactivity

The interview and testing situations (excluding the automatic battery) necessarily required the subject to make *verbal interpretations* of direct questions or of visual stimuli. This is not only the traditional method of acquiring descriptive information on humans, but the only method with a moderate degree of validity for those variables that contemporary theory regards as important.

Partly by accident and partly through a sensitivity to the language the subjects used, our attention was directed to the remarkable degree of intra-individual consistency in the way subjects dealt with the various test requirements. Regardless of the content of the interview questions or the stimulus character of the test situations, some subjects showed a consistent style of interpretation, a characteristic way of organizing stimulus input and of language expression. Subjects who were highly verbal and introspective during the interview produced Rorschach responses that were imaginative and contained dynamic content; they produced conceptual sorts of human figures that were based on emotional and motive states; and they emphasized the affect and ideational states of the TAT figures they described. On the other hand, subjects who had difficulty talking about their goals and conflicts during the interview produced popular and nonimaginative interpretations of ink blots; they did not group figures together on the basis of intra-psychic states; and they rarely mentioned the internal feelings or motive states of the people they described in TAT stories.

The people who preferred to conceptualize social stimuli in terms of affect and motive states were generally more introspective. They readily described their own motives and conflicts and evidenced more spontaneous affect during the interview. In effect, they entered into the verbal requirements of the interview with more emotional involvement. We speculated that these subjects might be more reactive autonomically, and this hypothesis was put to test.

Four instruments had been administered that could be scored for this style of conceptualization: modified Rorschach, 13-card TAT, figure-sorting task, and the tachistoscopic task.

ADMINISTRATION OF TESTS AND VARIABLES SCORED

Modified Rorschach

As described in Chapter Two, the subjects were administered the 32-item, ink blot test after the interview. Each stimulus in this series tended to be perceived as a unitary Gestalt, and, with one exception, each was either totally chromatic or achromatic. Over 90 per cent of the subjects produced 32 responses. The responses were scored for (a) ascription of action, motivation, or affect to human or humanlike stimuli (e.g., elves, witches), (b) ascription of action, motivation, or affect to animals, and (c) humans seen without any action or motivational component.

The median numbers of responses for these three categories were 3, 4, and 2, respectively. The relationships among these three variables (based on contingency coefficients with Yates' correction) indicated that human and animal movement were positively associated ($C = .47$; $p < .01$), and each was independent of human responses ($C = .11$ and .22).

Because of the positive correlation between human and animal movement these scores were pooled, and a variable, hereafter called *ink blot movement responses,* was obtained. The pooling of these two scores yielded a variable with a symmetrical distribution.

Thematic Apperception Test

A 13-card TAT was administered to each of the subjects after the interview but prior to the administration of the self-rating scale. The protocols were scored for several formal categories. The rater was instructed to score the first three phrases of each story. This limitation on length was intended as a control for general verbosity. The categories to be considered here include: (a) ascription of affect or feeling states to people (mad, happy, sad, tired), (b) ascription of ideational states to people (thinks, believes, wishes, wonders), and (c) ascription of social roles (farmer, mother, doctor) or abstract qualities (bad, good, competent, ambitious).

Each of the pictures had a differential tendency to elicit these categories and a separate weighting procedure was used for each variable for the male and female series of pictures. The four pictures with the greatest tendency to elicit each of these scores were given a score of "1." The four pictures with the least tendency were given a score of "3," and the five remaining pictures were given a score of "2." The subject's weighted score for each of these variables was a sum of his weights for all 13 pictures. Ascription of affect and ideational states were positively correlated ($C = .43$; $p < .10$, .44; $p < .10$ for males and females, respectively), and each was relatively independent of the ascription of role or abstract adjectives to TAT figures. For example, the correlation (contingency) between ascription of affect and role labels was $+.12$ for males and $-.34$ for females ($p < .05$).

The affect and ideational scores were pooled to obtain a variable hereafter called *TAT affect-ideation.*

Figure sorting

During the third test session, after the sessions in which the Rorschach and TAT were administered, the subjects were presented with three different arrays of human cardboard figures and asked to select groups of figures that went together on some common basis. During the course of the session, a total of 32 conceptual sorts was obtained; the order of administration of these arrays was described in Chapter Two. The subjects' responses fell into three major formal categories, and these are defined below.

Analytic-descriptive. This category included concepts that were based on similarity in objective, physical attributes among a group of stimuli. Examples of descriptive concepts were coatless people, people holding something with their arms up, people lying down, men with guns.

Relational. This category included concepts that were based on a functional relationship between or among stimulus members of a group. This functional relationship involved temporal, spatial, or inter-object relationships among the stimulus members. In this category, no stimulus was an independent instance of the concept and each stimulus derived its meaning from its relationship to other stimuli in the group. Examples of relational concepts were: a family, a married couple, a crime scene, mother giving food to child.

Categorical inferential. This category included concepts that were not directly based on any objective, physical attribute of the stimuli. In an inferential concept, as in a descriptive one, any stimulus in the group was an independent instance of the conceptual label. Examples of inferential concepts were: models, criminals, people who help mankind, poor people.

Affect concepts. This was a subcategory of the categorical inferential group in which people were grouped together on the basis of similarity in affect or motive state (e.g., these are mad, these are happy, these are sad, these people want to murder someone, these wish they were richer). The categorical inferential score (described above) did not contain these affect concepts.

The distributions for descriptive, categorical, and affect sorts were symmetrical with medians of 6, 12, and 3, respectively. The distribution for relational sorts was bimodal with one-quarter of the subjects producing no relational responses. For the present discussion we will omit this category. However, occurrence of relational sorts was negatively related to descriptive concepts ($\phi = -.49$; $p < .01$, and $-.25$ for men and women, respectively).

Tachistoscopic affect

Although the instructions for the tachistoscopic task emphasized the reporting of actions (What is each person on the picture doing?), some people ascribed affect states to these figures. This was true even though the scenes were presented at exposure speeds of less than one second. The protocols were scored for the number of scenes (98 in all) in which an affect state was attributed to the figures.

The inter-rater reliability (percentage of agreement) for the scoring for each of the above seven conceptual measures ranged from 90 to 96 per cent.

The intercorrelations among these seven variables were computed (product moment). The seven variables included ink blot movement, TAT affect-ideation, TAT role, figure-sorting affect, figure-sorting categorical, figure-sorting descriptive, and tachistoscopic affect. These intercorrelations appear in Table 4.

The data in Table 4 indicate moderate intra-individual consistency, among men, in the tendency to ascribe affect or motivational states to human figures. Of the six correlations involving affect labels, four were significant at the .05 level or better. For example, the correlation between figure-sorting affect and ascription of affect labels to tachistoscopic scenes was .59 ($p < .001$); the correlation between figure-sorting affect and TAT affect labels was .32 ($p < .05$). The tendency to ascribe intra-psychic states to social stimuli was independent of descriptive or categorical concepts on the figure-sorting task.

It seemed reasonable, on two accounts, to assume that those men whose style of conceptualization involved assumptions about motive and feeling states might be prone to become involved in the emotionally charged symbolic situations that were presented during the autonomic session. First, this class of responses was not popular and required a more reflective and motivated study of the stimuli. Second, subjects who characteristically thought in psychological terms (i.e., affect and motive labels) might more easily become emotionally and ideationally involved in the verbally presented motivational material contained in the tape-recorded monologues. Table 5 presents the correlations between each of these conceptual variables and heart rate and conductance increases to the monologues, physical stressors, and intellectual problems (total reactions, base to stress). In addition, the relationship to intelligence is also presented.

The results clearly indicate that increases in palmar conductance were highly related to the subject's tendency to ascribe affect or motive states to TAT figures in the opening sentences of his story or to sort human figures on the basis of affect or motive states—two variables

TABLE 4. INTERCORRELATIONS AMONG CONCEPTUAL VARIABLES

Variable	Rorschach Movement	TAT Affect	Fig. Sorting Affect	Tachistoscopic Affect	Fig. Sorting Descriptive	Fig. Sorting Categorical	TAT Role Abstract
Rorschach movement	–	.34**	.50***	.22	.00	.16	.26
TAT affect-ideation	.19	–	.32**	.25	.09	–.11	–.13
Figure sorting affect	.48****	.16	–	.59*****	–.40**	.23	.08
Tachistoscopic affect	.38**	–.13	.26	–	–.14	.06	.11
Figure sorting descriptive	.11	–.02	–.12	–.06	–	–.39**	–.06
Figure sorting categorical	.32*	.09	.00	–.07	.14	–	.46***
TAT role abstract	–.09	–.13	–.03	.41**	–.09	.11	–

* $p < .10$; two tails
** $p < .05$; two tails
*** $p < .01$; two tails
**** $p < .001$; two tails
Males to the right of the diagonal; females to the left of the diagonal

TABLE 5. RELATION OF CONCEPTUAL STYLE TO AUTONOMIC REACTIVITY

	Conceptual Categories						
	Fig. Sorting Affect	TAT Affect	Tachistoscopic Affect	Rorschach Movement	Fig. Sorting Descriptive	Fig. Sorting Categorical	TAT Role Abstract
Total Reaction Conductance							
Monologue: Control	.49****	.23	.18	.17	−.18	.00	−.03
Monologue: Harm	.45****	.04	.20	.02	−.12	.18	.04
Monologue: Aggression to peer	.52***	.06	.54***	.15	−.13	.20	.03
Monologue: Sex	.16	.00	.12	.19	−.02	.20	.07
Monologue: Aggression to mother	.17	.05	.01	.08	.02	.01	.23
Cold water	.58*****	.51***	.40**	.43**	−.05	.14	.03
Make-up sentences	.42**	.31*	.23	.10	−.09	.16	−.07
Noise	.40**	.31*	.48****	.01	−.13	.29	.21
Arithmetic	.41**	.38**	.15	.17	−.22	.29	−.02
Rules	.48****	.39**	.32*	.13	−.16	.12	−.06
Light	.37**	.29	.24	.10	−.09	.07	−.16
Spelling	.60****	.38**	.52***	.11	−.27	.12	.13
Heart Rate							
Monologue: Control	.37**	−.06	.20	.09	−.28	.28	.26
Monologue: Harm	.46****	−.07	.19	.11	−.10	.06	.01
Monologue: Aggression to peer	.29	−.05	.40**	.05	.09	.05	.04

Monologue: Sex	.16	.23	.05	.01	.16	.22	.17
Monologue: Aggression to mother	.31	.40**	.04	.49***	.12	.09	.22
Cold water	.23	.03	.00	.24	-.12	-.11	.04
Make-up sentences	.53***	.24	.45**	.25	-.03	.25	.02
Noise	.10	-.23	.08	.01	.11	-.21	.14
Arithmetic	.45**	.38**	.49***	.32*	.12	.15	.01
Rules	.37**	.38**	.30	.23	.22	.07	-.09
Light	.49****	-.01	.16	.40**	-.11	.19	.22
Spelling	.49****	.35*	.51***	.35*	.03	.29	.02
VS IQ	.07	.35**	.33**	.10	.51***	-.14	.07
PS IQ	.27	.23	.36***	.22	.37**	-.08	.05
FS IQ	.21	.30*	.37**	.21	.49***	-.11	.12

* $p < .10$; two tails
** $p < .05$; two tails
*** $p < .01$; two tails
**** $p < .001$; two tails

that are themselves highly related. The specificity of this type of conceptual style is indicated by the negligible correlations between autonomic change and the number of inferential conceptual sorts that did not involve affect states. Similarly, the tendency to ascribe abstract but nonmotivational adjectives to TAT figures was unrelated to autonomic reactivity.

Movement responses to the ink blots were much poorer predictors of conductance increases than the categories that dealt directly with the use of affect labels.

Heart rate increases were less consistently related to this conceptual style, especially when the stressors did not require any intellectual elaboration (cold water or noise). This finding is related to the previous statement that the degree of heart rate increase was consistent across tasks requiring intellectual effort or elaboration, but unrelated to cardiac changes to nonintellectual tasks. One reason for the positive correlation between affect sorts and cardiac acceleration to the flickering light task may be due to the fact that the subject was told he would see shapes and colors and would be asked to report them. Thus the task involved some degree of *mental effort and thoughtful elaboration.*

The positive relation between affect concepts and cardiac increase to the intellectual problems and selected monologues is interpreted as indicating that the production of affect labels was the consequent of an intellectually elaborative orientation. Such an orientation predisposed the subject to enter into the monologue or intellectual tasks with more affective involvement and a greater degree of ideational elaboration.

This conclusion is supported by the relation between affect conceptualization and behavior in the interview.

The tendency to use affect language in the conceptual tasks (figure sort, TAT, etc.) was associated with the interview rating of introspectiveness (i.e., tendency to elaborate on motives and conflicts). A composite and appropriately weighted index of the four affect measures (movement, figure-sorting affect, TAT affect, and tachistoscopic affect) was highly correlated with the interview rating of introspectiveness $(r = .47; \ p < .01)$ for males, $(.58; \ p < .01)$ for females, and $(.59; \ p < .001)$ for the entire sample. Thus subjects who easily and readily talked about conflictful material in the interview conceptualized social stimuli in terms of affect and motive states. Since these same subjects also showed large increases in palmar conductance and heart rate, it would appear that autonomic discharge in our laboratory situation was not an index of repressed conflicts. If anything, these reactions seem more closely related to lack of repression of these conflictful materials.

The tendency to use affect labels was unrelated to the subject's recognition thresholds for the tachistoscopic scenes. The correlations between figure-sorting affect responses and recognition threshold for the seven pairs of pictures ranged from −.33 to +.29, with a median correlation of +.02. Similarly, the correlations between TAT affect-ideation and recognition threshold ranged from −.40 to +.29, with a median correlation of .00. None of the conceptual variables had a significant relationship with recognition threshold for the control scenes. It appears that the processes responsible for autonomic change to conflictful communications were independent of the processes involved in early or late recognition of tachistoscopically presented scenes.

In summary, the tendency to manifest increases in palmar conductance to conflictful and nonconflictful stimuli appears to be a generalized characteristic of the individual. Many studies during the last decade have explicitly assumed that the amplitude of the GSR to stimuli designated as "anxiety arousing" was a reliable index of anxiety. The present data cast doubt upon this oversimplified assumption. It is possible that other aspects of the GSR might yield such an index (e.g., latency to maximal increase in conductance). However, in the light of existing data, it would appear that the amplitude of the GSR to conflictful verbal inputs should not be used as an index of anxiety without first controlling for the individual's general reactivity to both simple and complex stimulus material.

POSITION IDENTIFICATION

A third measure derived from the subject's descriptions of the tachistoscopic scenes has relevance for the concepts of active versus passive orientations. Each subject's verbatim protocol was scored for the figure that was first mentioned in the subject's description of the scene. Except for H-8 (person falling) there were two figures in each of the remaining 13 pictures. In picture H-9 one of the figures was a dog rather than a person. The subject had three alternatives in his initial labeling of the scenes. He could mention the figure on the right side of the picture, the figure on the left side of the picture, or he might label both figures as a unit (e.g., that's a couple, that's two men). This last category was infrequent for most of the scenes. Of the

13 scenes with two figures, 8 clearly involved one person doing something while the second figure was the passive recipient of the action; be it an aggressive, dependent, or sexual act. (Pictures A-1, 2, 13, 14, S-6, H-9, D-3, 4, 5). Pictures S-7, C-10, C-11, and C-12 did not clearly illustrate an active and passive pair. It was decided, therefore, to investigate the consistency and significance of any tendency to label initially the active person in the scene.

Each subject was assigned a score for each scene *indicating his preference to label the figure on the right* (i.e., number of times figure on the right was labeled first minus the number of times the figure on left was labeled first plus a constant).

The distributions for these scores were symmetrical for 5 of the 13 scenes (pictures A-1, A-2, A-14, D-4, H-9). The other scenes produced little variability in range. For pictures A-1, A-2, A-14, and D-4, the active figure was always on the right; for picture H-9, the active figure (the attacking dog) was on the left. Table 6 presents the average scores for right labeling preferences for the men and women.

TABLE 6. POSITION IDENTIFICATION: TENDENCY TO LABEL INITIALLY THE FIGURE ON THE RIGHT SIDE OF SCENE

Picture	Males	Females	p (two tailed)
A-1 Aggression to peer	10.0	9.4	–
A-2 Aggression to peer	9.4	7.8	$<.01$
A-14 Aggression to older man	8.2	5.4	$<.01$
D-4 Solicit older adult	10.0	8.3	$<.05$
H-9 Adult attacked by dog	8.6	10.9	$<.05$

On all 5 scenes the men had a greater tendency than the women to label the active figure first, and four of these five differences were significant. This result is not merely due to a tendency to label the figure on the right, for on picture H-9 (dog attacking man), the men labeled the dog more often than the women.

The intercorrelations among the scores for right labeling tendencies for these scenes appears in Table 7.

The tendency to name the active figure on the right for scenes A-1, A-2, A-14 and D-4 showed high consistency. The low nonsignificant correlation with picture H-9 (in which the active figure was on the left) supports the statement that this preference for labeling the active figure was not merely the result of a preference for naming the figure on the right.

TABLE 7. INTERCORRELATIONS AMONG POSITION IDENTIFICATION SCORES

Picture	A-1	A-2	A-14	D-4	H-9
A-1 Agg. peer	–	.67****	.40**	.45***	.28
A-2 Agg. peer	.37**	–	.69****	.77****	.26
A-14 Agg. older man	.10	.57****	–	.73****	.17
D-4 Solicit older adult	.44***	.59****	.66****	–	.21
H-9 Adult attacked by dog	–.10	.00	–.05	.06	–

  ** $p < .05$; two tails
  *** $p < .01$; two tails
  **** $p < .001$; two tails
Males to the right of the diagonal; females to the left of diagonal

In order to explore the significance of this tendency, two scenes were selected for further analysis—pictures A-2 and H-9. These particular stimuli were selected because (a) the figures on the right and left were most clearly separated, (b) picture A-2 had the active figure on the right while picture H-9 had the active figure on the left, and (c) there was no opportunity for the sex of one of the figures to facilitate a preference for naming the figure on the left or right.

Each subject's labeling score was then correlated with interview, child, and test variables. For picture A-2 a high score indicated a tendency to name the active figure first; for picture H-9 a high score indicated a tendency to name the passive figure first (i.e., the adult falling away from the attacking dog). Appendix 30 contains the correlations between the two labeling scores and selected interview ratings, child variables, and the tachistoscopic recognition thresholds.

The results suggest that the men who labeled the passive man on picture H-9 were, as adults, dependent on love objects ($p < .05$) and did not have masculine interests ($p < .10$). As adolescents (age 10 to 14) these men did not have masculine interest patterns ($p < .05$) and, for the first three years of life, were nonaggressive to mother and peers ($p < .05$) and passive in the face of frustration ($p < .01$). The ratings of aggression and passivity for 0 to 3 were better predictors of this tachistoscopic labeling preference than aggressive or passive behavior during the ages 3 to 14. In general, picture H-9 was a better predictor than A-2 of passivity, dependency, and lack of aggression for the males.

For women, the labeling of picture A-2 was a better correlate of an active orientation than was the labeling of picture H-9. The women who labeled the aggressive figure initially on picture A-2, in contrast to those who labeled the victim, were aggressive to mother during age 10 to 14 ($p < .01$), aggressive to peers during Periods III and IV ($p < .05$; $< .10$), and hyperkinetic during age 6 to 10 ($p < .05$).

There was no relationship between the initial labeling of pictures A-2 or H-9 and the recognition threshold for these scenes. Although these results are not as consistent or striking as we would have wished, they do suggest the potential value of attending to this class of behaviors. It is possible that such a response may be a sensitive index of the subject's tendency to identify with active or passive figures and consequently a reflection of his self-image.

It was not anticipated that this measure would be used in our analysis, and its study was undertaken after the fact. As in other results presented in this chapter, replication is necessary before confidence can be placed in these findings. However, if replication validates these results, it would be another instance of the usefulness of pretesting new measures on a longitudinal population for whom extensive behavioral information is available.

EVALUATIVE SUMMARY

The initial assumption that tachistoscopic thresholds and autonomic change might be measures of conflict and anxiety was not supported in any simple manner.

It is, of course, possible that our methods were inadequate. For example, the stimuli for the tachistoscopic task may have been inappropriate; or the use of threshold rather than above threshold exposures might have led to different results. Moreover, the conflictful monologues may have been an inappropriate and artificial method of arousing anxiety over sex, aggression, or physical harm, and perhaps we should have attempted to make the individuals angry or sexually excited through more direct techniques.[4]

However, the data obtained with these particular techniques suggest three tentative conclusions. First, delayed recognition of scenes depicting aggression, dependency, sexuality, and physical harm showed the highest correlations (and even then they were not high) for the group for whom repression of relevant content might be assumed to be strong. Delayed recognition of aggression and sexual scenes was more closely related to inhibition of these behaviors for women than for men.[5] Delayed recognition of dependency scenes was more closely related to inhibition of dependent behavior for men than for women.

It would appear that perceptual hypotheses involving sexual or aggressive action are weaker for women because these behaviors are inappropriate for the female sex role and related ideas have been repressed. These behaviors are more acceptable in men and it is reasonable to assume that sexual or aggressive associations are frequent and relatively strong for most males in our culture. Thus these tachistoscopic stimuli were not capable of differentiating differences in conflict among men.

There was no strong relationship between tachistoscopic thresholds and autonomic reactivity to conflictful stimuli in similar areas. Delayed recognition of conflictful scenes and autonomic reactivity to conflictful communications were not measures of any common process.

Finally, increases in palmar conductance or heart rate to different kinds of conflictful communications were not sensitive indexes of related anxiety or conflict.[6] In most instances increases in heart rate or conductance characterized the men whose behavior might be regarded as indicative of low conflict and high interest and involvement in the laboratory task.

The possibility that *one* important determinant of autonomic reactivity is degree of involvement in the measurement situation is both intuitively persuasive and concordant with the results of other investigations. For example, Berry and Martin (1957) found that instructions designed to produce maximum apprehension over anticipated electric shock produced *less effective GSR conditioning* in college women than instructions designed to minimize anxiety over the forthcoming shock administrations. It is possible that the high anxiety instructions led to psychological withdrawal from the task and consequently less efficient autonomic conditioning.

In another study (Westie and DeFleur, 1959), students designated as prejudiced and unprejudiced toward Negroes were exposed to pictures of Negro and white males and females. The greatest degree of autonomic reactivity (as measured by finger pulse) occurred when prejudiced white male subjects viewed pictures of white females (a situation that would be likely to facilitate high interest and involvement in the stimulus).

Pictures of males (Negro and white), on the other hand, produced the lowest skin-resistance levels. These data support the notion of the relative independence of skin resistance and cardiovascular reactions as well as the hypothesis that the *interest value of the stimulus* is a primary determinant of autonomic discharge.

In a recent and more elegant study (Mandler, Mandler, Kremen, and

Sholiton, 1961), college males were presented with phrases suggesting sexual, aggressive, and dependent content and asked to complete them while their autonomic reactions were being measured. One of the major findings was that subjects who avoided personal involvement in the stimulus showed less autonomic reactivity than those who became personally involved in the task.

These experimental findings, like the present ones, argue strongly for the conclusion that stimuli that psychologists classify *a priori* as anxiety arousing do not always elicit autonomic reactions in individuals who are presumed to have anxiety in that area.[7] It appears, rather, that a primary determinant of autonomic discharge is the degree to which the subject displays an *interest in* the material presented. It is obvious that degree of *interest* is not synonymous with degree of anxiety or conflict.

It is clearly possible that *absence* of autonomic discharge to stimuli that are designated as conflict arousing is a more sensitive index of repression of conflictful ideas than the occurrence of autonomic reactions to these situations.

The high positive relation between a preferred mode of conceptualization (i.e., sorting figures on an affect-motive basis) and autonomic reactions to varied stimuli give further support to the idea that a person's cognitive attitude to a task influences his physiological reactions. In sum, increases in autonomic activity, like most responses, are the final products of a series of complex cognitive transformations that occur between stimulus presentation and response output. Autonomic reactivity does not provide the investigator with a peek into his subject's unconscious, for it is too dependent on the individual's willingness (perhaps even his ability) to become involved in the situation.

Footnotes

1. This evidence of greater aggressive conflict for women than for men is supported by a study of college men and women. Buss & Durkee (1958) found that women were less likely than men to produce intensely hostile responses in a situation in which they were requested to select one of three verbs (neutral, mildly hostile, intensely hostile) and make up a sentence.

2. The reader will recall from Chapter Five that fear of harm among young boys was positively associated with adult involvement in intellectual mastery.

3. Analysis of the incidence of increases in conductance and heart rate for the alerting and stress periods revealed several trends that the reader should bear in mind as he studies this chapter. For the base-to-alert comparison, the majority of the men showed an increase in both conductance and heart rate to most of the stressors. For the base-to-stress comparison, however, conductance and heart

rate behaved somewhat differently. Most men showed greater conductance levels during each of the stress episodes (be it monologue, noise, or problem) than they did during the base or alert period. Occurrence of heart rate increases was more dependent on the nature of the episode. For tasks requiring continuous attention to external input information (e.g., the tape-recorded monologues, flickering light), many men showed a decrease in heart rate during the stress period, compared to the base or alert rate. For the tasks requiring mental concentration (intellectual tasks), the dominant trend was for most men to show an increase in heart rate in comparison to the base rate.

In the analyses to follow, we will be discussing the relation between heart rate increases to each of the 12 stressors and the interview and child ratings. For the intellectual tasks, individual differences in heart rate change do indeed reflect different degrees of cardiac *increase*. For the taped monologues, however, where the natural reaction was a slight decrease in rate, individuals with high scores are often those who showed the *least* decrease in heart rate or a minimal increase in heart rate while listening to the monologue. Individuals with low heart rate change scores showed cardiac decelerations while listening to the monologues.

4. Reiser (1961) has recently argued that autonomic reactions to laboratory situations may not be sensitive indexes of anxiety or conflict variables. He suggests that the subject's perception of the situation and his involvement in the tasks may be important determiners of degree of reactivity. He writes . . . "the clinical and laboratory data suggest that the soil has to be right for deep visceral changes to be activated. How often we encounter appropriate conditions for such responses in acute psychophysiologic experiments is open to question." (Reiser, 1961, p. 438.)

5. In a recent study with college students (Kagan & Moss, 1961a) it was found that the availability of aggressive ideas (as measured by the production of undisguised aggressive interpretations of ink blots) was positively correlated with ease of acquisition of the concept "angry" (using a standard concept acquisition task) for women but not for men. It was argued that aggressive associations are much more common among men and, therefore, measures of repression of aggression less sensitive for men than for women. This study, together with the present tachistoscopic data, suggest that experimental measures of degree of repression of conflictful ideas are apt to be most sensitive for groups having a fair proportion of individuals with generally high conflict and concomitant repression.

6. Buss (1961), after reviewing the literature on the autonomic correlates of aggressive communications, also concludes that it is difficult to differentiate the physiological reactions to aggressive communications from those that occur to other emotionally arousing situations.

7. Martin (1961) also suggests that if an area is successfully defended against, it is unlikely that anxiety is present (i.e., conflict relevant stimuli will not elicit autonomic reactions).

CHAPTER NINE

Summary and Conclusions

We found this an exciting project to execute and an equally exciting book to write. Some of our hunches were verified; others were clearly refuted. Equally important, however, were the unexpected discoveries that suggested provocative leads for future research and pointed to fallacies in current methodological practices. We do not intend to summarize all of the results in this short and final chapter. There are, however, five conclusions, which are relevant for developmental theory or for current methodological issues, that will be singled out for special attention. These statements must be regarded as tentative and limited by the many special characteristics of these data and of this longitudinal population.

DIFFERENTIAL STABILITY OF BEHAVIOR AS A FUNCTION OF SEX TYPING

The most dramatic and consistent finding of this study was that many of the behaviors exhibited by the child during the period 6 to 10 years of age, and a few during the age period 3 to 6, were moderately good predictors of theoretically related behaviors during early adulthood. Passive withdrawal from stressful situations, dependency on family, ease-of-anger arousal, involvement in intellectual mastery, social interaction anxiety, sex-role identification, and pattern of sexual behavior in adulthood were each related to reasonably analogous behavioral dispositions during the early school years. Figure 4 summarizes the differential stability of these seven classes of responses from childhood to adulthood. These results offer strong support to the popular

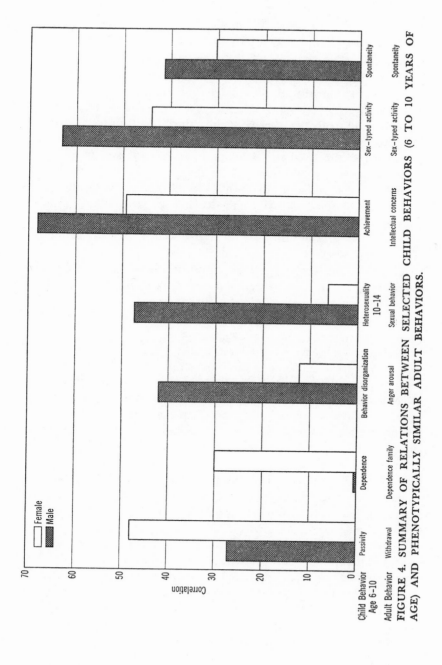

FIGURE 4. SUMMARY OF RELATIONS BETWEEN SELECTED CHILD BEHAVIORS (6 TO 10 YEARS OF AGE) AND PHENOTYPICALLY SIMILAR ADULT BEHAVIORS.

notion that aspects of adult personality begin to take form during early childhood.

However, the degree of continuity of these response classes was intimately dependent upon its congruence with traditional standards for sex-role characteristics. The differential stability of passivity, dependency, aggression, and sexuality for males and females emphasizes the importance of cultural rules in determining both behavioral change and stability.

Passive and dependent behavior are subjected to consistent cultural disapproval for men but not for women. This disapproval is communicated to the child through the direct rewards and punishments issued by peers and adults as well as the behavior of role models, be they real or the product of the public media. It is not surprising, therefore, that childhood passivity and dependency were related to adult passive and dependent behavior for women, but not for men, and that the men had greater difficulty than the women in recognizing the tachistoscopically presented dependency scenes.

A low threshold for anger, direct aggressive retaliation, and frequent sexual behavior, on the other hand, are disproportionately punished in females, whereas males are given greater license in these areas. The data revealed that childhood rage reactions and frequent dating during preadolescence predicted adult aggressive and sexual predispositions, respectively, for men but not for women. As might be expected, the women had greater difficulty than the men in accurately describing the tachistoscopically presented aggressive pictures and described themselves as less aggressive than the men on the self-rating questionnaire.

Intellectual mastery and adoption of appropriate sex-typed interests are positively sanctioned for both sexes, and both of these behaviors showed a high degree of continuity for males and females from the early school years through adulthood. In selected instances even preschool behavior was related to a similar disposition in adulthood. For example, the preschool girl's involvement in achievement tasks predicted her concern with intellectual mastery in adulthood ($r = .44$; $p < .05$).

Even the children who were reared by families that did not consciously attempt to mold the child in strict concordance with traditional sex-role standards responded to the pressures of the extrafamilial environment. The aggressive girls learned to inhibit direct expression of overt aggressive and sexual behavior; the dependent boys gradually placed inhibition on urges toward dependent overtures to others.

Moreover, the occurrence of derivatives of child behavior was related to the sex-role appropriateness of the childhood response. Passivity among boys predicted noncompetitiveness, sexual anxiety, and social apprehension in adult men, but not direct dependent overtures to parents or love objects. A tendency toward rage reactions in young girls predicted intellectual competitiveness, masculine interests, and dependency conflict in adult women, but not direct expression of aggression. It appears that when a childhood behavior is congruent with traditional sex-role characteristics, it is likely to be predictive of phenotypically similar behaviors in adulthood. When it conflicts with sex-role standards, the relevant motive is more likely to find expression in theoretically consistent substitute behaviors that are socially more acceptable than the original response. In sum, the individual's desire to mold his overt behavior in concordance with the culture's definition of sex-appropriate responses is a major determinant of the patterns of continuity and discontinuity in his development.

Not all of the childhood reactions displayed long-term continuity. Compulsivity and irrational fears during childhood were not predictive of similar responses during adulthood. Moreover, task persistence and excessive irritability during the first three years of life showed no relation to phenotypically similar behaviors during later childhood.

However, when a response displayed long-term stability, it was likely to be congruent with sex-typed behavior standards. The relevance of sex-role identification in directing behavioral choices is supported by investigations indicating that the child begins to differentiate the culture's definition of masculine and feminine characteristics and activities very early in development. Hartup and Zook (1960) have reported that even 3-year-olds are aware of the interests and objects that comprise the exterior decor of males and females in this culture. Other investigators (Kagan, 1956b; Kagan and Lemkin, 1960c; Kagan, Hosken and Watson, 1961b; Gardner, 1947) have reported that children from 5 to 10 years of age view the male, in relation to the female, as more competent, more aggressive, and more fear arousing, but less nurturant. The belief that aggressive behavior is more appropriate for males than for females is apparently acquired early in development and no doubt contributes to the girls' suppression of overt aggressive responses.

Osgood's (1957) work with the semantic differential suggests that adults categorize most objects and qualities with respect to their position on three dimensions: good-bad, potent-impotent, and active-passive. The qualities that define the potency and activity demensions resemble, in large measure, the stereotyped conceptions of male and female sex-typed traits. For example, the adjectives *large, strong, loud, heavy, bass, rough,* and *rugged* have the highest factor loadings on the potency factor. The adjectives *agitated, sharp, ferocious, tense, hot, angular, active,* and *fast* have the highest loadings on the activity factor. The above sets of adjectives are more commonly applied to males, whereas their polar opposites are typically attributed to females. Aggressive behavior is closely related to the potent and activity dimensions, whereas passive-dependent behavior is allied with impotence and inactivity.

Comprehension of the world is much like the game of twenty questions, with the child attempting to understand new experiences through successive categorizations from broad to narrow labels. It would appear that the masculine or feminine quality of an activity or object is one of the first questions implicitly asked by the child. Having determined the answer to this question, his behavior toward it (i.e., approach or avoidance) will depend on his sex-role identification.

The universe of appropriate behaviors for males and females is delineated early in development, and it is difficult for the child to cross these culturally given frontiers without considerable conflict and tension.

One of us recalls a conversation between a female college student (S) and his 3½-year-old daughter (D).

D: "What are you studying?"
S: "Psychology, for your daddy."
D: "Are you going to be a psychologist?"
S: "Yes."
D: "Are you going to be a mother?"
S: "Yes, I think so."
D: (After a puzzled pause) "Well, you can't be a psychologist and a mother too."

Social-class membership is an additional variable of constraint with respect to the specific sex-role values adopted by the child. Certain behaviors (e.g., interest in art and music) would be more acceptable to middle-class than to lower-class males, and vocational aspirations are, of course, highly dependent on social-class position. Thus knowledge of the sex and social class of a child allows one to make an unusually large number of predictions about his future interests, goals, vocational choice, and dependent, aggressive, sexual, and mastery behaviors. The behavioral face that is typically exposed to the social environment derives much of its topography from the cultural rules for sex and social class appropriate behaviors.

Sex-role identification as a governor of behavior

The preceding discussion places the construct of sex-role identification in a central position in directing the selective adoption and maintenance of several behavior domains. The expression of aggression, competitiveness, passivity, dependency, or sexuality is determined, in part, by the individual's assessment of the congruence of the behavior with traditional sex-role standards. For many individuals are motivated to behave in a way that is congruent with a hypothetical ego ideal or idealized model that embodies the essential qualities of masculinity or femininity.

This motive—like Festinger's (1957) construct of cognitive dissonance vs. consonance—locates both the goal state as well as the incentive conditions in the cognitive system of the individual rather than in the outside world. The motive paradigm chosen by psychologists in the behavioral tradition is derived from the hunger, thirst, pain model used with animals. In this model, the conditions that create motives (or drives) as well as the reward stimuli that gratify motives are defined primarily in terms of external stimulus events (e.g., frustration, rejection, or loss of loved one as motive arousing conditions; perception of injury in another or receipt of love as goal states).

We do not reject the usefulness or validity of this orientation. It seems necessary, however, to acknowledge the relevance of a need— perhaps unique to humans—to act and to believe in ways that are congruent with previously established standards. The incentive and goal stimuli for this motive are not always external events but evaluations of the match between a belief or proposed response and an internalized standard. Each individual has a cognitive picture of the person he would like to be and the goal states he would like to command—an idealized model of himself. Any behavior or belief that increases the discrepancy between the individual's evaluation of himself and his idealized model provokes anxiety and is likely to be shunned; any behavior that decreases the discrepancy between the evaluation of self and model is rewarding and is likely to be practiced.

It would appear that the desire to be an *ideal male* or *ideal female*, as defined by the individual, comprises an essential component of everyman's model. Thus the position of a response on a cognitive dimension ranging from *highly masculine* to *highly feminine* is a primary determinant of its acceptability and, therefore, of its probability of occurrence.

The early school years as a critical period

The continuity between child and adult behavior generally became manifest during the first four years of school. This relation was clearest for the behavior of withdrawal (for women), involvement in task mastery, social spontaneity, and degree of adoption of traditional sex-typed interests.

The poorer predictive power of behavior during the preschool years suggests that developments during the age period 6 to 10 induce important changes in the child's behavioral organization. The primary events of this period include (a) identification with parents and the concomitant attempt to adopt the values and overt responses of the parent, (b) the realization that mastery of intellective skills is both a cultural requirement as well as a source of satisfaction, and (c) the encounter with the peer group. The latter experience forces the child to accommodate, to some degree, to the values and evaluations made by peers. For some children, peer experiences strengthen patterns of dominance, social spontaneity, and positive self-evaluation. For others, peer rejection and a perception of marked deviation from peer-valued attributes lead to social anxiety, social submission, and a sense of ineffectiveness. Some children in the latter group develop compensatory domains of competence not involving peer interactions. Those who are unable to do so continue to anticipate failure when faced with task or social challenges.

It would appear that, for some children, the first four years of contact with the school and peer environments (i.e., during ages 6 to 10) crystallize behavioral tendencies that are maintained through young adulthood.

The present findings argue that those children who display intense strivings for mastery during the early years of school are likely to maintain this behavioral posture. The strategy of selecting bright, highly motivated fourth graders for special educational programs implicitly assumes that these children will not suddenly cease to exert efforts at task mastery. The results of this study support this assumption.

However, these data also suggest that withdrawal from anticipated task failure, among girls especially, grows rapidly during the early school years, and remedial or theraupetic intervention should be applied earlier in the curriculum than is now the case.

Behavior and motives

These conclusions about developmental continuities refer primarily to *behaviors*, not to *motives*. It is not suggested, for example, that the lack of relation between child and adult dependent behavior for men implies no continuity of dependency motivation. The longitudinal material did not allow for the reliable assessment of purely motivational constructs, and we have tried to avoid stating conclusions about motive states. This is an unfortunate lacuna but an unavoidable one. The difficulty in assessing motivational variables from overt behavior is not merely a function of the inhibiting influence of motive-related conflict and anxiety upon expression of goal-related behavior. The evidence presented in Chapters Four and Six indicated that aggressive or sexual behavior in boys and men might occur in the service of strengthening the individual's sex-role identification rather than be directed toward goal states traditionally regarded as endpoints for an aggressively or sexually motivated act. Thus absence as well as presence of certain forms of aggressive or sexual behavior are ambiguous as indexes of motive intensity. The valid assessment of motive constructs is one of the most perplexing and exasperating problems facing contemporary psychology and one that may not be solved until we discover lawful relations between the child's history of social experiences and his behavior. It is hoped that the results from this project are a small step in that direction.

SEX DIFFERENCES IN PATTERNS OF RELATIONSHIPS

A frequent but not always welcome finding in psychological research involves sex differences in the pattern of correlations among similar or identical variables. We found many such differences in our material.

There were striking sex differences in ease of recognition of the tachistoscopically presented scenes and in scores on some of the self-rating scales. Moreover, delayed recognition of the dependency scenes was related to independent indexes of conflict for men but not for women. Delayed recognition of aggressive scenes showed the opposite pattern. Independent indexes of aggressive conflict predicted delayed recognition for women but not for men.

The intercorrelations among the interview variables yielded dramatic sex differences.[1] For women, for example, dependency on love object and parents was positively associated, but each was independent of dependency on friends. For men, however, dependency on love object was unrelated to parental dependency but positively associated with dependency on friends. Competitiveness, retaliation, and anger arousal were all positively intercorrelated for the adult men. For the women, on the other hand, competitiveness was independent of both retaliation and anger arousal.

One of the clearest examples of the divergent meanings of phenotypically similar traits occurred with the correlations involving intellectual mastery (interview variable 35). Our intellectually oriented men, in contrast to the intellectual women, were less competitive, more likely to withdraw to stress. The differences between the correlations for the men and women for competitiveness and withdrawal were both significant (p < .01).

Dependency, aggression, sexuality, and achievement conflict differentially with the standards for sex-typed behaviors and, therefore, are in different hierarchical organizations for the sexes. Thus we should not expect the intercorrelations among these related behaviors to be similar for men and women. It is suggested, furthermore, that many phenotypically similar behaviors may be *of different psychological significance for males and females.* To illustrate, aggressive behavior in a group of school-age children (hitting, pushing, verbal taunts) is typically regarded as evidence of hostile motivation. However, these responses could be the product of different motives in boys and girls. Traditional sex-typed values regard some forms of aggression as a critical attribute of masculinity. Thus boys who are striving to identify with a masculine ideal will be prompted to push a peer, to grab a toy, to jeer at a teacher. These behaviors may not necessarily reflect hostile needs but may be the child's way of announcing to the social environment, "I am a boy, I am capable of executing those behaviors that help to define my role." Thus a boy may employ a shove or verbal taunt as a way of greeting a peer—a "hello" if you wish. *This use of aggression in a girl is unlikely.* For this reason, aggressive behavior with peers is probably a more accurate index of hostile motivation in girls than in boys.

Similarly, initiation of sexual behavior among adolescents and adult males is often used as a way of supporting a traditional masculine identification. The positive relation, for men, between traditional masculine interests in early childhood and frequency of sexual behavior in adolescence and adulthood supports this statement. Women are less likely to initiate sexual behavior as a means of strengthening their self-image as women.

This discussion suggests a more general statement. Overt aggressive, sexual, dependent, and mastery behaviors can serve different purposes (i.e., have different motivational bases for men and women). This is not an original conclusion, for psychology has long acknowledged that the same class of behavior in two individuals may have different causes. But we have occasionally ignored this axiom in interpreting empirical data.

It is more difficult to explain the sex differences in intercorrelation patterns obtained from test scores (e.g., perceptual performance, projective tests, etc.) that are not related directly to sex-typed behaviors. On the basis of what we know of sex-typed characteristics, it is possible that the hierarchy of motives in a psychological testing situation differs for the sexes. Let us assume, for example, that females are generally more concerned with gaining the examiner's acceptance, giving socially appropriate responses, and avoiding failure, in the broad sense of the term. Males are probably more concerned with the accuracy of their responses and with displaying their cognitive skills and efficiency at analyzing conceptual materials. These sex differences in orientation to examiner, approach to test material, and motive for accurate performance might lead to similar responses which were provoked by different motives and, consequently, were of different psychological significance.

For example, females who perform well on problems requiring analysis and complex reasoning tend to reject a traditional feminine identification. Males with high performance scores, on the other hand, do *not* reject a masculine identification. Thus men and women with masculine interests and values achieve high scores on complex intellective problems (Milton, 1957). Since degrees of identification with one's sex-role have implications for a variety of behavioral dispositions, we would not except the correlations between problem-solving ability and scores derived from personality tests to be similar for the sexes.

One tentative conclusion is suggested. It may be unwise to pool data for males and females without first examining the data for sex differences. This means more than merely computing means and standard deviations, for many of our variables showed no significant differences in these two parameters *but yielded different patterns of intercorrelations.* If the data had been pooled, many of the relationships between child and adult behavior would have been negligible. For the positive correlation for one sex would have been diluted by the zero order relationship for the other. It is likely that many studies in the literature or in a file drawer would have led the investigator to draw different conclusions if separate analyses had been made for males and females.

THE SIGNIFICANCE OF EARLY PASSIVITY

A tendency toward passivity during the first three years was linked to selected aspects of adolescent and adult personality. For example, the boys who were extremely passive at age 3 were nonaggressive, socially inhibited, dependent, and conforming during adolescence. As adults they were dependent on love objects, adopted nonmasculine interests, initially identified the passive man in the tachistoscopic scene of the attacking dog, and had low levels of cardiac arrhythmia at rest. Moreover, the related variables of lack of hyperkinesis and fear of harm, which were each positively correlated with passivity for the boys, had similar predictive consequents. Although passivity in the school-age girl predicted adult dependency on love object and family, and withdrawal from problem situations, a passive orientation during the first three years did not have any clear derivatives in the adult behavior of women. However, passivity was highly stable for girls over the first 10 years of life, and the replication study on an independent group of 26 girls revealed moderate stability for passivity over the first six years of life.

It was suggested earlier (see Chapter Three) that constitutional variables might have an indirect influence on degree of behavioral passivity. One specific argument put forward was that infants with low muscle mass might be initially predisposed to withdraw in the face of personal attack, strange social situations, or difficult instrumental problems. This initial avoidant disposition would become strengthened with further practice. Evidence was presented that tentatively suggested an association between passivity and low muscle mass during the first three years.

Beginning with the preschool years, however, the presumed relation between derivatives of passivity and muscle mass becomes more indirect and applies specifically to the boys' development. Boys with small muscle mass are likely to have more difficulty perfecting the gross motor and self-defense skills encouraged and rewarded by young boys and, therefore, less likely to gain acceptance by same sex peers. Moreover, a boy with little muscle and small frame perceives that he deviates markedly from the culture's definition of a masculine physique, and he is apt to anticipate difficulty in obtaining acceptance from men and love from women.

It is reasonable to assume that these beliefs might lead to apprehension in social situations, avoidance of heterosexual interaction, and failure to adopt masculine interests. Although the passive boy may eventually learn to inhibit blatant withdrawal to problems or direct dependent overtures to dependency, the early passivity may be manifested in excessive social and sexual anxiety and a withdrawal from the competitive requirements that characterize traditional masculine vocations and avocations.

The present findings argue for the hypothesis that early passivity (during the first five years) influences salient aspects of the child's future development. Whether this tendency is the complete product of early learning or partly the indirect consequence of constitutional factors is a question that needs to be answered. Maternal protection of boys during the first three years was positively related to school-age passivity, and one could argue that these early reinforcement experiences are sufficient to explain the boy's behavior in adolescence and adulthood. However, the authors feel that early passivity and its potential relation to constitutional variables warrant more intensive study. Such research may provide substance to the cliché, "Personality is the result of an interaction between the environment and the constitutional characteristics of the individual."

THE SLEEPER EFFECT

One of the major characteristics of psychological phenomena is their long-time course. The bombardment of atomic nuclei or the reaction of hydrochloric acid with a base leads to effects that are immediate—sometimes even too fast to measure. In psychological development, however, the effects of specific early experiences are often not evidenced for long periods of time. There may be a lag between a cause and open manifestation of the effect. For example, theory suggests that severe maternal deprivation during the first year will severely impair the child's self-esteem, ego identity, and level of intellectual development. Verification of these hypotheses may require the development of specific responses before one can assess the child's level of self-esteem or intellectual skills. Similarly, the assumption that physical contact and reciprocal stimulation between mother and infant are necessary for the development of satisfactory interpersonal relations cannot be verified until the child is 6 or 7 and beginning to enter into a variety of peer and adult relationships. In these illustrative examples, some of the critical antecedent events underlying a complex response occurred many years prior to the manifestation of the behavior—there was a time lag between cause and effect.

One way to detect such a lag is to uncover a stronger relation between a variable measured early and one measured late in development than between similar variables measured contemporaneously or more contiguously in time. We have called this set of circumstances the "sleeper effect." The phrase "sleeper effect" is purely descriptive, for such an effect could occur for a variety of reasons.

We noted this effect twice in our material. In one instance, passivity and fear of bodily harm for age 0 to 3 and the related variable of minimal hyperkinesis for age 3 to 6 were each better predictors of love-object dependency in adult men than later assessments of these childhood variables. A second example of this "sleeper effect" occurred when selected maternal practices during the first three years of life were more sensitive indexes of the child's preadolescent and adult behavior than evaluations of "similar" parental practices in later childhood. These findings require different explanations.

It is possible that manifestations of passivity and fear of harm in the young boy are less disguised during the preschool and school years. During the later age periods the boy learns to inhibit open expression of passivity and fear, for these are immature reactions that are subject to disapproval. Thus an assessment of basic predispositions to passivity or bodily harm anxiety from behavioral observations at age 6 is likely to be less sensitive than an evaluation of these tendencies during the second and third year of life. During the earlier period the child's defenses are weaker, and he is less able or less highly motivated to prevent these immature and anxiety-based reactions from gaining direct expression in overt behavior. However, a covert predisposition to passivity may be present during the school years and may find expression in adolescent and adult derivative reactions.

The reasons for the "sleeper effect" with the maternal variables are more complicated. It will be recalled from Chapter Seven, for example, that a critical maternal attitude toward daughters during age 0 to 3 predicted adult achievement behavior ($r = .59$; $p < .01$), while a critical attitude during ages 3 to 6 or 6 to 10 showed a negligible relationship with achievement behavior in adult women ($r = .18$ and $.22$). Similarly, maternal protection of a daughter during age 0 to 3 predicted adult withdrawal from stress ($r = .52$; $p < .01$), whereas protection during ages 3 to 6 or 6 to 10 showed no relation to adult withdrawal ($r = -.01$, $-.14$).

One explanation for these and related results, summarized in Chapter Seven, rests on the assumption *that the reciprocal nature of the mother-child interaction changes with time.* Specifically, the child's stimulus salience (i.e., his ability to provoke relatively permanent changes in specific maternal reactions toward him) increases with age. For a 6-year-old is more likely to produce a major alteration in the mother's characteristic behavior toward the child than is a 2-year-old. The mother-child dyad is a feedback system, and the degree to which the child's actions have the power to change the mother's behavior increases with development.

A mother typically establishes expectations as to what her child should be like; the standards to which his behavior should conform. The greater the discrepancy between her expectations and her evaluation of the child's behavior, the greater the likelihood that she will modify her behavior and exert pressure on the child in an attempt to direct him toward greater congruence with her expectations.

During infancy the child's "personality" is relatively ambiguous, and the discrepancy between her standard and what she perceives in the child is necessarily small. The mother sees the child as she would like to see him, and *he is an object primarily to be acted upon.* The form and content of many maternal behaviors toward an infant, therefore, are not as contaminated by the effect of the child's behavior on her as her behavior toward a 10-year-old. To illustrate, a mother's concern with the intellectual achievement of her 2-year-old (i.e., her level of satisfaction with his development and her encouragement of intellectual mastery) is more likely an index of her basic needs and values than her degree of concern with the performance of her 10-year-old who might be failing in school.

Some mothers change their expectations and values as the child develops, and a mother's lack of concern with the school achievement of her 10-year-old daughter who is failing could be a recently acquired defensive maneuver to protect the mother from disappointment. Similarly, encouragement of independence, a critical attitude, or overprotection toward a 10-year-old may be newly developed reactive measures to a child's excessive dependence, excessive rebelliousness, or fragile defenses, respectively. Excessive permissiveness or protection toward a 3-year-old is more likely a reflection of more fundamental maternal attitudes.

Thus the high correlation between maternal hostility or protection during age 0 to 3 and adult behavior in women could be due to the fact that these practices during the first three years—in comparison with similar practices at age 10—provided a more sensitive index of the mother's basic attitudes toward her child and, hence, her more lasting effect on the child's developing behavior.

The mother who was hypercritical during Period I was usually dissatisfied with her daughter's level of intellectual development and lack of autonomy. These mothers often resented the child's excessive dependency and rewarded mastery and independence. When the child began to achieve intellectually and to display autonomy at age 9 or 10, the mother became less critical. Thus the girl's adoption of the traits valued by the mother led to a decrease in the mother's overt criticism of the child. Those mothers who were hypercritical during the school years, on the other hand, were usually dissatisfied with the child cleanliness habits, excessive aggression, or disobedience. In many cases the mother's criticism was provoked by a sudden increase in these behaviors when the child started school.

The Period I maternal behaviors that displayed the "sleeper effect" in clearest form were maternal protection and hostility toward daughters. Maternal restriction during Period I was not a markedly better predictor of adult behavior than later assessments of this attitude. Moreover, maternal protection of girls showed a low degree of stability over the first 10 years, indicating that some mothers modified the degree of protection they displayed toward their daughters over the first 10 years of life. An extremely protective attitude was characteristic of mothers who wished to infantilize their children. A critical attitude was characteristic of mothers who wanted early autonomy and independence for their daughters. The daughters of these two groups of mothers developed personalities that were congruent with their mother's expectations. The daughters of protective mothers were, as adults, passive, afraid of social interaction, noncompetitive, and involved in traditional feminine interests. The daughters of critical mothers achieved early independence from the family and retained this orientation through adolescence and adulthood.

These findings suggest that the elucidation of cause-effect relations in personality development may require, for selected questions, a longitudinal design. For example, a cross-sectional investigation of the relation between maternal protection and passivity in a 10-year-old girl might yield a negligible association between these variables. However, if the maternal behavior had been assessed when the child was 3 years old, a positive relation might have emerged.

It is not suggested that all research on parent-child relations should be longitudinal. There are, however, certain classes of parent-child interaction variables that are particularly vulnerable to this sleeper effect. For example, maternal behaviors that are likely to change in frequency and intensity over the first decade (e.g., physical affection, reward of dependency, physical punitiveness) are more likely to show this effect than attitudes and patterns of reward that tend to be stable (e.g., attitude toward sexuality, attitude toward the appropriateness of traditional sex-typed traits).

Furthermore, maternal behaviors that are often specific reactions to the child's behavior during the school years (e.g., concern with academic achievement, punishment of aggression) may give misleading correlations between contemporaneous assessments of both maternal and child behavior.[2] For the degree of criticism, praise, restriction, or acceleration directed at the child is dependent, in part, on his contemporaneous behavior. More studies are needed to determine the extent of these phenomena and the classes of maternal and child behaviors for which they are most relevant. The initiation of a series of six-year studies in which the mother's behavior during the first three years would be correlated with the child's behavior during the first six might turn out to be a wise and profitable research strategy.

CONCEPTUAL STYLE, AUTONOMIC REACTIVITY AND THE MEASUREMENT OF CONFLICT

The data on the significance of preferred styles of categorization and autonomic reactivity have little to do with the longitudinal material, but they have potentially important implications for a theory of psychological assessment procedures. Adults develop preferred ways of organizing and interpreting stimuli, and some of these conceptual preferences are consistent over a wide variety of situations. It is likely that these conceptual styles influence, to some degree, the form and content of many samples of verbal behavior.

The data summarized in Chapter Eight indicated that individuals differ in their characteristic categorizations of social stimuli. The conceptualization of social stimuli in terms of affect and motive states is one approach that shows consistency across a variety of situations. Individuals who adopt this approach generally talk about motives and feelings in an interview, produce movement responses to an inkblot, ascribe motives and feelings to TAT heroes, and are highly introspective. Moreover, an introspective tendency (as measured by interview behavior and production of human movement responses) was moderately stable from adolescence through adulthood.

Other investigators also report that test indexes of introspection (e.g., human movement) are associated with behaviors involving the ready availability of motivational and conflictful ideas. For example, subjects who produce many human movement responses to ink blot stimuli, in contrast to those with few movement responses, are more likely to (a) think about their motives and conflicts (King, 1958; Singer, Wilensky and McCraven, 1956), (b) remain in therapy rather than terminate early (Gibby, Stotsky, Miller and Hiler, 1953; Affleck and Mednick, 1959), (c) have high test anxiety scores (Cox and Sarason, 1954), and (d) have conflictful concepts like aggression and sexuality available for cognitive manipulation (Kagan and Moss, 1961a; Kagan, 1961). Morover, the ascription of affect states to TAT figures, which is positively associated with the occurrence of human movement responses, is related to the production of undisguised aggressive responses to ink blot stimuli (Kagan and Moss, 1961a).

In sum, some individuals have a characteristic conceptual approach in their description of people that results in the use of language referring to motives, feelings, anxieties, and conflictful ideas. *It is tempting but possibly fallacious to regard these verbal responses as a measure of motive strength or intensity of conflict.*

Moreover, this conceptual preference was positively associated with the tendency to react autonomically to a variety of stressor episodes. The men who organized human figures on the basis of similarity in affect and motive states had the largest increases in palmar conductance to both neutral and conflictful tape-recorded monologues as well as to nonsymbolic stimuli (loud noise, flickering light). Changes in skin resistance or heart rate to conflictful monologues did not mirror the hidden ideas of the unconscious or reflect the individual's intensity of "anxiety." [3] As a matter of fact, the data in Chapter Eight suggested that independent estimates of anxiety over intellectual competence during childhood and adulthood were associated with *minimal* autonomic reactivity when intellectual challenges were presented. Similarly, the men who described themselves as nonaggressive on the self-rating scale or in the interview showed minimal increases in palmar conductance while listening to the monologue depicting anger at a friend.

Increases in heart rate or conductance to intellectual problems or conflict-related monologues were most frequent for those men whose behavior was suggestive of low anxiety in the area in question.

It appeared that autonomic discharge to simple stimuli or complex communications was a result of *interest* or *involvement in* and *ideational elaboration* of the communication. Recent research on behavioral correlates of autonomic reactivity (mentioned in Chapter Eight) supports this contention. Since repression of conflictful material should lead to minimal ideational elaboration of a conflictful stimulus, it seems unlikely that autonomic reactivity in experimental situations will provide an easy or simple index of the presence or intensity of unconscious conflicts.

The relation between interest and arousal

The contemporary concept of arousal (Duffy, 1957; Malmo, 1958, 1959) is related to, but not synonymous with, the present notion of interest. The arousal theorists assume that the organism is at different levels of activation at different times and that muscle potential, heart rate, skin resistance, finger volume, respiration, and electroencephalographic data may be used as indexes of degree of arousal or activation. However, the arousal that accompanies *interest* in a stimulus event is not necessarily associated with apprehension or joy over an event. Thus arousal includes interest but encompasses a variety of other phenomena.

The major implication of the present argument, which is not explicit in the writings of the arousal theorists, is that reactivity of one or more autonomic target organs *to new stimuli* is dependent on and must follow cognitive involvement in the situation. This statement implies that autonomic discharge to, say, a series of sexual stimuli will occur only among those individuals who become interested in and cognitively elaborate on the stimuli. If we admit the concept of repression into our theoretical system (and some psychologists may not wish to do so), then it is eminently reasonable to conclude that individuals who have repressed sexual ideas will not cognitively elaborate upon the sexual stimuli and, therefore, will show no autonomic reactivity.

This hypothetical sequence might well apply to real life situations (in contrast to the laboratory). That is, it is not unreasonable to assume that a woman who has repressed sexual ideas would show no autonomic reactivity when a young man put his arm around her *if she did not have sexual associations to the event and did not begin to think about the meaning of the stimulus.* The stimulus for autonomic discharge is not the external event but the associations resulting from cognitive elaborations on the stimulus. Thus the use of autonomic reactivity as an index of conflict requires a procedure that guarantees involvement in the test situation and the assurance that the test stimuli did indeed elicit the relevant associations.[4]

The existence of individual differences in autonomic reactivity to various *stimulus* situations has been demonstrated by other investigators (Lacey, 1950; Kling and Schlosberg, 1961; Lacey, Bateman, and Van Lehn, 1953), and our material corroborates these findings. Moreover, the present data indicate that heart rate and palmar conductance behaved differently to different kinds of inputs. When the experimental task required sustained attention to simple incoming signals, heart rate showed a deceleration while palmar conductance increased.

Thus an increase in level of reactivity in one autonomic channel is not necessarily correlated with increased reactivity in other channels (Lacey and Lacey, 1958b; Lacey, Bateman, and Van Lehn, 1953). However, some investigators arbitrarily choose the conditioned GSR as an index of "anxiety" in experimental work without regard for individual differences in autonomic reactivity or the response of other target organs.[5]

The moral of this discussion is that neither autonomic discharge nor dynamic interpretations of projective stimuli are sensitive measures for the assessment of conflict or anxiety variables. The heart, the palm, or the interpretation of an ink blot, like verbal report, are each subject to complex processing and censoring procedures. These responses are the final result of an intricate sequence of "black box" transformations and, as currently measured, are not shortcuts to the direct assessment of motive or anxiety constructs.

The privilege of writing this final paragraph was made possible through the efforts of many Fels staff members over the past 30 years. We have experienced occasional twinges of guilt over reaping the benefits of their wisdom and labor. Longitudinal research is difficult and taxes even a scientist's capacity to tolerate delay of gratification. We believe this project demonstrates the inestimable value of continuous study of the developing child. We need more standard measures, more rigorous theory, and the initiation of limited longitudinal studies (i.e., 5 to 10 years) aimed at specific developmental hypotheses. With these advantages we should become more adept at wresting from nature the secrets of human development.

Footnotes

1. Study of the intercorrelations among the interview variables (Appendix 33) reveals that there is one strong cluster of highly correlated variables for women,

involving competitiveness, achievement, intellectual mastery, masculine interests, low social anxiety, and reluctance to withdraw from stressful situations.

There is no such major cluster of highly correlated variables for the males. For men, there are two clusters of correlated variables. One includes competitiveness, retaliation, achievement, and reluctance to withdraw from stressful situations. The second involves intellectual mastery, achievement, and independence from family.

2. The possibility that maternal acceleration during the child's preschool years may have a greater effect on his intellectual mastery than acceleration later in the child's development led us to search for additional data in support of this idea. Information on 30 adolescent boys (none of whom were in the current sample but who were part of a separate, special investigation) was studied in an attempt to determine whether maternal acceleration during the years 2 to 4 had a greater effect on amount of increase in IQ score during the school years than maternal acceleration during the school years (age 4 to 7). Each of these boys had received the Stanford-Binet regularly, and the difference in IQ between 5½ and 9 years of age was used as the measure of IQ change. Since there was a slight negative relation between level of IQ at 5½ years and amount of increase in IQ score, pairs of boys were matched on IQ at age 5½, with one member of the pair increasing and the other member decreasing in IQ score. This procdure produced nine pairs of boys. The average gain for the IQ increase group was 16.2 points (range of 8 to 28). The average drop for the IQ decrease group was 6.1 points (range 1 to 14), but every member in this group decreased in IQ score. The mothers of these boys had been rated semiannually on the Fels Parent Behavior Rating Scales for the degree to which they encouraged their sons to master developmental skills; the degree to which they accelerated the boys' mental and motor development. The scores on maternal acceleration were averaged for two separate age periods, age 2 to 4 and age 4 to 7, and the average scores on acceleration were compared for the two groups. For the age period 2 to 4, the boys who showed an increase in IQ experienced more maternal acceleration than the boys decreasing in IQ.

However, for the age period 4 to 7, the means were reversed. The boys with drops in IQ experienced more acceleration than the boys rising in IQ. When the scores on maternal acceleration were compared for the two periods, it was found that the mothers of sons with IQ increases displayed less acceleration as the child matured, whereas the mothers of boys who lost in IQ increased their acceleratory pressures as the child grew older. The difference between these trends almost reached statistical significance. These results suggest that maternal acceleration during the school years may be a reaction to the child's lack of motivation with respect to intellectual mastery.

3. A summary of the evidence bearing on the relationship between autonomic responses and the construct of anxiety appeared in a recent paper by Martin (1961), who stated ". . . one cannot conclude . . . that any clearcut pattern of physiological-behavioral responses, associated with anxiety arousal, distinguishable from other arousal patterns, has been demonstrated" (Martin, 1961, p. 251).

4. This conclusion holds mainly for situations in which one wishes to measure the presence of a conflict produced by the individual's natural life experiences. When a conflict or conditioned anxiety reaction is established *de novo* in a laboratory setting, then interest in the anxiety-arousing stimulus is presumably high for all subjects and autonomic discharge may then be a more sensitive index of the anxiety potential of the conditioned stimulus.

5. In some cases investigators draw conclusions about central nervous system processes from data on the conditioned GSR. For example, in a recent investigation (Halberstam, 1961) subjects were classified as hysterics or psychasthenics on the basis of their MMPI responses. The GSR was conditioned to the word "cow" through the use of electric shock. The hysterics required more trials than the psychasthenics before the conditioned GSR appeared and fewer trials to extinction. The author did not restrict his conclusions to GSR conditioning but implied that hysterics condition more slowly *in most situations* and that these findings have implications for the cerebral functioning of hysterics. Since the data in Chapter Eight suggested that nonintrospective adults (perhaps hysterics) were less likely to have GSR changes to *any stimulus* (be it stressful or neutral) it is reasonable to conclude that the results of the above study, and of similar investigations, do not demonstrate that hysterics condition more slowly *in general* but that they are less likely to have large GSR changes. If a different response system had been chosen, there might not have been any relation between hysteria and number of conditioning or extinction trials.

References

Affleck, D. C., and Mednick, S. A., 1959. The Rorschach test in the prediction of the abrupt terminator in individual psychotherapy. *J. consult. Psychol.*, 23, 125–128.

Anderson, L. D., 1939. The predictive value of infancy tests in relation to intelligence at five years. *Child Develpm.*, 10, 203–212.

Baldwin, A. L., Kalhorn, Joan, and Breese, Faye H., 1945. Patterns of parent behavior. *Psychol. Monogr.*, 58, No. 3.

Baldwin, A. L., Kalhorn, Joan, and Breese, Faye H., 1949. The appraisal of parent behavior. *Psychol. Monogr.*, 63, No. 4.

Bayley, Nancy, 1949. Consistency and variability in the growth of intelligence from birth to eighteen years. *J. genet. Psychol.*, 75, 165–196.

Bayley, Nancy, 1954. Some increasing parent-child similarities during the growth of children. *J. educ. Psychol.*, 45, 1–21.

Bayley, Nancy and Schaefer, E. S., 1960. Relationships between socioeconomic variables and the behavior of mothers toward young children. *J. genet. Psychol.*, 96, 61–77.

Behnke, A. R., 1959. The estimation of lean body weight from skeletal measurements. *H. Biol.*, 31, 295–315.

Bell, R. Q., 1960. Relations between behavior manifestations in the human neonate. *Child Develpm.*, 31, 463–478.

Beller, E. K., 1955. Dependency and independence in young children. *J. genet. Psychol.*, 87, 25–35.

Beller, E. K., 1957. Dependency and autonomy achievement strivings related to orality and anality in early childhood. *Child Develpm.*, 28, 287–315.

Beller, E. K., 1959. Exploratory studies of dependency. *Transactions in New York Academy of Science*, 21, 414–426.

Bennett, E. M. and Cohen, L. R., 1959. Men and Women: Personality patterns and contrasts. *Genet. Psychol. Monogr.*, 60, 101–153.

Berry, J. L. and Martin, B., 1957. GSR reactivity as a function of anxiety, instructions, and sex. *J. abnorm. soc. Psychol.*, 54, 9–12.

Bolles, R. C., 1958. The usefulness of the drive concept. In M. R. Jones (Ed.), *Nebraska Symposium on Motivation*. Lincoln: University of Nebraska Press, pp. 1–32.

Bradway, K. P., 1945. An experimental study of factors associated with Stanford-

Binet IQ changes from the preschool to junior high school. *J. genet. Psychol.*, 66, 107–128.

Bradway, K. P., Thompson, C. W., and Cravens, R. B., 1958. Preschool IQs after twenty-five years. *J. educ. Psychol.*, 49, 278–281.

Bradway, K. P. and Robinson, N. M., 1961. Significant IQ changes in twenty-five years: A follow-up. *J. educ. Psychol.*, 52, 74–79.

Bronson, W. C., Katten, E. S., and Livson, N., 1959. Patterns of authority and affection in two generations. *J. abnorm. soc. Psychol.*, 58, 143–152.

Burks, B. S., Jenson, D. W., and Terman, L. M., 1930. *Genetic studies of genius, Vol. III. The promise of youth. Follow-up studies of 1,000 gifted children.* Stanford University Press, 1930.

Buss, A. H., 1961. *The psychology of aggression.* New York: John Wiley.

Buss, A. H. and Durkee, A., 1958. Conditioning of hostile verbalizations in a situation resembling a clinical interview. *J. consult. Psychol.*, 22, 415–418.

Castaneda, A., McCandless, B. R., and Palermo, D. S., 1956. The children's form of the Manifest Anxiety Scale. *Child Develpm.*, 27, 317–327.

Child, I. L., Potter, E. H., and Levine, E. M., 1946. Children's textbooks and personality development: An exploration in the social psychology of education. *Psychol. Monogr.*, 60, No. 279.

Cobb, H. V., 1954. Role wishes and general wishes of children and adolescents. *Child Develpm.*, 25, 161–171.

Cox, F. N. and Sarason, S. B., 1954. Test anxiety and Rorschach performance. *J. abnorm. soc. Psychol.*, 49, 371–377.

Crandall, V. J. and Preston, A., 1955. Patterns and levels of maternal behavior. *Child Develpm.*, 26, 267–277.

Dollard, J. and Miller, N. E., 1950. *Personality and psychotherapy.* New York: McGraw-Hill.

Duffy, E., 1957. The psychological significance of the concept of arousal or activation. *Psychol. Rev.*, 64, 265–275.

Dunlop, G. N., 1951. Certain aspects of children's fears. Unpublished doctoral dissertation, Columbia University, 1951.

Ebert, E. and Simmons, K., 1943. The Brush Foundation Study of child growth and development. *Child Develpm. Monogr.*, 8, No. 2.

England, A. O., 1946. Non-structured approach to the study of children's fears. *J. clin. Psychol.*, 2, 364–368.

Escalona, S. and Heider, G. M., 1959. *Prediction and outcome.* New York: Basic Books.

Festinger, L., 1957. *A theory of cognitive dissonance.* Evanston: Row, Peterson.

Foran, T. G., 1926. The constancy of the intelligence quotient: a review. *Cath. Univ. Amer. Educ. Res. Bull.*, 1, No. 10.

French, E. G., 1955. Some characteristics of achievement motivation. *J. exper. Psychol.*, 50, 232–236.

French, E. G., 1956. Motivation as a variable in work-partner selection. *J. abnorm. soc. Psychol.*, 53, 96–99.

Gardner, R. L., 1947. Analysis of children's attitudes toward fathers. *J. genet. Psychol.*, 70, 3–28.

Gardner, R. W., 1953. Cognitive styles in categorizing behavior. *J. Pers.*, 22, 214–233.

Gardner, R. W., Holzman, P. S., Klein, G. S., Linton, H. B., and Spence, D. P., 1959. Cognitive control: A study of individual consistencies in cognitive behavior. *Psychol. Issues*, 1, No. 4.

Garn, S. M., 1957. Roentgenogrammetric determinants of body composition. *H. Biol.*, **29**, 337–353.

Garn, S. M., 1958. Fat, body size, and growth in the newborn. *H. Biol.*, **30**, 265–280.

Garn, S. M., Clark, A., Landkof, L., and Newell, L., 1960. Parental body build and developmental progress of the offspring. *Science*, **132**, 1555–1556.

Gesell, A. et al., 1939. *Biographies of child development.* New York: Harper.

Gibby, R. G., Stotsky, B. A., Miller, D. R., and Hiler, E. W., 1953. Prediction of duration of therapy from the Rorschach test. *J. consult. Psychol.*, **17**, 348–354.

Gottesman, I. I., 1960. The psychogenetics of personality. Unpublished doctoral dissertation: University of Minnesota.

Halberstam, J. L., 1961. Some personality correlates of conditioning, generalization, and extinction. *Psychosom. Med.*, **23**, 67–76.

Hanfmann, E. and Kasanin, J., 1936. A method for study of concept formation. *J. Psychol.*, **3**, 521–540.

Harlow, H., 1962. The heterosexual affectional response system in monkeys. *Amer. Psychol.* (in press).

Hartup, W. W. and Zook, E. A., 1960. Sex-role preferences in three- and four-year-old children. *J. consult. Psychol.*, **24**, 420–426.

Holzman, P. S. and Gardner, R. W., 1959. Leveling and repression. *J. abnorm. soc. Psychol.*, **59**, 151–155.

Honzik, M. P., 1938. The constancy of mental test performance during the pre-school period. *J. genet. Psychol.*, **52**, 285–302.

Jenkins, J. J. and Russell, W. A., 1958. An atlas of semantic profiles from 360 words. *Amer. J. Psychol.*, **71**, 688–699.

Jersild, A. T., Markey, F., and Jersild, K. L., 1933. Children's fears, dreams, wishes, daydreams, likes, dislikes, pleasant or unpleasant memories. *Child Develpm. Monogr.*, No. 12.

Kagan, J., 1956a. The measurement of overt aggression from fantasy. *J. abnorm. soc. Psychol.*, **52**, 390–393.

Kagan, J., 1956b. The child's perception of the parent. *J. abnorm. soc. Psychol.*, **53**, 257–258.

Kagan, J., 1961. Stylistic variables in fantasy behavior: The ascription of affect states to social stimuli. In J. Kagan, and G. S. Lesser, (Eds.), *Contemporary Issues in Thematic Apperceptive Methods.* Springfield, Illinois: C. C. Thomas, pp. 196–220.

Kagan, J., Sontag, L. W., Baker, C. T., and Nelson, V. L., 1958. Personality and IQ change. *J. abnorm. soc. Psychol.*, **56**, 261–266.

Kagan, J. and Moss, H. A., 1959a. Stability and validity of achievement fantasy. *J. abnorm. soc. Psychol.*, **58**, 357–364.

Kagan, J. and Moss, H. A., 1959b. Parental correlates of child's IQ and height: A cross-validation of the Berkeley Growth Study results. *Child Develpm.*, **30**, 325–332.

Kagan, J. and Moss, H. A., 1960a. The stability of passive and dependent behavior from childhood through adulthood. *Child Develpm.*, **31**, 577–591.

Kagan, J., Moss, H. A., and Sigel, I. E., 1960b. Conceptual style and the use of affect labels. *Merrill-Palmer Quart. Beh. Develpm.*, 261–278.

Kagan, J. and Lemkin, Judith, 1960c. The child's differential perception of parental attributes. *J. abnorm. soc. Psychol.*, **61**, 440–447.

Kagan, J. and Moss, H. A., 1961a. The availability of conflictful ideas: A neglected parameter in projective test responses. *J. Pers.*, **29**, 217–234.

Kagan, J., Hosken, B., and Watson, S., 1961b. The child's symbolic conceptualization of the parents. *Child Develpm.*, 32, 625–636.

Kagan, J. and Garn, S. M., A constitutional correlate of early intellective functioning. *J. genet. Psychol.* (in press).

King, G. F., 1958. A theoretical and experimental consideration of the Rorschach human movement reseponse. *Psychol. Monogr.*, 72, whole No. 458.

Kinsey, A., Pomeroy, W., and Martin, C., 1948. *Sexual behavior in the human male.* Philadelphia: Saunders.

Kinsey, A., Pomeroy, W., and Martin, C., 1953. *Sexual behavior in the human female.* Philadelphia: Saunders.

Kling, J. W. and Schlosberg, H., 1961. The uniqueness of patterns of skin conductance. *Amer. J. Psychol.*, 74, 74–79.

Klopfer, B., Ainsworth, M. D., Klopfer, W. G., and Holt, R. R., 1954. *Developments in the Rorschach technique.* Vol. 1. New York: World Book.

Knop, C., 1946. The dynamics of newly born babies. *J. Pediat.*, 29, 721–728.

Kohn, M. L., 1959. Social Class and parental values. *Amer. J. Sociol.*, 64, 337–351.

Kounin, J. S., 1941. Experimental studies of rigidity. I. The measurement of rigidity in normal and feebleminded persons. *Character and Personality*, 9, 251–272.

Lacey, J. I., 1950. Individual differences in somatic response patterns. *J. comp. physiol. Psychol.*, 43, 338–350.

Lacey, J. I., 1956. The evaluation of autonomic responses: toward a general solution. *Annals of New York Academy of Sciences*, 67, 123–164.

Lacey, J. I., Bateman, D. E., and VanLehn, R., 1953. Autonomic response specificity. *Psychosom. Med.*, 15, 8–21.

Lacey, J. I. and Lacey, B. C., 1958a. The relationship of resting autonomic activity to motor impulsivity. *Res. Publ. Asso. nerv. ment. Dis.*, 36, 144–209.

Lacey, J. I. and Lacey, B. C., 1958b. Verification and extension of the principle of autonomic response stereotypy. *Amer. J. Psychol.*, 71, 50–73.

Lesser, G. S., 1958. Conflict analysis of fantasy aggression. *J. Pers.*, 26, 29–41.

Levy, D. M., 1943. *Maternal overprotection.* New York: Columbia University Press.

Lipsitt, L. P. and Levy, N., 1959. Electrotactual threshold in the neonate. *Child Develpm.*, 30, 547–554.

Littman, R. A., 1958. Motives, history and causes. In M. R. Jones (Ed.), *Nebraska Symposium on Motivation.* Lincoln: University of Nebraska Press, pp. 114–168.

McClelland, D. C., Atkinson, J. W., Clark, R. A., and Lowell, E. L., 1953. *The achievement motive.* New York: Appleton-Century-Croft.

McCulloch, H. J. and Stewart, J. C., 1960. Sexual norms in a psychiatric population. *J. nerv. ment. Dis.*, 131, 70–73.

McKinnon, K. M., 1942. Consistency and change in behavior manifestations. *Child Dev. Monogr.*, No. 30.

Maccoby, E. E. and Gibbs, R. K., 1954. Methods of child rearing in two social classes, In W. E. Martin and C. B. Stendler (Eds.), *Readings in child development,* New York: Harcourt, Brace, pp. 380–396.

Malmo, R. B., 1957. Anxiety and behavioral arousal. *Psychol. Rev.*, 64, 276–287.

Malmo, R. B., 1958. Measurement of drive: An unsolved problem in psychology. In M. R. Jones (Ed.), *Nebraska Symposium on Motivation.* Lincoln: University of Nebraska Press, pp. 229–265.

Mandler, G., Mandler, J. N., Kremen, I., and Sholiton, R. D., 1961. The response to threat: Relations among verbal and physiological indices. *Psychol. Monogr.*, 75, No. 513, 1–22.

Martin, B., 1961. The assessment of anxiety by physiological behavioral measures. *Psychol. Bull.*, 58, 234–255.

Milton, G. A., 1957. The effects of sex role identification upon problem solving skill. *J. abnorm. soc. Psychol.*, 55, 208–212.

Mood, A. M., 1950. *Introduction to the theory of statistics.* New York: McGraw-Hill.

Moss, H. A. and Kagan, J., 1958. Maternal influences on early IQ scores. *Psychol. Rep.*, 4, 655–661.

Moss, H. A. and Kagan, J., 1961. The stability of achievement and recognition seeking behavior from childhood to adulthood. *J. abnorm. soc. Psychol.*, 62, 543–552.

Murray, H. A., 1943. *Thematic Apperception Test.* Cambridge: Harvard University Press.

Mussen, P. H., 1961. Some antecedents and consequents of masculine sex typing in adolescent boys. *Psychol. Monogr.*, 75, whole No. 506, pp. 1–24.

Mussen, P. H. and Jones, M. C., 1957. Self conceptions, motivations, and interpersonal attitudes of late and early maturing boys. *Child Develpm.*, 28, 243–256.

Mussen, P. H. and Jones, M. C., 1958. The behavior inferred motivations of late and early maturing boys. *Child Develpm.*, 29, 61–67.

Nash, H., 1958. Assignment of gender to body organs. *J. genet. Psychol.*, 92, 113–115.

Neilson, P., 1948. Shirley's babies after fifteen years: A personality study. *J. genet. Psychol.*, 73, 175–186.

Nelson, V. L. and Richards, T. W., 1938. Studies in mental development: I. Performance on Gesell items at six months and its predictive value for performance at two and three years. *J. genet. Psychol.*, 52, 303–325.

Nemzeh, C. L., 1931. Is the IQ constant? *Peabody J. Educ.*, 9, 123–124.

Osgood, C. E., Suci, G. J., and Tannenbaum, P. H., 1957. *The measurement of meaning.* Urbana: University of Illinois Press.

Peck, R. F., 1958. Family patterns correlated with adolescent personality structure. *J. abnorm. soc. Psychol.*, 57, No. 3, 347–350.

Peck, R. F. and Havighurst, R. J., 1960. *The psychology of character development.* New York: Wiley.

Piaget, J., 1952. *The origins of intelligence in children.* New York: International Universities Press.

Reiser, M. F., 1961. Reflections on the interpretation of psychophysiologic experiments. *Psychosom. Med.*, 23, 430–439.

Richards, T. W. and Simons, M. P., 1941. The Fels child behavior scales. *Genet. Psychol. Monogr.*, 24, 259–309.

Rotter, J. B., 1954. *Social learning theory and clinical psychology.* New York: Prentice-Hall.

Sanford, R. N., Adkins, N. M., Miller, R. B., Cobb, E. A., et al., 1943. Physique, personality, and scholarship: A cooperative study of school children. *Monogr. Soc. Res. Child Develpm.*, 8, No. 1.

Sarason, S. B., Davidson, K. S., Lighthall, S. F., Waite, R. R., and Reubush, D. K., 1960. *Anxiety in elementary school children.* New York: John Wiley.

Schaefer, E. S., 1959. A circumplex model for maternal behavior. *J. abnorm. soc. Psychol.*, 59, 226–235.

Schaefer, E. S. and Bayley, N., 1960. Consistency of maternal behavior from infancy to preadolescence. *J. abnorm. soc. Psychol.*, **61,** 1–6.

Sears, R. R., 1961. Relation of early socialization experiences to aggression in middle childhood. *J. abnorm. soc. Psychol.*, **63,** 466–492.

Sears, R. R., Whiting, J. W. M., Nowlis, V., and Sears, P. S., 1953. Some child rearing antecedents of aggression and dependency in young children. *Genet. Psychol. Monogr.*, **47,** No. 234.

Sears, R. R., Maccoby, E. E., and Levin, H., 1957. *Patterns of child-rearing.* Evanston: Row, Peterson.

Sheldon, W. H., 1942. *The varieties of temperament: A psychology of constitutional differences.* New York: Harper.

Shneidman, E. S., 1949. *The Make-a-Picture-Story test.* New York: Psychological Corp.

Singer, J. L., Wilensky, H., and McCraven, V. G., 1956. Delaying capacity, fantasy, and planning ability: A factorial study of some basic ego functions. *J. consult. Psychol.*, **20,** 375–383.

Smith, M. E., 1952. A comparison of certain personality traits as rated in the same individuals in childhood and fifty years later. *Child Develpm.*, **23,** 159–180.

Sontag, L. W., Baker, C. T., and Nelson, V. L., 1958. Mental growth and personality development: A longitudinal study. *Monogr. Soc. Res., Child Develpm.*, **23,** No. 68, 1–143.

Stone, A. A. and Onqué, G. C., 1959. *Longitudinal studies of child personality.* Cambridge: Harvard University Press.

Terman, L. M., et al., 1925. *Genetic studies of genius: I. Mental and physical traits of a thousand gifted children.* Stanford University Press.

Terman, L. M., Burks, B. S., and Jensen, D. W., 1930. *Genetic studies of genius: III. The promise of youth: Follow-up studies of a thousand gifted children.* Stanford University Press.

Terman, L. M., and Oden, M., 1940. Status of the California gifted group at the end of sixteen years. *39th Yearbook, Nat. Soc. Stud. Educ.*, Part 1, 67–74.

Terman, L. M. and Oden, M., 1940. Correlates of adult achievement in the California gifted group. *39th Yearbook, Nat. Soc. Stud. Educ.*, Part 1, 74–89.

Terman, L. M. and Oden, M. H., 1947. *Genetic studies of genius: IV. The gifted child grows up. Twenty-five years follow-up on the superior group.* Stanford University Press.

Terman, L. M. and Oden, M. H., 1959. *Genetic studies of genius: V. The gifted group at mid-life.* Stanford University Press.

Thomas, A., Chess, S., Birch, H., and Hertzig, M., 1960. A longitudinal study of primary reaction patterns in children. *Comprehensive Psychiat.*, **1,** 103–112.

Thorndike, R. L., 1940. Constancy of the IQ. *Psychol. Bull.*, **37,** 167–186.

Thorndike, R. L. and Hagen, E., 1959. *10,000 careers.* New York: John Wiley.

Tuddenham, R. D., 1959. The constancy of personality ratings over two decades. *Genet. Psychol. Monogr.*, **60,** 3–29.

Wechsler, D., 1958. *The measurement and appraisal of adult intelligence.* Baltimore: Williams & Wilkins.

Westie, F. R. and DeFleur, M. L., 1959. Autonomic responses and their relationship to race attitudes. *J. abnorm. soc. Psychol.*, **58,** 340–347.

Whiting, J. W. M. and Child, I. L., 1953. *Child training and personality.* New Haven: Yale University Press.

Author Index[*]

Adkins, N. M., 83, **291**
Affleck, D. C., 282, **287**
Ainsworth, M. D., 36, **290**
Anderson, L. D., 6, **287**
Atkinson, J. W., 146, **290**

Baker, C. T., 6, 155, **289, 292**
Baldwin, A. L., 16, 207, **287**
Bateman, D. E., 284, **290**
Bayley, N., 6, 228, **287, 289, 292**
Behnke, A. R., 82, **287**
Bell, R. Q., 81, **287**
Beller, E. K., 51, **287**
Bennett, E. M., 139, **287**
Berry, J. L., 263, **287**
Birch, H., 80, **292**
Bolles, R. C., 14, **287**
Bradway, K. P., 6, **287, 288**
Breese, F. H., 16, 207, **287**
Bronson, W. C., 8, **288**
Burks, B. S., 5, **288, 292**
Buss, A. H., 264, 265, **288**

Castenada, A., 193, **288**
Chess, S., 80, **292**
Child, I. L., 189, **288, 292**
Clark, A., 82, **289**
Clark, R. A., 146, **290**
Cobb, E. A., 83, **291**
Cobb, H. V., 139, **288**
Cohen, L. R., 139, **287**

Cox, F. N., 282, **288**
Crandall, V. J., 207, **288**
Cravens, R. B., 6, **288**

Davidson, K. S., 193, **291**
DeFleur, M. L., 263, **292**
Dollard, J., 34, 229, **288**
Duffy, E., 230, 283, **288**
Dunlop, G. N., 189, **288**
Durkee, A., 264, **288**

Ebert, E., 6, **288**
England, A. O., 189, **288**
Escalona, S., 9, **288**

Festinger, L., 271, **288**
Foran, T. G., 6, **288**
French, E. G., 37, **288**

Gardner, R. L., 269, **288**
Gardner, R. W., 35, **288**
Garn, S. M., 82, 119, **289, 290**
Gesell, A., 7, **289**
Gibby, R. G., 282, **289**
Gottesman, I. I., 80, 84, **289**

Hagan, E., 153, **292**
Halberstam, J. L., 286, **289**
Hanfmann, E., 45, **289**
Harlow, H., 81, 119, **289**
Hartup, W. W., 269, **289**

[*] Boldface page numbers refer to pages where these authors can be found in the list of references.

293

Havighurst, R. J., 8, 9, 291
Heider, G. M., 9, 288
Hertzig, M., 80, 292
Hiler, E. W., 282, 289
Holt, R. R., 36, 290
Holzman, P. S., 35, 288
Honzik, M. P., 6, 289
Hosken, B., 139, 269, 290

Jenkins, J. J., 139, 289
Jensen, D. W., 5, 288, 292
Jersild, A. T., 189, 289
Jersild, K. L., 189, 289
Jones, M. C., 83, 291
Jones, M. R., 14, 290

Kagan, J., 6, 34, 35, 82, 83, 139, 146, 147, 151, 153, 196, 265, 269, 282, 289, 290, 291
Kalhorn, Joan, 16, 207, 287
Kasanin, J., 45, 289
Katten, E. S., 8, 288
King, G. F., 196, 282, 290
Kinsey, A., 171, 201, 290
Klein, G. S., 35, 288
Kling, J. W., 284, 290
Klopfer, B., 36, 290
Klopfer, W. G., 36, 290
Knop, C., 81, 290
Kohn, M. L., 170, 290
Kounin, J. S., 123, 125, 290
Kremen, I., 263, 290

Lacey, B. C., 81, 284, 290
Lacey, J. I., 81, 241, 284, 290
Landkof, L., 82, 289
Lemkin, J., 269, 289
Lesser, G. S., 34, 289, 290
Levin, H., 87, 207, 292
Levine, E. M., 288
Levy, D. M., 207, 290
Levy, N., 119, 290
Lighthall, S. F., 193, 291
Linton, H. B., 35, 288
Lipsitt, L. P., 119, 290
Littman, R. A., 14, 290
Livson, N., 8, 288
Lowell, E. L., 146, 290

Maccoby, E. E., 87, 99, 207, 290, 292

Malmo, R. B., 14, 230, 290
Mandler, G., 263, 290
Mandler, J. N., 263, 290
Markey, F., 189, 289
Martin, B., 263, 265, 285, 287, 291
Martin, C., 171, 201, 290
Martin, W. E., 290
McCandless, B. R., 193, 288
McClelland, D. C., 120, 146, 290
McCraven, V. G., 196, 282, 292
McCulloch, H. J., 171, 290
McKinnon, K. M., 7, 290
Mednick, S. A., 282, 287
Miller, D. R., 282, 289
Miller, N. E., 34, 229, 288
Miller, R. B., 83, 291
Milton, G. A., 275, 290
Mood, A. M., 154, 290
Moss, H. A., 6, 83, 146, 147, 153, 196, 265, 282, 289, 291
Murray, H. A., 12, 36, 146, 291
Mussen, P. H., 83, 291

Nash, H., 139, 291
Neilson, P., 7, 291
Nelson, V. L., 6, 155, 289, 291, 292
Nemzeh, C. L., 6, 291
Newell, L., 82, 289
Nowlis, V., 292

Oden, M., 5, 292
Onqué, G. C., 9, 292
Osgood, C. E., 269, 291

Palermo, D. S., 193, 288
Peck, R. F., 8, 9, 291
Piaget, J., 125, 291
Pomeroy, W., 171, 201, 290
Potter, E. H., 288
Preston, A., 207, 288

Reiser, M. F., 265, 291
Reubush, D. K., 193, 291
Richards, T. W., 6, 61, 291
Robinson, N. M., 6, 288
Rotter, J. B., 136, 291
Russell, W. A., 139, 289

Sanford, R. N., 83, 291
Sarason, S. B., 193, 282, 288, 291

Schaefer, E. S., 16, 228, **287, 291, 292**
Schlosberg, H., 284, **290**
Sears, P. S., **292**
Sears, R. R., 87, 99, 207, **292**
Sheldon, W. H., **292**
Shneidman, E. S., 37, **292**
Sholiton, R. D., 263, **290**
Sigel, I. E., 196, **289**
Simons, M. P., 61, **291**
Simmons, K., 6, **288**
Singer, J. L., 196, 282, **292**
Smith, M. E., 7, **292**
Sontag, L. W., 6, 149, 151, 152, 155, **289, 292**
Spence, D. P., 35, **288**
Stendler, C. B., **290**
Stewart, J. C., 171, **290**
Stone, A. A., 9, **292**
Stotsky, B. A., 282, **289**

Suci, G. J., 269, **291**

Tannenbaum, P. H., 269, **291**
Terman, L. M., 5, **288, 292**
Thomas, A., 80, **292**
Thompson, C. W., 6, **288**
Thorndike, R. L., 6, 153, **292**
Tuddenham, R. D., 7, 8, **292**

VanLehn, R., 284, **290**

Waite, R. R., 193, **291**
Watson, S., 139, 269, **290**
Wechsler, D., **292**
Westie, F. R., 263, **292**
Whiting, J. W. M., 189, **292**
Wilensky, H., 196, 282, **292**

Zook, E. A., 269, **289**

Subject Index

Achievement behavior, and achievement themes, 146–148, 154
and athletic mastery, 106, 120–124, 129–138, 148, 150–154, 157
and desire for mastery, 3, 7, 9, 14, 28, 30, 50, 77, 120–125, 129–138, 202–203, 221–223, 248–250, 267–268
and intellectual mastery, 106, 108, 120–125, 129–154, 248–250, 267–268
and mechanical mastery, 120–124, 129, 132–135, 138, 147–153
Active behavior, 81, 138
Aggression, 3, 7–9, 14–15, 17, 28, 30, 33–34, 37, 39, 58, 77, 79, 85–89, 93, 102, 118–120, 129, 138–139, 145, 152–154, 188, 199, 223–225, 233–234, 236, 242–244, 262–264, 267–269
and behavioral disorganization, 86–89, 93–98, 101–102, 106–112
Anxiety, 9, 13, 16, 33–34, 51, 53, 55–57, 64, 66–71, 82, 84–85, 95, 98–100, 104–105, 108–110, 118, 120, 130, 137, 142, 167, 172–183, 188–193, 226, 229–231, 236, 258–259, 262–264, 282–284
and fears, 2, 139–140, 142, 145–146, 189–193
over expectancy of failure, 15, 68–69, 122, 124, 130–138
over physical harm, 15, 28, 33–34, 37, 39–40, 79, 138–145, 156, 160, 188–193, 226, 233–234, 236, 246–248, 262–264
over social interaction, 15–16, 82, 156, 172–183, 197–198, 226, 267–268
Arousal, 282–284

Authority, attitude toward, 8–9
Autonomic reactions, 19, 33–34, 46–47, 81, 186, 238–242, 244–251, 256–259, 262–264, 281–284
and cardiac response, 34, 46, 81, 186, 238–242, 244–251, 256–259, 262–264
and palmar conductance, 34, 46, 81, 238–242, 244–251, 256–259, 262–264

Behavior, stability of, 7–9, 19, 49–58, 63–67, 72, 78–81, 84–89, 93–95, 98–99, 107, 112, 118–120, 123, 125, 129–130, 137, 146–147, 151–160, 266–269

Competitiveness, 6, 87–88, 94–96, 100, 111, 118, 122, 124, 129–135, 140, 143, 145, 149
Compulsivity, 28, 37, 156, 183–187, 226, 236
Conceptualization, and affect labels, 253–259, 262–264
and figure-sorting responses, 253, 256–259, 262–264
and position identification, 259–262
preferred mode, 34–35, 37–38, 45, 250–251, 254–259, 262–264, 281–284
Conflict, 13, 33–34, 39, 54, 56, 58, 67, 69, 70–71, 76, 84–85, 94–95, 98–100, 105, 108–112, 119–120, 130, 145, 160, 165, 167, 200–201, 229–231, 236, 258–259, 262–264, 282–284
Conformity, 79, 86, 88, 93, 96, 101, 106–111, 118, 160
Constitution, 81–83, 93, 119, 276–277

Defense (defensive), 9, 13, 15–16, 56, 84, 142

Dependency, 6, 15, 28, 30, 33–34, 37, 39–40, 49–85, 119–120, 152–154, 199, 212–215, 233–234, 236, 245, 262–264, 267–268

Derivatives of child behavior, 2, 79, 83, 93, 110, 199

Dominance of others, 16, 58, 77–78, 84, 86, 88, 93–96, 100–101, 107, 109, 111, 139, 157

Fels Parent Behavior Rating Scale, 13, 16, 21, 28

French Insight Test, 37

Frustration, 51–52, 69, 77, 86, 89, 93–94, 98, 100

Gesell Developmental Schedule, 12

Hanfmann-Kasanin Test, 45

Hyperkinesis, 28, 100, 156, 193–195, 197–198

Identification, 58, 98, 105, 112, 118, 136, 145, 153, 154, 157, 159, 161, 272
and sex role, 9, 15, 31, 54, 69, 76, 85, 93, 98, 100, 105–106, 110–120, 131, 136, 139, 145, 156–171, 200–203, 225, 262–264, 266, 271, 273–276
and sex-typed interests, 14, 76, 79, 82–83, 100, 148, 156–171, 200–203, 225, 266–271, 273–276

Impulsivity, 8–9, 15, 79, 185–187

Independence, 6, 51–58, 64, 66–72, 76, 145

Intelligence, 5–7, 11, 34–35, 125, 148–152, 155, 248–250, 256–258
and the Merrill-Palmer Test, 12, 82
and Primary Mental Abilities, 13
and the Stanford-Binet, 6, 12, 82, 125, 149, 155
and the Wechsler-Bellevue, 13, 19, 40, 45, 149, 155

Interaction, social, 13–16, 28, 37, 80, 87, 157

Introspectiveness, 156, 195

Involvement, 258–259, 262–264

Kuder Preference Test, 12

Longitudinal, 2–12, 17, 20, 27–29, 33, 47, 49, 50, 52, 75, 99, 121, 156

Maternal practices, acceleration, 3, 16, 153, 205, 228
acceptance and affections, 8, 15
hostility, 3, 16, 205, 228
protection, 3, 16, 205, 228
restrictiveness, 205, 228

Minnesota Multiphasic Personality Inventory, 12, 80, 84

Motive (motivation), 8–9, 13–16, 37, 56, 63, 67–68, 70–71, 85, 94, 98, 100, 106, 108, 110, 120, 123, 125, 129, 130–131, 136, 145, 151–152, 154, 273, 282–284

Motor coordinations, 9, 82

Nurturance of others, 14–15, 28, 49, 51, 53, 55–57, 63–71, 84, 156, 187–188

Observations, naturalistic, 6–13, 20–21, 24, 28

Passivity, 3, 28, 49, 50–59, 63–72, 75–83, 119–120, 136, 154, 197–199, 212–215, 233–234, 261–262, 267–268, 276–277
and withdrawal, 15, 28, 30, 51, 56, 68–70, 72, 76–84, 122, 124–125, 130–133, 136–139, 145, 172–183

Perception, tachistoscopic, 19, 33–34, 38–46, 58, 99, 119, 160, 231–236, 243, 245–247, 256–259, 262–264

Punishment, effects of, 3, 54, 58, 87, 94, 99, 100, 112, 152

Recognition-seeking behaviors, 8, 14, 28, 30, 37, 100, 120–124, 129, 135, 138, 147–153, 160, 236

Reward, function of, 3, 54, 58, 85, 87, 104, 112, 152

Rorschach (modified), 11–12, 19, 35–36, 186, 196, 251–252, 256–259

Self-rating scale, 19, 37, 193, 235

Sexual behavior, 14–15, 28, 30, 33–34, 37, 39, 40, 82, 156–171, 197–198, 225, 233–234, 236, 245–246, 262–264, 267–268

Sleeper effect, 3, 197–198, 277–281

Social class, 6, 10, 18, 75, 108, 118, 131, 152–154, 160, 170–171, 183, 187, 192, 195–196, 209, 211

Spontaneity, social, 8–9, 15, 79, 174–183

Thematic Apperception Test, 11–12, 19, 36, 146–148, 252, 256–259